Assessment and Management of Central Auditory Processing Disorders in the Educational Setting:

From Science to Practice

2nd Edition

A Singular Audiology Text

Jeffrey L. Danhauer, Ph.D.
Audiology Editor

Assessment and Management of Central Auditory Processing Disorders in the Educational Setting:

From Science to Practice

Second Edition

Teri James Bellis, Ph.D.

THOMSON

★

™

DELMAR LEARNING

Assessment and Management of Central Auditory Processing Disorders in the Educational Setting From Science to Practice, Second Edition

by Teri James Bellis

Executive Director, Health Care Business Unit:
William Brottmiller

Executive Editor:
Cathy L. Esperti

Developmental Editor:
Darcy M. Scelsi

Executive Marketing Manager:
Dawn F. Gerrain

Channel Manager:
Gretta Oliver

Editorial Assistant:
Maria D'Angelico

Executive Production Manager:
Karen Leet

Art/Design Coordinator:
Robert Plante

Production Coordinator:
Cathy Ciardullo

Project Editor:
Shelley Esposito

Library of Congress Cataloging-in-Publication Data
Bellis, Teri James.
  Assessment and management of central auditory processing disorders in the educational setting : from science to practice / by Teri James Bellis—2nd ed.
    p. cm.
Includes bibliographical references and index.
  ISBN 0-7693-0130-4
  1. Word deafness. I. Title.
  RC394.W63 B45 2003
  617.8—dc21
                            2002007157

NOTICE TO THE READER

Contents

Statistical Procedures • Meeting the Research
Challenge

Preface

When I wrote the first edition of this book nearly seven years ago, I predicted that our view of auditory processing disorders would undergo significant changes within the following decade. In some regards, that prediction was correct. We have witnessed a dramatic upsurge in awareness of the disorder on the part of professionals, parents, educators, and the general public. Numerous sites devoted to the subject of auditory processing have appeared on the World Wide Web (something, I might add, that was virtually inconceivable not that long ago). Clinical programs to address auditory processing and its disorders have sprung up like wild prairie grass throughout this country and in other countries as well, and I often receive communications and queries from such far-reaching lands as Egypt, India, South Africa, Brazil, The Netherlands, Australia, China, Germany, Russia, Italy, and Israel. Even in today's world of unsettled international relations, our scientific and audiologic communities remain united as one in the spirit of scientific inquiry and devotion to delivery of quality clinical services.

Our understanding of how the brain processes auditory input, especially spoken language, has improved, largely due to the advent of more advanced imaging technology and electrophysiologic techniques. Findings in neurogenesis and neuroplasticity have provided us with renewed hope that, once diagnosed, we can treat auditory processing and related disorders through actually changing the function of the neural pathways of the brain. And, although the profession of audiology is moving toward greater and greater autonomy, we can no longer fail to acknowledge the need for interdisciplinary collaboration with speech-language pathologists, cognitive neuroscientists, neuropsychologists, and professionals and scientists in countless other disciplines in our quest to define, understand, diagnose, and treat auditory processing disorders.

Yet, we still lack universal consensus regarding how to define, diagnose, and treat auditory processing disorders. Indeed, despite the proliferation of literature devoted to the subject, we still remain divided on such basic, fundamental subjects as how to label these disorders or even whether they exist at all. Despite the ever increasing evidence that auditory processing and its disorders are topics of unimagined complexity, it seems that we still search naively for the easy answer, the simple definition, the one method of diagnosis and treatment, the single phrase or descriptor that will somehow capture the essence of this disorder in a few short words.

As researchers continue to search for answers to these questions, clinicians in schools and clinics everywhere remain caught in the crossfire, trying to keep up with the constantly evolving literature and meet the rising demand for auditory processing services. I hope that this second edition helps in this regard by providing clinicians "in the trenches" with the latest information on this subject—information that, no doubt, will once again undergo dramatic transformations in the near future, perhaps even by the time this book comes to press.

A Word About Terminology

At a recent consensus conference convened at the University of Texas–Dallas, it was recommended that the term *auditory processing disorder* (APD) be used to emphasize that the auditory system—and disorders involving that system—involve far more than just the central auditory pathways. Much debate has ensued over the appropriateness of the removal of the word *central* from the label, particularly as relates to the potential danger of broadening the scope of the disorder to such a degree that it holds little or no clinical utility. As we come to a greater understanding of the scope of auditory processing and the interrelationship among audition, language, learning, and information processing in general, our label for this disorder may change yet again. Perhaps we will choose to conclude that, because different types of auditory processing disorders exist, different labels may be indicated. Perhaps we will acknowledge that, at least in some cases, what we are really dealing with are the "auditory manifestations of information processing disorders." In this book, I have chosen to use the previous term *central auditory processing disorders* (CAPD), primarily to remain consistent with the first edition, but also to emphasize that we are, indeed, referring to disorders that occur central to the peripheral auditory system. Therefore, the term *CAPD* will be used throughout this text.

New to This Edition

In preparation for writing this second edition, I naturally scanned the current literature to ensure the most up-to-date coverage of this topic. I also surveyed the opinions of users of the first edition as well as comments and input received worldwide from colleagues, practitioners, and families of children with CAPD. I believe that these issues have been addressed in this edition and that they serve to enhance the quality of the product, and I thank those who provided valuable input. Although this second edition is substantially updated, the book follows the general format of the first edition. Part One presents an overview of the science of central auditory processing, including neuroanatomy and neurophysiology of the central auditory nervous system, mechanisms of auditory and spoken language processing, and a discussion of neuromaturation and neuroplasticity. Part Two provides readers with detailed information regarding screening for and diagnosing CAPD, including administration and interpretation of diagnostic tests of CAPD. Part Three discusses management and intervention for CAPD and also provides readers with guidance regarding service delivery issues, including collection of normative data and documentation of program efficacy and treatment outcomes. Readers familiar with the first edition will recognize that the majority of this text has been completely rewritten, and presents information not included in the previous edition. Most of these additions and updates were made in response to the hundreds of requests, queries, and suggestions I received from colleagues around the world. They include:

- Expanded information on the neurophysiologic bases of speech encoding in the central auditory pathways
- In-depth discussion of the underlying mechanisms of selected auditory processes, top-down factors in auditory processing, and the relationship between auditory processing and language, memory, cognition, and other higher-order functions
- Updated information on maturation of the central auditory pathways and implications of recent findings in neuroplasticity for treatment of CAPD
- Step-by-step guidance in multidisciplinary screening for CAPD for the purposes of determining the need for a diagnostic evaluation and reducing over-referrals for central auditory services
- Administration and interpretation of behavioral and electrophysiologic tests of central auditory processing, including the addition of several "new" measures and normative values from age 7 to adult for the majority of commonly used central auditory tests
- Expanded and completely revised procedures for interpreting results of central auditory diagnostic findings

- Expanded and completely revised management chapters, including highly prescriptive guidance for developing deficit-specific intervention programs for children with CAPD and areas of needed research in CAPD treatment
- The latest issues in service delivery, including the need for documenting program efficacy and treatment outcomes

I hope that this second edition assists clinicians practicing in schools and clinics everywhere in better serving the children with whom they work every day.

Teri James Bellis
April 2002

Acknowledgments

With heartfelt thanks to Jeff Danhauer, who has been a guiding force in my life for almost two decades, from teaching me principles of amplification and providing advice as to where I should go for my CFY experience (remember that?), to involving me in research and allowing me to see my name appear in print as co-author of a published article for the very first time in the mid-1980s, and now to holding my hand through this latest project. Without you, neither the current nor the previous edition of this book would exist. You have provided exemplary editorial input, invaluable personal and professional support and advice, and much-needed encouragement. If not for you, I would still be staring at a blank page in a vague state of panic, wondering where to go next.

Thanks also to my infinitely patient and loyal graduate assistants, Alexia Georgas Gillen and Stacey Hesse, who assisted in revising the answers to the review questions and performed countless additional tasks critical to the production of this book. You'll both go far along whatever path life takes you!

As in everything I do, I am profoundly grateful for the support of my family—Tim, Jennie, Chris, and especially Danny, who was "as yet unnamed" when I wrote the first edition. All that I accomplish is with you in mind, even if it doesn't always seem that way.

This book is dedicated to my colleagues throughout the world who toil in the trenches every day, all the while searching for illumination, understanding, and better ways to serve our children.

About the Author

Teri James Bellis, PhD, professor of audiology at The University of South Dakota, received her doctorate in audiology and hearing sciences with a specialty certification in language and cognition from Northwestern University. The author of *When the Brain Can't Hear: Unraveling the Mystery of Auditory Processing Disorder* (2002, Pocket Books), Dr. Bellis has been involved in the development, management, and implementation of audiologic and neurodiagnostic programs in clinical and educational settings, including multimodality evoked potentials programs and central auditory processing service delivery programs. She is an internationally recognized expert in auditory processing disorders, and has lectured and published widely on the subject of central auditory processing assessment and management. Her writings have been featured in numerous audiology and medical journals, including the prestigious *Journal of Neuroscience*.

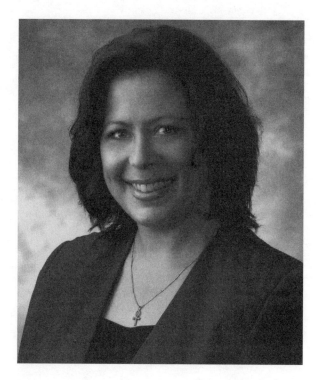

PART

ONE

The Science of Central Auditory Processing

C H A P T E R

ONE

Neuroanatomy and Neurophysiology of the Central Auditory Nervous System

I t is essential for the clinician involved in the assessment and management of auditory processing and its disorders to have an understanding of the underlying anatomical and physiological bases and neuropsychological principles. According to information processing theory (Massaro, 1975), ultimate comprehension relies on the extraction of information at various stages of processing. In addition, complex interactions between sensory and higher-order cognitive/linguistic operations occur both simultaneously (parallel) and sequentially (distributed) throughout the system, or processing network. In this chapter, we consider the primary principles governing the neurophysiologic encoding of auditory signals from the auditory nerve to the brain, referred to as "bottom-up" factors in information processing theory. Here, the term *bottom-up* is used to denote those mechanisms and processes that occur in the auditory system prior to higher-order cognitive and linguistic operations at the cortical level.

It is logical to assume that if the fundamental bottom-up encoding of auditory signals is disrupted at any point along the central auditory pathways, the final auditory percept will be affected adversely. However, it should be remembered that such bottom-up factors are, themselves, influenced by higher-order factors such as attention, memory, and linguistic competence through the presence of complex feedback and feedforward mechanisms. That is, the brain is not organized as a merely hierarchical system, in which information moves in only one direction and is processed sequentially at ascending levels of the central nervous system (CNS). Rather, there are multiple representations of sensory information throughout the system, with each area connected reciprocally to many other areas. The presence of backward and lateral, as well as forward, connections allows for a distributed network that includes both parallel and hierarchical processing and that involves extremely complex operations to arrive at a cohesive percept of the world around us.

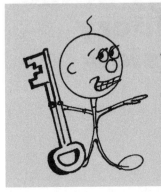

KEY CONCEPT

According to information processing theory, both bottom-up and top-down factors determine an individual's ability to process auditory information.

The tests of central auditory nervous system (CANS) function that will be discussed in this book are based directly on the underlying neurophysiologic principles that will be discussed in this and subsequent chapters, as are test interpretation and management of auditory processing disorders. Without knowledge of the functioning of the CANS, the full clinical value of central tests may go untapped.

This chapter provides an overview of the anatomy and physiology of the CANS, particularly as it relates to encoding and processing of speech stimuli. A discussion of higher-order cognitive, linguistic, and related "top-down" influences on auditory processing will be presented in Chapter 2. Although it is not within the scope of this book to provide a complete review of these subjects, the topics discussed here will provide a basic understanding of the functions of the CANS as well as direction for further study. There are numerous sources available in which more detailed analyses of neuroanatomy, neurophysiology, neuropsychology, and information processing theory can be found. Readers are directed to the References at the end of this book for further resources.

Finally, when one considers bottom-up influences on auditory processing, the importance of the peripheral auditory system cannot be overemphasized. At its most basic level, bottom-up processing in the CANS relies on the integrity of auditory signals provided to it by the ears and the auditory nerve. Thus, anything that has a negative effect on an auditory signal at the level of the ear will also adversely affect the individual's ability to process auditory information. Perhaps the most obvious example of this situation involves individuals with hearing impairment. The hearing loss will have a deleterious effect on the quality of auditory signals even before they enter the CANS. As a result, deaf individuals almost certainly will be poor auditory processors; however, their auditory processing difficulties can be ascribed mainly to peripheral factors. Therefore, when addressing auditory processing and its disorders, one must consider the entire auditory system, from the ear to the brain. Although this chapter will not discuss the function of auditory structures that are peripheral to the auditory nerve, readers should keep in mind the importance of peripheral auditory system integrity to an individual's overall ability to process auditory information.

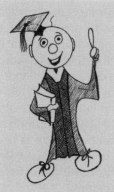

Learning Objectives

After studying this chapter, the reader should be able to:

1. Define technical terms related to planes of brain section and directional reference.
2. Identify the primary lobes of the brain and discuss the general function of each.
3. Discuss the general mechanism of synaptic transmission.

(continued)

(*continued*)

4. Discuss the physiologic representation of auditory stimuli in the auditory nerve.
5. Identify primary central auditory nervous system brainstem structures and discuss their functions relating to encoding and processing of auditory (especially speech) signals.
6. Discuss the encoding and processing of auditory (especially speech) signals in the auditory cortex.
7. Discuss the structure and function of the corpus callosum, particularly as it relates to auditory function.
8. Discuss current theory relating to the function of the central auditory nervous system efferent pathways and the olivocochlear bundle.

Terminology

Specific terminology is used in neuroscience to indicate the direction and position of various structures in relation to other structures in the brain. In this section, we discuss terminology related to *planes of brain section* and *directional reference*.

The human brain can be sectioned into three primary planes: *sagittal*, *coronal*, and *horizontal*. The term *sagittal* refers to a cut in which the brain is divided into right and left sides. A midsagittal section is one in which the brain is divided at midline, or center, thus separating the brain into two equal halves (Figure 1-1a). A coronal section divides the brain into front (anterior) and back (posterior) sections (Figure 1-1b), whereas a horizontal section divides the brain into upper (superior) and lower (inferior) portions (Figure 1-1c). Another important term relating to planes of section is *transverse*. A transverse cut is one that is diagonal to the horizontal plane (Figure 1-1d). Because of the curvature of the brainstem and other structures, transverse sections are often necessary to view internal landmarks adequately.

Neuroscience also uses terminology relating to directionality in the brain as well as the location of a given structure in relation to other structures. The term *rostral* refers to locations toward the head and away from the tail, whereas *caudal* indicates the opposite—toward the tail and away from the head. For example, in gross terms, the brainstem is caudal to the cerebrum, but rostral to the spinal cord. The terms *lateral* or *distal* indicate a structure that is to the side or away from the midline, while the terms *medial* or *proximal* refer to a structure that is toward or near the midline. For example, the cochlea is lateral to the VIIIth nerve, but medial to the tympanic membrane. Finally, the terms *ventral* and *dorsal* are used to mean toward the belly and toward the back, respectively. They are synonymous with the terms *anterior* and *posterior* in the human, but convey different meanings for animals in which the anatomical position is not upright.

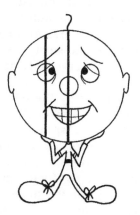

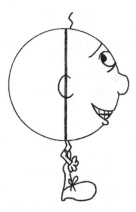

a. sagittal and midsagittal section   b. coronal section

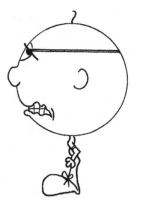

c. horizontal section   d. transverse section

Figure 1-1. Planes of brain section.

Although there are other common terms relating to neuroanatomy, these are the primary ones that will be used throughout this chapter.

Gross Anatomy of the Brain

The adult human brain weighs approximately 2 lb and represents 2% of the total body weight. The cerebrum consists of the two cerebral hemispheres and makes up the largest portion of the brain. The surface of the brain is referred to as the *cortex* and consists of gray (unmyelinated) matter. The cortical surface is convoluted, forming ridges (*gyri*) and valleys (*sulci*) that serve as landmarks for important primary structures. The number and size of gyri and sulci vary greatly from individual to individual; therefore, they serve only as rough frames of reference.

The two cerebral hemispheres are separated by the *longitudinal fissure* (Figure 1-2). Each cerebral hemisphere is essentially a mirror image of the other, although, as will be discussed later in this chapter, there exist some significant asymmetries in terms of size and length of cerebral landmarks. Moreover, the relative functions of the right and left hemispheres of the brain differ, although the right/left dichotomy is not quite so circumscribed as popular writings on the subject would have us believe. Nevertheless, it cannot be denied that each hemisphere exhibits some degree of specialization for certain types of tasks. For example, in the vast majority of individuals, the storage of lexical information (i.e., association of words with meaning), generation of syntax, and phonological processing are subserved primarily by the language-dominant (usually left) hemisphere. The right hemisphere does have some linguistic processing abilities, but they tend to be both more simple and more randomly organized than those of the left hemisphere. Furthermore, typically only the left hemisphere has the capability of producing speech.

Similarly, the right hemisphere appears to be more adept at detection and recognition of faces, especially unfamiliar ones, and for the interpretation of many involuntary facial expressions associated with emotions. In contrast, only the left hemisphere is able to generate voluntary facial expressions.

Regarding spatial attention and visual search abilities, the left hemisphere appears to be quite organized and systematic in detecting a visual target in a background of foils, whereas the right hemisphere tends to examine a visual environment in a far less organized manner. Yet the right hemisphere appears to be better at disengaging, shifting, and reengaging attention, or allocation of attention, than the left.

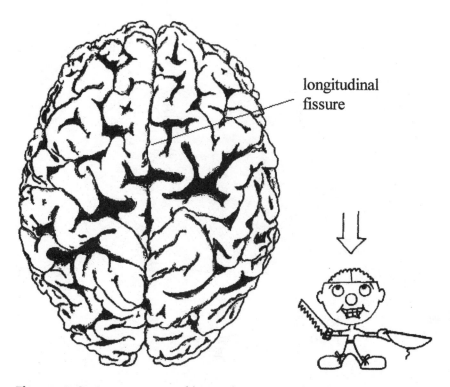

longitudinal
fissure

Figure 1-2. Superior view of brain showing cerebral hemispheres separated by longitudinal fissure.

In general, the right hemisphere is dominant for part-to-whole gestalt synthesis, sequencing, visual-spatial abilities, mathematics calculation, art and music skills, processing of nonlinguistic aspects of communication, abstract reasoning, and similar types of tasks. Conversely, the left hemisphere appears to be more analytic, better at breaking down a whole into its constituent parts, more phonologic and linguistically oriented (particularly relating to semantics and syntax), and better able to engage in concrete thought processes. For an excellent review of topics related to hemispheric specialization, as well as an overview of fundamental principles of cognitive neuroscience, readers are referred to Gazzaniga, Ivry, and Mangun (1998).

Each cerebral hemisphere consists of four primary lobes named for the bones of the skull that cover them: the *frontal, parietal, temporal,* and—most posterior—*occipital* (Figure 1-3). Although general functions can be ascribed to each lobe in the typical brain, a tremendous amount of cross-modality integration and interplay occurs in all

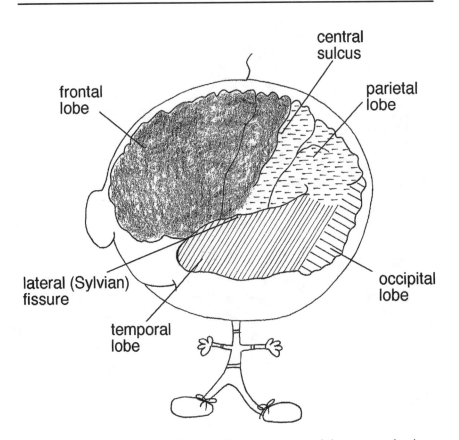

Figure 1-3. Lateral view of brain showing primary lobes, central sulcus, and lateral (Sylvian) fissure.

areas. For example, although the temporal lobe is generally considered to "house" the auditory portions of the brain, auditory responsive regions are found throughout the brain and subcortical structures. Therefore, the following discussion provides merely a general overview of the primary functions of each lobe and should be considered a very simplistic view of brain function.

The frontal lobe lies anterior to the central sulcus and superior to the lateral (or Sylvian) fissure. This lobe governs the planning and carrying out of motor actions. The precentral gyrus, or primary motor cortex, governs voluntary motor movement for the entire body. Additional motor areas include the premotor cortex and the supplementary motor cortex. Finally, the anterior-most portion of the frontal lobe, the prefrontal cortex, is concerned with executive function, or higher-order planning and execution of behavior.

The parietal lobe is located between the frontal and occipital lobes and above the temporal lobe. It is concerned primarily with perception and elaboration of somatic sensation and integration of multimodality or cross-modality information. Perception of pain, temperature, touch, and other somatosensory information is subserved by the parietal lobe. In addition, posterior portions of the parietal lobe, along with thalamic and prefrontal structures, play an important role in selective attention, specifically relating to switching attention from one location to another for purposes of detecting a target and in determining spatial relationships between objects. As such, the parietal lobe is implicated both in allocation of attention and in a variety of visual-spatial tasks.

The temporal lobe is located inferior to the frontal and parietal lobes and anterior to the occipital lobe. The Sylvian (lateral) fissure marks the superior boundary of this lobe. The temporal lobe is the site of the primary auditory cortex and auditory association areas, including Wernicke's area (or Brodmann area 22). In addition, along the medial surface of the temporal lobe is the *hippocampal formation*, which plays a role in emotional processing and memory. Auditory functions of the temporal lobe will be discussed further later in this chapter.

Only a small portion of the occipital lobe can be seen on the lateral surface of the brain. The majority of this lobe lies along the medial surface of the cerebral hemisphere. This lobe contains the primary and secondary visual cortices.

Upon midsagittal sectioning of the brain, further structures can be viewed (Figure 1-4). Most notable for our purposes is the *corpus callosum*. Present only in mammals, the corpus callosum is the largest fiber tract in the primate brain. Heavily myelinated (white matter), it is located at the base of the longitudinal fissure and connects most cortical areas of the two cerebral hemispheres. Because of its importance in central auditory processing, the corpus callosum will be discussed further later in this chapter.

Other structures of the brain seen in the midsagittal view include the *cerebellum* (located below the occipital lobe and posterior to the brainstem; it is concerned primarily with coordination of motor activities and maintenance of equilibrium); the *diencephalon*, which consists of both the *thalamus* (concerned with relay of sensorimotor information to the cortex and some speech/language and auditory functions) and the *hypothalamus* (regulates various autonomic functions such as

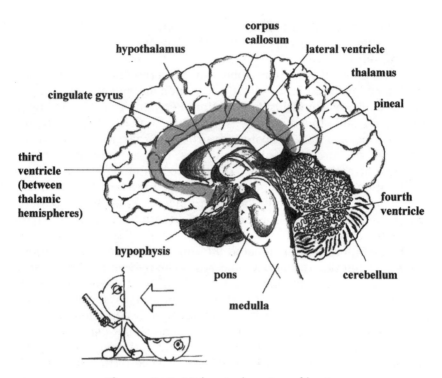

Figure 1-4. Midsagittal section of brain.

body heat production, hormone production, and reproduction, among others); the *pineal body* (appears to contribute to circadian rhythm and sexual reproduction cycles); and the *hypophysis (pituitary gland)*—called the "master gland" of the body—which secretes hormones that regulate a variety of functions, including metabolism, sexual drive, pain, emotion, temperature, and electrolyte control.

Two additional cerebral structures are worthy of mention: the *insula* and the *limbic system*. The *insular cortex*, also known as the *isle of Reil*, is located within the lateral fissure and cannot be viewed from the surface without spreading or removing portions of the frontal, parietal, and temporal lobes (Figure 1-5). As will be discussed later, the insula has important implications for audition.

The *cingulate gyrus* is located along the most medial margins of the frontal, parietal, and temporal lobes. This structure, along with the hippocampal formation and associated structures, forms the *limbic system*. The limbic system is thought to provide emotional drive to a

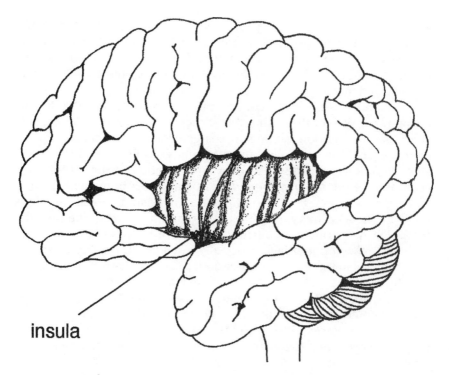

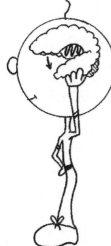

insula

Figure 1-5. Lateral view of brain with temporal lobe displaced to expose insula.

variety of functions necessary for survival, including instinctual reflexes, aggression, defensive behaviors (e.g., the "fight or flight" response), mating, and other primitive functions and emotional processing. More recently, the limbic system has also been implicated in learning and memory.

The *brainstem*, which will be considered in depth later in this chapter, consists of three structures: the *midbrain*, *pons*, and *medulla oblongata*. In addition, some sources consider the structures of the diencephalon (thalamus and hypothalamus) to be part of the brainstem (Bhatnagar & Andy, 1995). A good portion of the midbrain is composed of the *reticular formation*, which serves to mediate arousal and consciousness. It is also implicated in basic survival functions related to heart activity, respiration, and motor reflexes. The reticular formation is a principal contributing source to the middle and late auditory evoked potentials, especially in children, leading to significant changes in these potentials related to states of arousal and sleep. This topic will be discussed more fully in later chapters.

There are four *ventricles* (or cavities) within the brain that function to circulate cerebrospinal fluid: two *lateral ventricles*, a *third ventricle*, and a *fourth ventricle*. The body of the lateral ventricle is formed by the corpus callosum and the floor is formed by the superior surface of the thalamus. The lateral ventricle extends from the frontal lobe (anterior horn) to the occipital lobe (posterior horn). The third ventricle is located between the two hemispheres of the thalamus and connects superiorly to the lateral ventricle through Monro's foramen and inferiorly to the fourth ventricle of the brainstem through the cerebral aqueduct. The floor of the third ventricle is formed by the nuclei of the hypothalamus. The floor of the fourth ventricle is located in the brainstem at the level of the pons and medulla. Because of its location, hydrocephalus of the fourth ventricle can result in abnormal findings on auditory brainstem evoked potential testing due to compression of structures that give rise to the auditory brainstem response. The fourth ventricle contains openings through which cerebrospinal fluid can access the subarachnoid space surrounding the CNS.

The *basal ganglia* are subcortical (gray matter) structures that help to regulate muscle tone and motor functions (Figure 1-6). The primary structures of the basal ganglia are the *caudate, putamen,* and *globus pallidus*. The putamen and globus padillus lie between the *internal capsule* and the *external capsule*, which are pathways composed of white matter. The internal capsule is of particular interest, as it is the pathway through which auditory information is transmitted from the brainstem to the auditory cortex. The external capsule contains fibers that carry auditory (as well as somatic and possibly visual) information from the internal capsule to the insula. Within the external capsule lies a thin strip of gray matter, the *claustrum*, which also seems to be highly responsive to acoustic stimulation. Overall, the basal ganglia have been found to serve a function in motor control as well as in short-term memory and executive function.

The brain is protected within the head by the *meninges* (three fibrous tissue membranes that surround the CNS), cerebrospinal fluid, and the bones of the skull. These are only a few of the important structures of the brain, and readers are referred to the References at the end of this book for further, more detailed study.

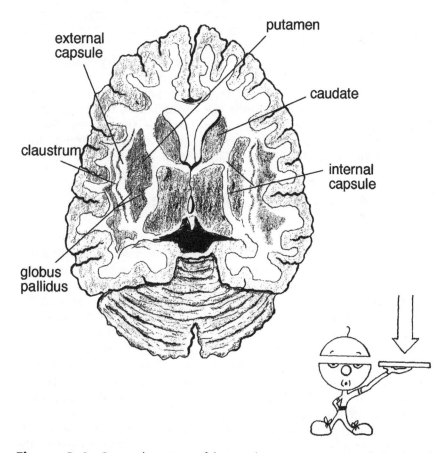

Figure 1-6. Coronal section of brain showing structures of the basal ganglia, internal and external capsules, and claustrum.

Bases of Neural Transmission

Nerve cells communicate through nerve impulses that are mediated by *neurotransmitters*, chemical substances that are released at the synapse and cause specific events to take place. The synapse is the point at which nerve cells interact. There are two primary effects of neurotransmitters: *excitatory* and *inhibitory*.

Excitatory neurotransmitters lower the postsynaptic cell's membrane potential or threshold, thus allowing the cell to fire and propagate the nerve impulse. Inhibitory neurotransmitters work in the opposite way by raising the threshold of the postsynaptic cell and making it less likely to fire. Both excitatory and inhibitory neurotransmitters are critical to appropriate functioning of the nervous system. Speed of transmission is related to the diameter of the nerve cell and amount of myelination, among other factors.

Although a complete discussion of neurochemistry is not within the scope of this chapter, it should be noted that the chemical composition at the synapse site is affected by a variety of drugs. Therefore, pharmacologic intervention holds great promise for the treatment of many auditory and vestibular complaints, either by increasing excitability of the postsynaptic neurons or by encouraging inhibition (Musiek & Hoffman, 1990; Sahley, Kalish, Musiek, & Hoffman, 1991).

Brainstem Auditory Pathways

Figure 1-7 is a diagram of the anterior surface of the brainstem. The most caudal portion of the brainstem is the *medulla*. Proceeding in a caudal to rostral direction, the next portion is the *pons*, and the most rostral portion is termed the *midbrain*. In order to view the posterior surface of the brainstem, the cerebellum must first be removed. A diagram of the posterior surface of the brainstem is shown in Figure 1-8. Although a few structures essential to auditory function can be seen on the surface of the brainstem, many cannot; transverse sectioning of the brainstem is required in order to view them adequately. Several brainstem structures comprise the ascending auditory pathway. These include the *cochlear nuclei, superior olivary complex, lateral lemniscus*, and *inferior colliculus* (Figure 1-9).

The auditory nerve and brainstem structures are frequently thought of as relay stations that simply pass information along from the ear to the brain. However, this view is overly simplistic and does not acknowledge the truly exquisite nature of processing and information

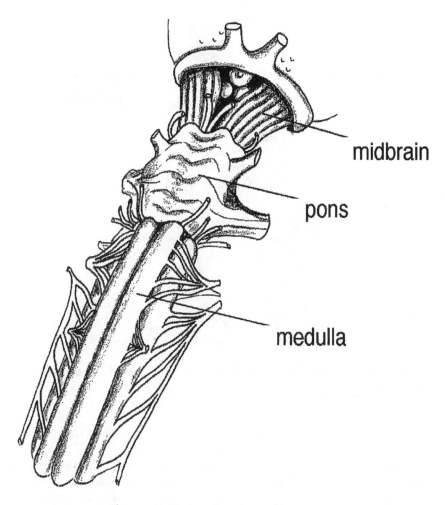

midbrain

pons

medulla

Figure 1-7. Anterior view of brainstem.

extraction that takes place at each point along the central auditory pathways. This having been said, readers should be cautioned that the neural mechanisms underlying the encoding of complex signals, including speech, are not fully understood. Rather, the majority of research in this area has focused on the encoding of relatively simple stimuli, and attempts have been made to extrapolate characteristics of such encoding that may have relevance for the processing of speech. In addition, our understanding of complex signal processing is more complete at

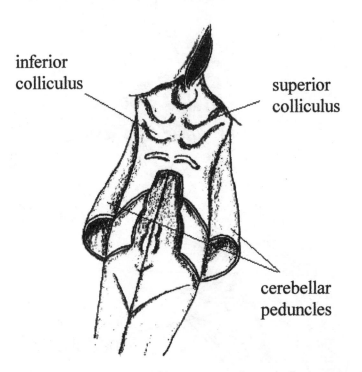

inferior
colliculus

superior
colliculus

cerebellar
peduncles

Figure 1-8. Posterior view of brainstem with cerebellum removed.

lower levels of the auditory pathways (e.g., auditory nerve) and decreases as we ascend in the auditory system.

Despite these drawbacks, it behooves us to examine what is known currently about neural encoding in general at each level of the CANS so that we may develop models of auditory processing that are consistent with the information available from neuroscience. Therefore, the following discussion will serve to acquaint readers with the various structures in the auditory pathways and to provide an overview of what is known about how auditory signals, particularly speech, are encoded at each level. Only in this way can an appreciation of the enormous complexity of the auditory system be facilitated.

Auditory Nerve

Although not a brainstem structure, and considered in some texts to be part of the peripheral auditory system, the synapse between the

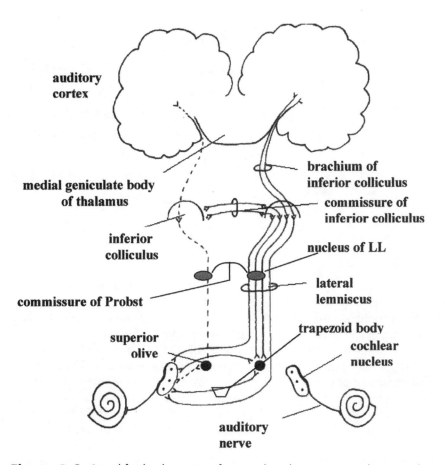

Figure 1-9. Simplified schematic of ascending brainstem auditory pathways.

hair cells of the cochlea and the *auditory nerve fibers* (*ANFs*) is where the neural transmission of auditory signals begins. As such, the auditory nerve serves a critical role in auditory processing, and disorders of the nerve have a significant impact on audition.

Single-unit recordings of ANFs have provided us with a reasonably clear idea of signal encoding at the level of the auditory nerve. The properties of the auditory nerve mirror the mechanical properties of the cochlea, particularly that of basilar membrane tuning. Therefore, ANFs demonstrate sharp frequency tuning, with the frequency to which each fiber responds optimally determined by the inner hair cell

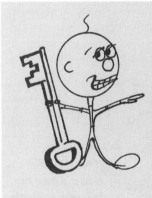

KEY CONCEPT

Rather than serving as simple relays, each level of the ascending auditory pathways contributes a significant amount of processing that results in extraction and enhancement of important speech features.

(IHC) of the cochlea with which the fiber synapses. In other words, ANFs with high-frequency tuning contact the IHCs in the basal portion of the cochlea while low-frequency ANFs contact the IHCs in the apical portion of the cochlea, resulting in tonotopic organization of ANFs.

Another important characteristic of ANFs is their ability to represent periodicities in the auditory signal via *phase-locking*. Through this mechanism, spectral peaks in the signal (e.g., fundamental and formant frequencies, modulations representing syllabic information) can be represented by ANF firing patterns up to approximately 4000 Hz.

Finally, for low to moderate intensities, ANFs represent intensity via increases and decreases in firing rate. Additional nerve fibers are recruited for the representation of high-intensity signals. The various combinations of which ANFs fire and at what rate, combined with the phase-locking capability mentioned above, allow the auditory nerve to represent faithfully the information in the auditory signal presented to the inner ear. What, then, does this mean for the encoding of speech signals themselves?

Delgutte (1997) listed three primary characteristics of continuous speech. First, continuous speech is characterized by relatively strong vowels alternating with relatively weak consonants (i.e., syllables), resulting in a modulation of the amplitude of the stimulus waveform at a frequency of approximately 3 to 4 Hz. Second, the spectral envelope of speech exhibits pronounced maxima that correspond to fundamental and formant frequencies. Third, speech stimuli exhibit both periodic and aperiodic components, with periodic components corresponding to voiced consonants and steady-state vowels, and aperiodic components corresponding to fricatives and stop consonants.

As such, **speech may be characterized by continuous, rapid alterations in amplitude envelope, spectral envelope, and fine spectral structure.**

Characteristics of ANFs that are critical for the encoding of running speech include their ability to phase-lock to periodicities, which is important for the representation of fundamental and formant frequencies found in steady-state vowels. Likewise, ANFs increase their firing rate to maxima in the amplitude envelope of the signal, thus representing overall syllabic structure. Spectral information, or the frequency components of both consonants and vowels, also can be represented by a place code, or which ANFs fire at a given point in time.

Two final, critical characteristics of ANFs are those of *short-term adaptation* and *suppression*. In response to signals that exhibit rapid changes in amplitude, such as very short tone bursts, ANFs display a maximal discharge rate shortly after the onset of the stimulus, then the rate decays gradually. This characteristic of ANF response patterns appears to play several roles in speech encoding. First, it increases the temporal resolution with which stimulus onsets, important for the perception of transient stimuli such as stop consonants, are encoded. Second, adaptation serves to enhance spectral contrasts between successive segments of the signal by decreasing the responsiveness of ANFs to successive stimuli that share spectral characteristics with preceding stimuli while, at the same time, continuing responsiveness to novel spectral characteristics. In this manner, the auditory nerve's response to spectral contrasts is enhanced. Furthermore, the nature of the spectral contrast will result in different patterns of adaptation in the auditory nerve. For example, the abrupt onset of affricate consonants results in a more prominent adaptation peak than does the more gradual onset of fricative consonants (Delgutte & Kiang, 1984). Thus, the peaks in discharge rate provided by adaptation help point to regions of the speech signal that are rich in phonetic information. The term *suppression* refers to the reduction in response of an ANF to a signal in the presence of another signal. This mechanism also serves to enhance contrasts in the auditory nerve and assists in the encoding of a signal in the presence of ongoing noise.

These basic characteristics of ANFs—phase-locking, tonotopicity, adaptation, and suppression—allow for the representation of both tonic (ongoing) and phasic (rapidly changing) components of the incoming acoustic signal. Because of the ongoing periodic nature of steady-state vowels, vowel encoding in the auditory nerve is relatively straightforward. The fundamental and formant frequencies of vowel stimuli are represented through a combination of phase-locking and place coding (i.e., a rate-place code).

Consonant stimuli present a more complex picture, primarily because of their inherent differing spectral components and rapid changes combined with a lack of periodicity. As discussed above, the tonotopicity of the auditory nerve allows for a place code for spectral, or frequency, components of consonants. Furthermore, short-term adaptation in the auditory nerve results in activity of ANFs at any given point in time being highly dependent on the immediately preceding context. This adaptation increases contrasts between successive speech segments, and also enhances cues related to consonant rise/fall time. For example, the response of ANFs to the speech sound [ch] demonstrates a very abrupt rise in discharge rate at the onset followed by a rapid decay, whereas the response to [sh] demonstrates a more gradual increase in average discharge rate commensurate with the longer rise time of [sh]. Therefore, the adaptation peak for [sh] is much less pronounced than is that for [ch] (Delgutte & Kiang, 1984). In this manner, profiles of absolute discharge rate allow for differential encoding of consonants that share essentially the same spectral characteristics, but differ in terms of stimulus rise time, such as voiceless fricatives. Finally, voice-onset time (VOT), or the delay between the release of stop consonants and the onset of voicing, is represented by accurate temporal representation of the onset of both the release and the voicing, thereby allowing for differential coding of contrasts such as /p/ versus /b/, which differ in VOT.

In summary, **the primary role of the auditory nerve is to break down the incoming acoustic signal into its components and to relay accurately all information to the CANS for further processing and extraction of relevant, perceptually salient, components.** Speech encoding at the level of the auditory nerve can be explained adequately by a combination of rate/place and temporal encoding along with methods of contrast enhancement. As a result, auditory nerve integrity is critical to the initial encoding of all characteristics of the speech signal. As a consequence, auditory nerve dysfunction can have a devastating impact on an individual's ability to process incoming auditory information.

Cochlear Nucleus—Pons

The cochlear nucleus, the most caudal structure in the CANS, may be considered the first level of the central auditory pathways in which actual processing of the signal occurs. In other words, whereas the auditory nerve breaks down the incoming signal into its characteristic components and relays this information to higher centers, the primary function of the cochlear nucleus appears to be the enhancement of certain features within the neural signal. This is accomplished, at this level and at higher levels in the central auditory system, via patterns of *divergence*, in which one neuron sends information to several other neurons, and *convergence*, in which input from several neurons converges upon one neuron, in combination with the presence of nerve cells that are specialized for specific functions.

There are three main cochlear nuclei (CN): the *anterior ventral* (AVCN), *posterior ventral* (PVCN), and *dorsal* (DCN). The CN are located on the posterolateral surface of the pontomedullary junction, where the pons, medulla, and cerebellum meet. This area is also known as the *cerebellopontine angle* and is a common site of tumors.

Upon entering the CN, ANFs diverge and send complementary information to different portions of the CN for differential processing of the signal. The cells within the CN complex are tonotopically arranged, with response patterns of those in the AVCN most resembling those of the auditory nerve. That is, many of the cells in the AVCN tend to demonstrate the precise phase-locking and sharp tuning of the ANFs with which they share large, secure synapses. Thus, there is a one-to-one relationship between tonotopic organization of the hair cells within the cochlea and tonotopic organization of the cells within the AVCN. Cells in the AVCN appear to function as simple relays, sending the information to higher centers without significant alterations. Consistent with this view, the AVCN receives ANFs that carry information from the entire cochlea—from base to apex—encompassing the entire frequency range. It should be noted that all areas of the CN exhibit tonotopic organization, with high-frequency information represented more ventrally and low-frequency information represented more dorsally within each division. This provides the beginning of parallel representation of information in the CANS in which the tonotopic organization of the cochlea is repeated throughout the ascending auditory pathways (Kiang, 1975).

In other areas of the CN, simple relay of unaltered signals does not occur. Rather, cells in the PVCN and DCN are designed to extract specific, perceptually salient information from the input provided by the auditory nerve. For example, within the PVCN, there are cells that respond robustly to the onset of stimulation, then demonstrate decreased activity for the remainder of the stimulus. These *onset units* are particularly useful in enhancing temporal information in the signal relating to onsets, which is very important for the perception of VOT, short duration consonant stimuli such as affricates, segmental aspects of the speech signal, and similar characteristics of speech stimuli. In contrast, *chopper units* in the PVCN respond to sinusoidal stimuli at regular intervals that are dependent on stimulus frequency and phase. As such, they provide information regarding absolute signal duration.

In the DCN, certain cells respond with one or two initial spikes at stimulus onset, followed by a silent period, then a gradual build-up of response for the duration of the stimulus. These *pauser units* are instrumental in the encoding of both stimulus onsets and duration. Similarly, *build-up units* in the DCN also respond to the duration of the signal with a gradual build-up in firing rate over time, but without the initial onset spikes. Finally, some units in the DCN exhibit excitatory responses to wideband noise and inhibition to tones, whereas others exhibit the opposite pattern of responses. Therefore, units in the DCN are implicated in enhancement of signals in noise. Additional signal enhancement is thought to occur in a top-down fashion through inhibitory influences of the efferent auditory system, which will be discussed later in this chapter.

The previous discussion provided a general overview of the main types of cell responses found in the CN. It should be noted, however, that several subtypes of each category of responses are seen as well. The proliferation of different response types in the CN, combined with divergence and convergence of input from ANFs, allows for the extraction of spectral features and enhancement of contrasts necessary for speech perception. For example, frequency encoding in the CN occurs in much the same manner as in the auditory nerve because primary units in the AVCN closely mirror the response patterns of ANFs. Intensity coding in the CN, although not fully understood, may well be accomplished by the presence of chopper units that demonstrate wide dynamic ranges and receive convergent input from ANFs of varying frequency, resulting in the encoding of wide variations in intensity, irrespective of frequency.

As previously suggested, **a key function of the CN appears to be contrast enhancement.** One particular characteristic of the auditory signal that undergoes significant enhancement within most areas of the CN is *amplitude modulation*. Amplitude modulation refers to the peaks and troughs in amplitude/intensity found in the spectral envelope of ongoing signals. Many of the cells in the CN enhance this modulation of the spectral envelope, making the peaks higher and the troughs lower. Thus, important portions of the speech signal, such as syllable structure, are rendered more prominent and, therefore, more accessible perceptually.

In addition to the enhancement of modulation in the spectral envelope, the diversity of response types in the CN allows for what may be the first stage of extraction of specific features within the auditory stimulus that ultimately will hold importance for speech perception. For example, units in the AVCN are particularly suited for the preservation of fine temporal aspects of the stimulus. Likewise, onset units are critical for the coding of onsets and transient changes. Therefore, even at this first brainstem level, we begin to see the effects of divergence and convergence of neurons that carry different information and the assumption of various roles by different regions and cells within the structure while, at the same time, maintaining the tonotopicity characteristic of the entire auditory system.

The importance of these response characteristics in the CN to speech perception is clear. For example, vowel encoding at the level of the CN occurs in much the same way as in the auditory nerve. Furthermore, at the level of the CN, we begin to see the beginnings of a rate/place code for vowels, which will become important as the ability to phase-lock decreases as the signal ascends in the CANS.

Not much is known about consonant encoding in the CN; however, because of the response characteristics of various units in this region of the brainstem, it is possible to hypothesize about the importance of different cell types to the encoding of consonant stimuli. For example, onset units likely play a critical role in the coding of transients, including VOT, rapid rise times, and frication. As previously discussed, the enhancement of modulation in the signal has likely implications for the overall encoding of syllabic information. Finally, because cells in the AVCN essentially mirror response patterns of ANFs, consonant encoding in this region likely occurs in the same manner as in the auditory nerve.

No discussion of the CN would be complete without some mention of the output pathways, each of which appears to subserve different purposes. Neurons in the CN project to more rostral structures by way of three main tracts: the *dorsal acoustic stria*, the *intermediate stria*, and the *ventral stria*. Although the majority (80%) of auditory fibers from the CN cross the midline (decussate) and project contralaterally, some of the fibers remain ipsilateral. The fibers of the dorsal stria project to the contralateral superior olivary complex, lateral lemniscus, and inferior colliculus. Fibers of the intermediate stria communicate with the contralateral lateral lemniscus and inferior colliculus. The ventral stria, by far the largest fiber tract, project to both the ipsilateral and contralateral superior olivary complex, which has profound implications for binaural hearing. The fact that the CN are located on the posterolateral surface of the brainstem makes it particularly susceptible to pathological effects of tumors such as acoustic neuromas. Finally, **because this is the first level in the CANS at which decussation occurs, dysfunction below this level will result primarily in ipsilateral abnormalities, whereas dysfunction at or above the level of the CN likely will result in bilateral or contralateral abnormalities. This concept is critical to any discussion of CAPD diagnosis and treatment that will occur in this text.**

In conclusion, the primary function of the CN appears to be contrast enhancement, particularly of modulation in the input signal and preliminary feature extraction for use by higher centers. At this level, as in subsequent levels of the CANS, convergence of disparate information onto a single cell along with divergence of complementary information to several cells with different response characteristics allows for feature extraction, enhancement, and integration of auditory input.

Superior Olivary Complex—Pons

The superior olivary complex (SOC) is medial to the cochlear nucleus in the caudal pons and cannot be viewed on the surface of the brainstem. It receives information from both ipsilateral and contralateral cochlear nuclei. Although specific processing of speech has not been studied in the SOC, **this structure is fundamental to the processing of binaural input, important for localization of auditory stimuli, and essential for hearing in the presence of background noise.** In addition, this level of the CANS provides a good illustration of the utility of convergence and divergence in the ascending central auditory pathways.

Coding of binaural cues in the SOC occurs in two primary ways. First, cells within the *medial superior olive* of the SOC are innervated by successive branches of incoming neurons from both the ipsilateral and contralateral CN. In other words, as a neuron enters the SOC, it sends branches to several cells in succession. This divergence of input from a single fiber results in a *delay line* of information, in which successive SOC cells are activated one after the other, resulting in an interaural time delay. In addition, branches of some CN fibers from both ears converge on single SOC cells at different times. Finally, some cells within the SOC respond preferentially to specific timing differences from the two ears. As a result, a population of cells in the SOC provides information regarding the localization of a sound source via interaural time/phase differences. It may even be logical to hypothesize that one reason that the periodicity information from the auditory nerve is preserved in the CN and passed on to the SOC is for the determination of interaural timing and phase differences because as the signal ascends in the auditory pathways beyond the level of the SOC, this information either does not appear to be as necessary or is coded in different ways.

A second method of binaural coding in the SOC occurs via differential patterns of excitation and inhibition. In this situation, information from the ipsilateral ear arrives at the *lateral superior olive* of the SOC directly from the CN, whereas information from the contralateral ear detours first through the medial nucleus of the *trapezoid body*, which appears to serve an inhibitory function. Therefore, binaural stimulation results in excitatory input from the ipsilateral ear and inhibitory input from the contralateral ear, in effect canceling one another out and resulting in no response from these SOC cells. Unilateral stimulation or intensity differences between ears, such as that seen in high-frequency localization, however, would result in differential patterns of excitatory and inhibitory input converging onto single SOC cells. As a result, those cells on the side ipsilateral to the stimulus would tend to respond in an excitatory fashion, whereas those contralateral to the stimulus would tend to be inhibited. This pattern of response enhances those cues that are important for localization of auditory stimuli.

Therefore, the SOC is implicated in successful localization, lateralization, and binaural integration using patterns of divergence and convergence of differential information from both ipsilateral and contralateral CN. This provides an excellent example of how successive levels of the CANS utilize the information provided by lower structures to extract and integrate relevant information from incoming signals. These functions of the SOC hold significant implications for binaural hearing in general, including those that aid in speech-in-noise skills.

Lateral Lemniscus—Pons

Composed of both ascending and descending fibers, **the lateral lemniscus (LL) is the primary ascending auditory pathway.** It extends from the SOC to the inferior colliculus in the midbrain. Like the SOC, the LL cannot be seen from the surface of the brainstem. It contains cell bodies (nuclei) along its length that receive crossed and uncrossed projections from more caudal auditory structures, thus continuing bilateral representation of auditory stimuli and possibly contributing further to feature extraction and enhancement. Tonotopic organization is present in the nuclei of the LL. Fibers from the nuclei of the LL can cross from one side to the other by way of the *commissure of Probst* or via the reticular formation.

Inferior Colliculus—Midbrain

The inferior colliculus (IC) is located on the posterior surface of the brainstem and is easily viewed following removal of the cerebellum. Both ICs are connected by commissural fibers, called the *brachium*. As a result, **the IC is another structure that has profound implications for the ability to localize sound sources and other binaural processes.**

The IC exhibits a *nucleotopic* organization in which different subdivisions receive multiple (parallel) sets of input from lower brainstem structures, resulting in partial segregation of neurons with different patterns of input. This is referred to as "patchy" organization—or the organization of patches of neurons with similar response characteristics separated from other patches of neurons with different response characteristics—and will become one of the fundamental organizational principles of the CANS.

In addition, the tonotopicity seen at every level of the CANS is also present in the IC in the form of *isofrequency laminae*, or sheets of cells, each of which corresponds to a single point on the cochlear basilar membrane. Within each lamina, a finer degree of organization is seen in which the sharpness of frequency tuning, threshold and latency of firing, and sensitivity to amplitude modulation differ among individual nerve fibers.

The sharpness of frequency tuning in the IC is also arranged tonotopically, with the sharpest tuning located in more central regions of each isofrequency lamina. This allows for continued place representation of frequency such as was seen in the auditory nerve and in lower areas of the brainstem. The ability of IC neurons to phase-lock to mid- to high-frequency stimuli is poor, although temporal representation of low frequencies and amplitude modulation remains robust.

Coding of specific speech stimuli has not yet been studied in the IC. However, the responses of IC neurons to complex amplitude- and frequency-modulated signals have been given some attention, and **it appears that the primary contribution of the IC to speech encoding is the further enhancement of modulations in the acoustic signal.**

As previously mentioned, the encoding of binaural signals is also strong in the IC. Specifically, many IC neurons demonstrate sensitivity to ongoing phase delays in the signal while others are sensitive to interaural intensity information obtained via converging input from lower centers. Therefore, the IC is involved in additional processing of binaural information from the CN. The diffuse pathway is implicated specifically in binaural hearing and in the establishment of a map of auditory space.

It is at the level of the IC that the ascending central auditory pathway appears to divide into two main pathways. The *primary (cochleotopic) pathway* originates in the central nucleus of the IC and is characterized by sharp tuning and tonotopic organization. The *diffuse (noncochleotopic) pathway* originates in the pericentral nucleus and exhibits broader frequency tuning and little or no tonotopicity. These two pathways most likely subserve different functions and ultimately project onto different areas within the auditory cortex. Some of the auditory information received by the IC is projected to the superior colliculus, reticular formation, and cerebellum for coordination of eye, head, and body movements in reflexive localization toward a sound source. In addition, the IC projects to both the ipsilateral and contralateral thalamus as well as directly to the ipsilateral cortex. It is possible that this direct projection from the IC to the cortex may be responsible for the preservation of some localization abilities in cases of thalamic or cortical lesions.

In conclusion, throughout the brainstem auditory pathways, we see both parallel and hierarchical processing of auditory stimuli. This means that progressive levels of convergence and divergence give rise to enhancement of specific spectral features and integration of input from the two ears. This information is represented redundantly via ipsilateral and contralateral projections to higher structures, possibly for differential processing of identical information by higher-order structures in the CANS.

The Thalamus

As **the primary way station for information between the brainstem and the cortex,** the thalamus consists of several nuclei with vastly different functions. Our discussion here will be concerned with the *medial geniculate body* **(MGB), the auditory nucleus of the thalamus.**

The MGB is located on the inferior surface of the thalamus, medial to the auditory cortex. Cell types within the MGB exhibit a wide variety of acoustic properties that tend to reflect the highly selective patterns of ascending and descending connectivity among the IC, MGB, and cortex. In other words, different regions within the MGB may derive acoustic input from the same source, yet respond in different manners. The incredible degree of convergence and divergence seen in the MGB results in the ability of a very small number of MGB cells working together to affect vast areas of the auditory cortex while, at the same time, processing and integrating information from lower levels. Furthermore, some regions of the MGB receive information from nonauditory areas such as the perirhinal cortex in the limbic system in addition to virtually every division of the IC. These regions, in turn, project to various nonauditory cortical areas as well as to each subdivision of the auditory cortex, both tonotopic and nontonotopic. Thus, **the MGB may play a significant role in multimodality integration.**

The ability of cells in the MGB to phase-lock to periodicities in the acoustic signal is, for the most part, poor, with *locker units* able to phase-lock only up to approximately 100 to 200 Hz. This low-frequency phase-locking ability has also been referred to as *entrainment*. Thus, the auditory system is unable to maintain a temporal code for frequency representation at this level. It is likely that this low-frequency entrainment serves an entirely different function, such as contributing to the encoding of fundamental frequency for pitch perception and amplitude-modulation coding for spectral information. The fact that tonotopic organization continues in regions of the MGB renders a rate-place code for continued higher frequency representation highly likely. Intensity coding in the MGB is not fully understood; however, the presence of cells that exhibit sound pressure levels to which they respond preferentially suggests that a rate-place code for intensity may be present as well.

A proliferation of response types may be seen throughout the auditory thalamus that allow for feature extraction in response to speech and other complex input signals. For example, certain cells respond preferentially to novel stimuli, providing a further mechanism for the encoding of onsets and transitions. Amplitude modulation in the signal continues to be enhanced in the MGB, and some cells exhibit a "best modulation frequency" to which they respond preferentially, or demonstrate directional sensitivity to either the maxima or minima in the spectrum. Therefore, it can be hypothesized that the modulation enhancement seen in the CN and the IC is put to use for the extraction of specific features of the modulation at the thalamic level. How this information ultimately is used in speech perception, however, remains a matter of speculation.

The encoding of specific consonant and vowel stimuli has not yet been studied in the thalamus. Indeed, because of the degree of complexity at this level of the CANS and the inability to predict the response of a single unit to complex stimuli from its response to simple stimuli, it is unlikely that single-unit recordings of MGB neurons would shed significant light on the processing of complex stimuli. It is more likely that **complex stimuli such as speech are coded over a population of neurons, with the response of a single unit at any instant in time being affected significantly by the context immediately preceding, as well as by convergent input from other neurons.** Therefore, a more useful method of investigating the coding of complex stimuli at the level of the MGB is through the use of multiple unit recordings and evoked potentials.

Kraus and colleagues at Northwestern University (King, McGee, Rubel, Nicol, & Kraus, 1995; Kraus, McGee, Carrell, King, Littman, & Nicol, 1994; Kraus, McGee, Littman, Nicol, & King, 1994; McGee, Kraus, King, & Nicol, 1996) have described the investigation of discrimination of acoustic contrasts via electrophysiologic recording. Results of their studies in the animal model suggest that **stimuli with slowly varying acoustic parameters such as /ba/ versus /wa/, in which the primary difference is in the duration of the formant transition, appear to be coded adequately at the thalamic level.** A particularly interesting finding is that neural representation of such segments may actually occur in nonprimary thalamus rather than in areas considered to be primary auditory thalamic regions. **In contrast, stimuli that consist of rapid spectral-acoustic changes in which a precise integration of both onset and frequency is required, such as /da-ga/, require integration across a neuronal pool, a task more suited to the auditory cortex.** Furthermore, tone-burst discrimination encoding appears to occur at the subcortical (i.e., thalamic or lower) level as well. These findings are consistent with reports of impaired consonant discrimination, especially stop consonants that exhibit rapid changes, combined with intact vowel discrimination, in which the stimuli are of longer duration, in cases of cortical damage (Phillips & Farmer, 1990).

Finally, the issue of binaural processing in the auditory thalamus should be addressed. It is important to note that cells within the MGB differ in their responses to monaural and binaural stimuli. Cells that respond to binaural stimuli, logically referred to as *binaural responders*, relay integrated information from the two ears obtained from both the ipsilateral and contralateral IC to the ipsilateral cortex where, as we will see, ear dominance bands exist that exhibit characteristic responses to input from the ipsilateral versus the contralateral ear.

In conclusion, **a vast amount of processing of the input signal occurs at the thalamic level, including contrast and amplitude modulation enhancement, extraction of features, encoding of binaurality, and additional complex signal processing.** Indeed, it appears that some speech signals, such as vowels and slowly changing consonant stimuli, may be encoded sufficiently well at the level of the thalamus so as to demonstrate preservation even in cases of cortical damage. Certainly, further investigation into the role of the thalamus, as well as other areas of the CANS, in complex speech encoding is needed. However, from the information presently available, it is clear that a great deal of processing of auditory signals occurs at each level of the CANS prior to ever arriving at the level of the auditory cortex.

Auditory Areas of the Cerebrum

Neurons that respond to auditory stimuli have been found in virtually every region of the cerebrum, including the parietal, frontal, and occipital cortex in addition to the expected temporal lobe regions. This discussion, however, focuses on the two main auditory areas of the temporal lobe: the *primary auditory cortex* (*cochleotopic; AI*) and the *auditory association cortex* (*noncochleotopic or diffuse; AII*). Additional auditory areas of the temporal lobe exist, including the anterior and posterior auditory fields; however, these will not be discussed in this chapter.

Primary Auditory Cortex

The primary auditory cortex, also referred to as *Heschl's gyrus*, or AI, is located approximately two-thirds of the way posteriorly on the upper surface of the temporal lobe. This upper surface also is referred to as the *supratemporal plane*. Heschl's gyrus cannot be observed on the lateral surface of the cortex; instead, the temporal lobe must be removed or displaced inferiorly in order to expose the supratemporal plane (Figure 1-10). The primary auditory cortex receives projections from the MGB via the *internal capsule, insula,* and *external capsule* and, like all levels of the CANS, retains the tonotopic organization of the cochlea. In fact, although the auditory cortex has been viewed historically as consisting of one primary, tonotopically organized area surrounded by secondary areas, recent findings have shown that several tonotopic areas exist within the auditory cortex, and these areas are interconnected anatomically (Phillips, 1995). Although the various tonotopically organized auditory fields appear to exhibit differences in response characteristics, the actual perceptual implications of such differences for speech perception are not yet understood.

In this section, we summarize general findings regarding stimulus encoding in the tonotopically organized primary (usually left hemi-

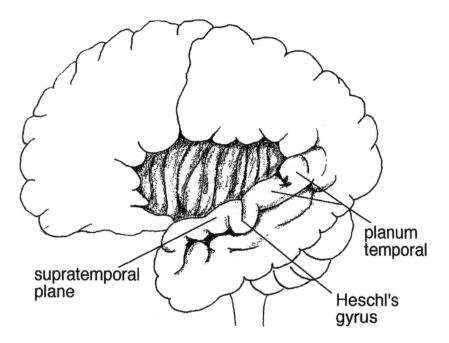

Figure 1-10. Lateral view of brain with temporal lobe displaced to expose Heschl's gyrus.

sphere) auditory cortex (AI), and suggest possible implications of such response characteristics for speech perception in general. It should be noted that the complexity of auditory cortical organization precludes a simple description of response characteristics to simple or complex stimuli. Indeed, **even frequency and intensity representation in AI appear to occur via aggregate input from a population of neurons rather than from simple single-unit responses.** As a result, the following discussion will be based on studies using both single- and multiple-unit electrophysiologic recordings.

The middle layers of AI are tonotopically organized, with low frequencies represented posteriorly and high frequencies represented anteriorly. Cells with similar frequency responses appear to be arranged along isofrequency contours in AI. Furthermore, as discussed by Schreiner (1995), the size of the receptive fields of individual fibers varies along the isofrequency axis, with the most narrow bandwidths located in the medial portion of each contour and wider bandwidths observed at the ends. Adding further to the complexity of the organization in AI, fibers are organized in *ear-dominance bands* as well, so that different patterns of response to ear-specific stimulation exist within each band, regardless of frequency (Schreiner & Mendelson, 1990). It is likely that these bands are the result of converging input from the auditory thalamus, as well as from the contralateral cortex via interhemispheric connections. Therefore, binaural representation continues to be particularly strong at the cortical level.

It has been suggested that stimulus intensity may be represented in AI in two possible ways (Phillips, 1990). First, cells exist that exhibit preferential responses to certain intensities while, at the same time, other cells continue to speed up firing rate with increasing intensity in a monotonic, or relatively linear, fashion. Second, it is possible that stimulation of different populations of neurons across a neuronal ensemble with differences in signal intensities occurs, resulting in an "amplitopic," or place code for intensity. In this situation, firing rates of the neurons themselves would remain relatively stable regardless of intensity, but different populations of neurons would respond to different stimulus intensities. It should be noted, however, that it is not clear whether either or both of these mechanisms adequately explains the coding of intensity in AI.

As mentioned several times previously, the ability of neurons to phase-lock to frequency components in the signal decreases as the signal ascends in the CANS. At the level of AI, locker units such as those seen in the thalamus continue to be present, but their phase-locking or entrainment capability is limited to very low frequencies (i.e., approximately 50 to 100 Hz). Therefore, it is unlikely that a temporal code based on phase-locking is possible for frequency representation in AI. Syllabic information, however, continues to be represented adequately.

On the other hand, a place code for frequency representation appears to be highly likely due to the exquisite tonotopic organization of AI. Furthermore, populations of neurons with similar frequency response characteristics have been shown to demonstrate remarkable synchronization in firing that continues throughout the duration of the stimulus (DeCharms & Merzenich, 1996). This characteristic of AI response patterns may provide a basis for extraction of the time course and frequency of an ongoing stimulus via coordination of spikes across populations of neurons working together.

As we have seen, convergence of ascending input results in an enhancement of modulations in the auditory signal as higher levels of the CANS are reached. Responses of AI fibers to amplitude-modulated signals exhibit sensitivity to both direction and rate of amplitude change, as well as to carrier signal level (Phillips & Hall, 1987). AI neurons most efficiently represent modulation frequencies up to approximately 50 to 100 Hz. Although the significance of this fact for general speech perception is not clear, it is important to note that this frequency range does encompass the modulation range seen in the envelope of running speech.

A common misconception regarding the auditory cortex is that neurons at this level demonstrate poor temporal encoding. This certainly is true when one defines *temporal encoding* as the ability to phase-lock to periodicities in the signal. However, **when temporal coding is considered in terms of precision of spike response timing, the temporal resolution of neurons in AI is quite excellent.** Indeed, it has been shown that the ability of neurons in AI to discharge precisely to the onset of a stimulus is nearly as good as that seen in the auditory nerve (Phillips & Hall, 1990). Therefore, cortical neurons are able to represent faithfully the timing of phonetically important components of speech, such as VOT, place of articulation, and rapid spectro-temporal transitions.

In contrast, the type of temporal encoding necessary for vowel representation—phase-locking to fundamental and formant frequencies—appears to be virtually nonexistent in AI. It is possible, however, that the population place code for frequency, as discussed previously, may be instrumental in vowel representation at the cortical level. Indeed, it appears that **the cortex exhibits a specialized role in the coding of rapid acoustic events necessary for fine-grained acoustic discrimination, such as that necessary for discrimination among stop consonants. These findings hold particular implications for the effects of cortical pathology on different types of speech signals, with consonant discrimination more vulnerable to disruption by cortical dysfunction than vowel discrimination.** A second key function of the auditory cortex appears to be in the development of a concept of auditory space in the contralateral field and in the coordina-

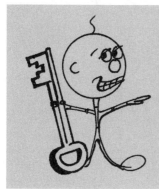

KEY CONCEPT

Temporal encoding of stimulus onsets and other rapid transient events is excellent at the level of the primary auditory cortex.

tion of behavioral responses in relation to localization via multimodality integration.

Auditory Association Cortex

The primary and association auditory cortices are connected by an extensive axonal bundle. Structurally, the *planum temporal* extends along the cortical surface from the most posterior portion of Heschl's gyrus back along the *lateral (Sylvian) fissure* to its end point. The *supramarginal gyrus* curves around the most posterior aspect of the lateral fissure. This area, along with the *angular gyrus* (located immediately posterior to the supramarginal gyrus) is the approximate region of *Wernicke's area*, and is referred to as the auditory association cortex, or AII (Figure 1-11).

Wernicke's area is concerned with recognition of linguistic stimuli and comprehension of spoken language and contributes to language formulation. Specifically, Wernicke's area is instrumental in recognizing words and other language stimuli, interpreting their meaning on the basis of previous auditory memory and linguistic experience, and comprehending spoken language. In addition, the portion of Wernicke's area that extends into the inferior parietal lobe is also

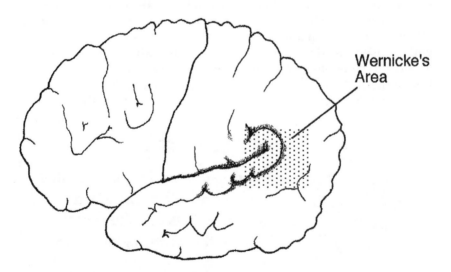

Wernicke's Area

Figure 1-11. Lateral view of brain.

implicated in reading and written language. As such, this area involves a good deal of multimodality as well as multifunction integration and, therefore, will be discussed more comprehensively in Chapter 2, when we consider top-down factors in auditory processing.

Asymmetries of Auditory Areas of the Cerebrum

Geschwind and Levitsky (1968) initially discovered that the planum temporal was larger on the left side than on the right in the majority of the subjects they studied. The implications of this finding are significant when theories of hemispheric dominance for language are considered. In addition, Musiek and Reeves (1990) reported a relationship between the length of the Sylvian fissure and the length of the planum temporal, with both structures being significantly longer on the left side in all specimens studied. Heschl's gyrus was also found to be longer on the left side. **It is possible that these cerebral asymmetries contribute to left-hemisphere dominance for functions involving binaural listening, and provide a basis for greater language development potential for the left side** (Musiek & Reeves, 1990).

Regarding functional asymmetries in auditory areas of the cerebrum, for the majority of people (96% to 98.3%), **the left hemisphere is dominant for language function, including analytic syntactic and semantic linguistic processing, phonological analysis and discrimination, word retrieval, and the like** (Gazzaniga et al., 1998; Kolb & Whishaw, 1996; Rasmussen & Milner, 1977). In contrast, for most individuals, **the right hemisphere typically subserves perception of nonlinguistic stimuli, including rhythm, stress, and other nonlinguistic acoustic parameters; the perception of acoustic contours within a linguistic or nonlinguistic signal; discrimination and ordering of tonal stimuli; and prosodic elements of speech.** For example, when listening to musical pieces that have lyrics, it has been shown that the perception of a song's words is subserved by the left hemisphere, whereas perception of the melody is subserved by the right hemisphere (Gazzaniga et al., 1998). It should be remembered, however, that hemispheric specialization is not absolute and that both hemispheres may contribute somewhat to all auditory functions. Furthermore, a small percentage of normal right-handed individuals exhibit reversed cerebral dominance for language with no ill effects whatsoever. Lastly, it has been estimated that, although the majority of left-handed individuals exhibit typical left-hemisphere dominance for language, approximately 15% exhibit either reversed or bilateral cerebral dominance. Therefore, the finding of reversed cerebral dominance in a given individual may or may not be indicative of cortical dysfunction. These findings underscore the necessity for recognizing the existence of normal variations in brain organization.

It is of particular interest to note that functional asymmetry in the neurophysiological representation of speech stimuli is not restricted to the auditory cortex. Indeed, **such asymmetries have been shown to be present even at the thalamic level, indicating that laterality of some auditory functions may be a fundamental principle of elemental sensory representation of speech** (King, Nicol, McGee, & Kraus, 1999).

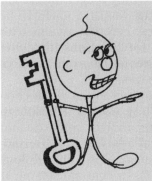

KEY CONCEPT

Functional asymmetry and left-sided dominance for speech-sound encoding is present even at the level of the auditory thalamus.

Additional Auditory-Responsive Areas of the Cerebrum

The inferior portions of the parietal and frontal lobes are also responsive to acoustic stimulation, as are some portions of the anterior occipital lobe. In addition, as mentioned previously, the insula has a large number of fibers that respond to acoustic input. This is not surprising, as the posterior aspect of the insula is immediately adjacent to Heschl's gyrus.

There are two primary pathways through which auditory information is transmitted from the MGB in the thalamus to the auditory cortex. The first is via the internal capsule to Heschl's gyrus. The second is through the internal capsule, under the putamen to the external capsule, and to the insula.

Finally, Wernicke's area in the temporal lobe connects to Broca's area in the frontal lobe via the *arcuate fasciculus,* a large fiber tract. Broca's area is considered to be responsible for motor speech output and this area has been shown to be activated during auditory comprehension tasks. Therefore, audition is not a simple process involving auditory cortical areas in the temporal lobes alone. Rather, the overall skill of processing auditorily presented information involves a complex network of integrative activity encompassing areas within virtually every region of the brain in addition to lower CANS structures.

Summary of Auditory Signal Encoding in the CANS

The information presented in the previous sections of this chapter reveals some general organizational principles and encoding characteristics of ascending CANS levels. **One fundamental organizing principle of the CANS is its tonotopicity.** At every synaptic level, neuronal fibers are arranged to represent specific places on the basilar membrane of the cochlea. This organization may serve as the basis for a variety of perceptual phenomena, including frequency representation, binaural processing, and cortical representation of steady-state components across neuronal populations.

A second key organizing principle of the CANS is its pattern of convergence and divergence. At every level, from the CN upward, convergence of disparate information onto single cells forms the basis for integration and enhancement of afferent input. In addition, divergence of complementary information onto physiologically segregated cell regions allows for the extraction of specific acoustic features of the signal and for parallel representation of important auditory information. Because of this, **assigning a single role to any CANS structure would be impossible. Instead, each level of the CANS serves multiple functions, and these functions likely are both anatomically and physiologically segregated.**

The auditory nerve apparently functions to break down the signal arriving at the cochlea into its constituent parts for relay to and further processing by higher CANS levels. Therefore, it is critical for fibers in the auditory nerve to be able to respond in a relatively homogeneous and predictable fashion so that all information needed by higher CANS levels is represented faithfully. Because of this, one can

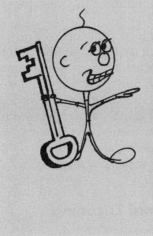

KEY CONCEPT

General CANS organizational principles include parallel and distributed networks, tonotopicity, patterns of divergence and convergence, and "patchy" organization. At higher levels, phase-locking decreases and feature extraction and enhancement increase.

readily see why dysfunction at the level of the auditory nerve that disrupts the precise synchrony of firing can have disastrous consequences for ultimate speech perception.

As the auditory signal ascends in the CANS, the ability of neurons to phase-lock to periodicities in the signal decreases. Indeed, after the extraction of periodicity-related temporal information necessary for the determination of interaural phase differences important for localization occurs at the level of the SOC, the representation of such information is not noted as precisely at higher levels. On the other hand, an increase in enhancement and extraction of phonetically relevant characteristics of the signal, such as modulations and onsets, is seen with ascending levels of the CANS. **By the time the signal reaches the cortical level, much processing has already been accomplished and, in AI, convergence and divergence of ascending input allows for a cortical representation of auditory space and, most important, the precise temporal encoding of transients critical to auditory discrimination of consonants.** Therefore, far from being merely relay centers that pass information from the cochlea up to the cortex unchanged, each level of the CANS plays a significant role in speech perception. Information regarding auditory signal encoding at each level of the CANS is summarized in Table 1-1.

The Corpus Callosum

The auditory cortical areas in both hemispheres are connected to one another via the corpus callosum. As mentioned previously, the corpus

Table 1-1

Summary of Auditory Signal Encoding and Contribution to Auditory Processing of Each Level of the Ascending Auditory Pathways

Auditory Structure	Key Contributions to Auditory Processing
Auditory Nerve	Breakdown of incoming signal from cochlea into constituent components via phase-locking, tonotopic organization, adaptation, and suppression for relay to higher CANS structures
Cochlear Nuclei	Contrast enhancement of modulations and transients in the signal and preliminary feature extraction via convergence and divergence and differential cell responses
Superior Olivary Complex	Coding of binaural cues via convergence and divergence from ipsilateral and contralateral cochlear nuclei for localization, lateralization, and binaural integration
Inferior Colliculus	Further enhancement of amplitude modulations and binaural cues; division of ascending pathway into primary and diffuse auditory systems
Medial Geniculate Body	Primary way station for information between brainstem and cortex; coding of stimuli with slowly changing acoustic parameters such as vowels and syllable contrasts differing in duration; additional binaural encoding, contrast and modulation enhancement, feature extraction, and complex signal processing; multimodality integration
Primary Auditory Cortex	Coding of rapid acoustic events necessary for fine-grained discrimination, especially of consonant stimuli; development of the concept of auditory space for localization
Auditory Association Cortex	Recognition of linguistic stimuli, comprehension of spoken language, some language formulation capacity

callosum is the largest commissural fiber bundle and connects the two cerebral hemispheres.

The corpus callosum consists of five main parts. They are, moving in an anterior to posterior direction, the *anterior commissure, rostrum, genu, body*, and *splenium* (Figure 1-12). Within the corpus callosum, some areas of the cortex project to the same (*homotopic*) functional region in the opposite hemisphere. Conversely, some areas project to both homotopic and *heterotopic* regions, or regions subserving differ-

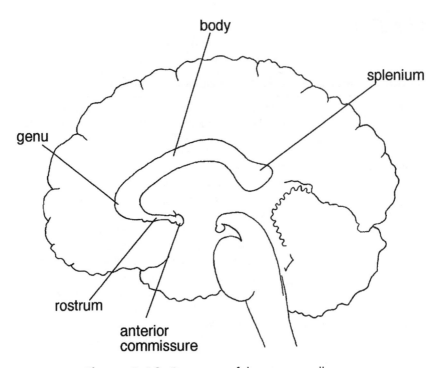

Figure 1-12. Five parts of the corpus callosum.

ent functions, in the opposite hemisphere. For example, the primary sensory cortex projects to primary sensory, associative, and supplemental sensory cortices in the opposite hemisphere (Pandya & Kuypers, 1969). On the other hand, interhemispheric connectivity of the visual cortex is confined primarily to the splenium of the corpus callosum. Furthermore, some bidirectionality, or back-and-forth transmission, can be seen in the connectivity of certain cortical fibers, including those of the auditory cortex (Pandya, 1995). Thus, **interhemispheric connectivity via the corpus callosum is extremely complex, with a significant amount of overlap of fibers from different cortical regions existing in many portions of the structure.** Finally, it appears that some regions of the cortex exhibit virtually no interhemispheric connectivity whatsoever.

Although most cortical fibers do not traverse the corpus callosum in a purely horizontal direction, contacting the homolateral region in the opposite hemisphere via the shortest possible route, it is a general rule that interhemispheric fibers project to the contralateral cortex via the section of the corpus callosum adjacent to the cortical region from which they arise. Therefore, fibers of the primary motor cortex in the frontal lobe project to the contralateral hemisphere via the anterior portion of the callosum, while, as previously mentioned, fibers of the visual cortex in the occipital lobe project via the splenium, or posterior portion of the corpus callosum. It should be noted that **a rich network of *intra*hemispheric, or connections among various areas of the same hemisphere, exists as well, resulting in a remarkable degree of connectivity among virtually all areas of the cortex and allowing for multimodality integration.**

The auditory segment of the corpus callosum is confined primarily to its posterior portion. Baran, Musiek, and Reeves (1986) found that although anterior sectioning of the corpus callosum resulted in essentially no change in central auditory function, posterior commissurotomy significantly altered auditory function. Specifically, the posterior two-thirds of the callosum has been shown to be critical for auditory, as well as visual and tactile, interhemispheric transfer of sensory information (Musiek, Reeves, & Baran, 1985; Musiek & Reeves, 1986; Myers, 1959; Myers & Ebner, 1976; Sauerwein & Lassonde, 1997). Interhemispheric projections of the primary auditory cortex exhibit finer organization; areas of similar tonotopic arrangement and binaural sensitivity are connected, possibly providing a mechanism for midline auditory fusion and conceptualization of auditory space necessary for tracking an object and localization. The role of the anterior portion of the corpus callosum is less clear; however, it appears that this region may play a role in cognitive, rather than sensory, interaction, including the transfer of semantic information between the hemispheres (Sidtis, Volpe, Holtzman, Wilson, & Gazzaniga, 1981).

Damage or dysfunction anywhere along the transcallosal pathway can have a significant effect on the interhemispheric exchange of sensory information. In addition, **because the corpus callosum has contact with such a large part of the brain, lesions of the cortex, which is very thin, also may affect fibers of the corpus callosum.**

The corpus callosum is primarily responsible for the communication and integration of information from the two cerebral hemispheres. In the case of auditory processing, the left hemisphere is dominant for functions such as syntactic and semantic aspects of language, phonological discrimination, and whole-to-part analysis. The right hemisphere is dominant for music perception and other acoustic contour recognition tasks, and for part-to-whole gestalt synthesis. For an individual to perform certain auditory tasks—such as dichotic listening, which will be discussed in Chapter 2—the two cerebral hemispheres must be able to communicate. Lesions affecting the corpus callosum will significantly affect individuals' ability to perform these auditory tasks.

The function of the corpus callosum described above may be thought of as being *facilitatory* in nature. That is, integration of information between hemispheres relies on bilateral excitation of neurons. It has been suggested, however, that the corpus callosum serves an *inhibitory* function as well (Dennis, 1976; Gazzaniga & Hillyard, 1973; Preilowski, 1972, 1975). Ringo and colleagues (Ringo, Doty, Demeter, & Simard, 1994) have presented a model in which the inhibitory function of the corpus callosum leads to lateralization and hemispheric dominance for certain tasks during development. In their model, the authors suggested that the time lag that occurs during conduction of information from one hemisphere to the other is, in many cases, too long to permit interhemispheric integration of neural impulses. Rather, the authors suggested that the delays associated with interhemispheric communication via the corpus callosum actually may serve to inhibit neural responses to competing stimuli in the opposite hemisphere, resulting in a greater degree of laterality and hemispheric specialization.

Such a view holds important implications for assessing callosal integrity in that **dysfunction in the corpus callosum may result in *more* laterality for tasks that require the callosum to serve in a facilitatory fashion (e.g., dichotic listening tasks, in which disparate information to the two hemispheres must be integrated). Conversely, callosal dysfunction may result in *less* laterality on tasks that require the callosum to serve an inhibitory function (e.g., when the same information is presented to both hemispheres simultaneously).** Indeed, recent electrophysiologic studies of interhemispheric dysfunction in aging populations have yielded just such a pattern, with dysfunction resulting in greater laterality during conditions of dichotic stimulation (Jerger, Moncrieff, Greenwald, Wambacq, & Seipel, 2000), whereas neurophysiologic representation of noncompeting speech signals demonstrated bilateral symmetry, or less laterality (Bellis, Nicol, & Kraus, 2000).

Although the importance of the facilitatory function of the callosum has obvious real-world applicability in the integration of disparate information processed by the two hemispheres both within and across modalities into a unitary percept, the purpose of inhibition in the corpus callosum beyond the developmental years is more subtle. Moscovitch (1992) provided a theory that directly relates inhibition in the corpus callosum to successful language processing and production. In this theory, the nondominant (usually right) hemisphere retains some language processing abilities as a fail-safe mechanism in case of irreversible damage to the dominant hemisphere.

However, in the normal brain, the language capabilities of the non-dominant hemisphere must be suppressed, because, if both hemispheres processed verbal input at the same time, they would compete for control of motor speech output pathways. Furthermore, because speech sounds require very rapid processing in terms of both reception and production, and because the time required for interhemispheric integration of input and output far exceeds the fine time resolution necessary for perception and production, a lack of nondominant hemisphere suppression would result in competition between the two hemispheres, thus increasing distortion.

A final argument in support of the need for callosal inhibition may be found from the performance of right-handed individuals who develop right-hemisphere dominance for language as a result of left-hemisphere damage at birth. Many of these individuals demonstrate poorer performance on visual-spatial tasks than do typical right-handers (Miller, 1971; Nebes, 1971). Therefore, it is possible that language, visual-spatial, and other nonverbal abilities may compete in the nondominant hemisphere if restriction of language to the dominant hemisphere does not occur.

It should be emphasized, however, that **there is no direct evidence that inhibition actually occurs in the corpus callosum.** In fact, physiologic evidence suggests that the neurons of the callosum are primarily, if not exclusively, excitatory (e.g., Swadlow, 1979). Furthermore, there is a marked absence of inhibitory neurotransmitter in the corpus callosum (Voigt, LeVay, & Stamnes, 1988). These findings have led to the development of alternative theories of corpus callosum function that allow for the presence of "slow" and "fast" channels that result in adaptive behaviors such as the slowing down of the hand controlled by the dominant (faster) hemisphere and the speeding up of the hand controlled by the nondominant (slower) hemisphere for tasks requiring synchronized bimanual coordination. **Such a dynamic model of corpus callosum function would permit the presence of fast *inter*hemispheric channels that could, in theory, be faster than slow *intra*hemispheric channels, thus having the same effects that have been attributed to callosal inhibition.**

Whether the corpus callosum functions in an excitatory fashion with differentially speeded channels, or exerts inhibitory influences as well, it is clear that the functions of the corpus callosum traverse a wide variety of domains. The structure is implicated in functions ranging from basic sensory perception of different stimuli presented to the two hemispheres to general executive functions such as bilateral arousal and attention. Modality-specific functions, including those directly related to audition, may be affected adversely by callosum dysfunction, as may multimodality functions requiring integration

Table 1-2
Overview of Selected Cognitive and Sensory Functions to which the Corpus Callosum Contributes

Cognitive/Sensory Domain	Corpus Callosum Contributes To:
Audition	Binaurality and localization; verbal labeling of nonverbal auditory stimuli; auditory figure-ground abilities; verbal labeling of left-ear dichotic stimuli; phonological processing; perception of midline fusion
Language	Linking of prosodic and linguistic input for judging communicative intent; development of hemispheric specialization and lateralization of function; other syntactic, semantic, and pragmatic functions
Other Sensory	Bilateral comparison of tactile stimuli; verbal labeling of objects in nondominant hand or visual field; binding of stimulus attributes for object formation; visuospatial and visuoperceptual skills; perception of tactile and visual midline fusion
Motor	Bimanual and bipedal coordination
Higher-Order Cognition	Selective and sustained attention; mediation of bilateral arousal levels; multimodality integration; sound-symbol association for reading and spelling; linking of orthographic symbols and linguistic meaning for reading comprehension and written language; auditory-verbal learning and memory; all tasks requiring interhemispheric integration

between the two hemispheres. Abilities in which the corpus callosum appears to play a role are summarized in Table 1-2.

Efferent Auditory Pathways

In recent years, much attention has been given to the *efferent*, or *centrifugal*, auditory pathway; however, the function of this pathway is still not fully understood. It is known that an efferent system runs from the auditory cortex to the cochlea and parallels the afferent system.

Available information indicates that the efferent auditory system includes both excitatory and inhibitory activity, and has significant implications in functions such as detection of a signal in a background of noise (Noback, 1985).

The *olivocochlear bundle* (*OCB*) has received the majority of the focus of the research into the efferent auditory pathways. As its name implies, the OCB extends from the superior olivary complex (SOC) to the fibers beneath the hair cells of the cochlea. The OCB apparently has inhibitory effects on the hair cells themselves as well as on the acoustic reflex. In addition, it has been hypothesized that the OCB may play a role in auditory attention (Musiek, 1986). Additional hypotheses regarding the role of the OCB include, as previously stated, the improvement of detection of signals in noise, particularly when discrimination of two sounds is required; maintenance of optimal mechanical function of the cochlea; and assistance in the proper coding of transients and other brief stimuli. For more comprehensive, albeit quite technical, reviews of efferent auditory system function, readers are referred to Berlin (1999) and Sahley, Nodar, and Musiek (1997).

Summary

Familiarity with the anatomy and physiology of the central auditory nervous system is critical for appropriate assessment and management of auditory processing and its disorders. Information processing theory states that both bottom-up factors (or sensory encoding) and top-down factors (or cognition, language, and other higher-order functions) work together to affect ultimate processing of auditory input. The human brain consists of two cerebral hemispheres separated by the longitudinal fissure. The cerebrum can be divided into four primary lobes—the frontal, parietal, occipital, and temporal—each of which subserves different functions. The brainstem consists of three major divisions: the pons, medulla oblongata, and midbrain. The ascending central auditory nervous system extends from the auditory nerve to Heschl's gyrus, the primary auditory cortex. Patterns of convergence and divergence and the presence of cells that exhibit differential response characteristics result in the enhancement and extraction of features in the auditory signal that are important for binaural hearing and speech perception. The corpus callosum serves to integrate information between the two hemispheres both within and across modalities, and may also serve in an inhibitory fashion to diminish the possibility of interhemispheric competition in selected tasks. The efferent central auditory system parallels the ascending system and is thought to be instrumental in the detection of auditory signals in noise and auditory attention, as well as in performing other inhibitory and excitatory activities.

Review Questions

(Answers to all review questions are provided in the Appendix.)

1. Define the following terms related to planes of reference and directional orientation within the brain:

   sagittal   coronal
   horizontal   transverse
   anterior   posterior
   rostral   caudal
   lateral/distal   medial/proximal
   dorsal   ventral

2. Using the following diagram, identify and discuss the anatomical significance of the following cerebral landmarks and lobes:

   longitudinal fissure   central sulcus
   lateral (Sylvian) fissure   frontal lobe
   parietal lobe   temporal lobe
   occipital lobe

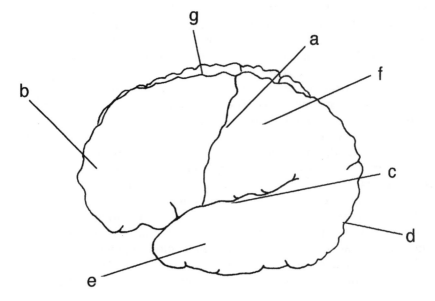

3. Discuss the general function of the following structures:

limbic system   ventricles
meninges

4. Using the following diagram, identify the following structures:

caudate   globus padillus
putamen   internal capsule
external capsule   claustrum

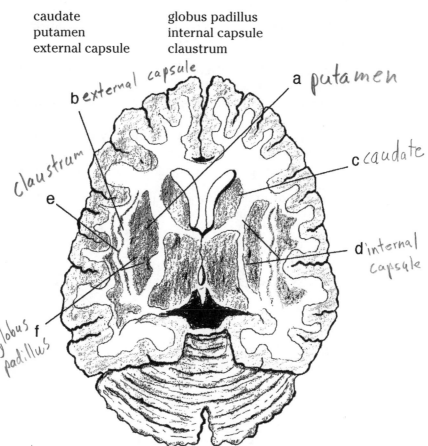

5. Discuss the two primary effects of neurotransmitters.

6. Identify the three divisions of the brainstem.

7. Discuss the primary characteristics of acoustic signal
encoding in the auditory nerve.

8. Identify the three primary characteristics of continuous
speech.

9. Discuss the primary functions of the following auditory brainstem structures:

    cochlear nucleus   superior olivary complex
    lateral lemniscus   inferior colliculus

10. Discuss the primary characteristics of acoustic signal encoding in the auditory thalamus (medial geniculate body).

11. Contrast the primary (cochleotopic) and nonprimary (noncochleotopic, diffuse) auditory systems.

12. Discuss the significance related to auditory function of the following cerebral structures:

    supratemporal plane   Heschl's gyrus (primary auditory cortex, AI)
    planum temporal   supramarginal gyrus
    angular gyrus   insula
    arcuate fasciculus   associative auditory cortex (AII)

13. Using the diagram below, identify the five main parts of the corpus callosum.

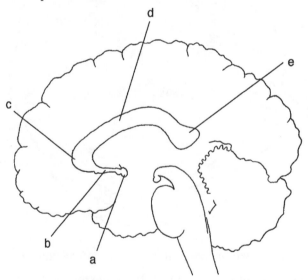

14. Discuss the function of the corpus callosum as it relates to (a) audition and (b) multimodality integration.

15. Discuss the probable significance of the efferent auditory system.

CHAPTER

TWO

Mechanisms of Selected Auditory and Related Processes

The act of hearing does not end with the mere detection of an acoustic stimulus. Rather, several neurophysiological and cognitive mechanisms and processes are necessary for the accurate decoding, perception, recognition, and interpretation of auditory input. As seen in the previous chapter, the CANS is a highly complex, redundant system, and its optimal functioning is critical to the recognition and discrimination of even the most simple, nonverbal acoustic stimuli as well as of highly complex messages such as spoken language.

Much of what is considered to be central auditory processing is preconscious; that is, it occurs without the listener being aware of it. However, even the simplest auditory event is influenced further by higher-level cognitive factors such as memory, attention, and learning. What is ultimately experienced by listeners, then, depends on the interaction between bottom-up and top-down factors. That is, although analysis of an acoustic signal relies initially upon detection and processing within the CANS, higher-level neurocognitive and behavioral factors greatly influence listeners' ultimate ability to recog-

51

nize, decode, and interpret the acoustic signal and, therefore, what they actually perceive.

This chapter explores the mechanisms of and pathological effects on selected auditory phenomena presumed either to underlie more complex auditory perceptual behaviors or to identify areas of dysfunction in the CANS. This chapter also briefly explores higher-order, top-down influences that affect auditory processing ability and comprehension of spoken language. Only by having a thorough understanding of these concepts can clinicians appropriately interpret tests of central auditory function used to evaluate these processes.

Readers should be aware that, although certain studies are reviewed here in order to illustrate relevant concepts, this chapter is not intended to be a comprehensive treatment of the literature. Therefore, many relevant studies in these areas are not mentioned here. Readers are referred to the references cited in this chapter for further information.

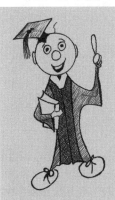

Learning Objectives

After reading this chapter, the reader should be able to:

1. Discuss the presumed anatomic and physiologic bases of dichotic listening.
2. Identify mechanisms underlying various types of temporal processing.
3. Delineate types of auditory tasks that rely on temporal processing.
4. Discuss the presumed anatomic and physiologic bases of auditory pattern recognition.
5. Identify the physiological structures most crucial to binaural interaction.
6. Delineate types of auditory tasks that rely on binaural interaction.

7. Discuss basic principles of the mechanisms underlying speech-sound discrimination.
8. Delineate the effects of various pathological conditions on these selected auditory processes.
9. Discuss the influence of top-down factors such as attention, memory, and cognition on auditory processing.

Definition of Central Auditory Processing

The ASHA Task Force on Central Auditory Processing (ASHA, 1996) suggested the following definition of central auditory processing: central auditory processes are the auditory system mechanisms and processes responsible for the following behavioral phenomena:

- sound localization and lateralization
- auditory discrimination
- auditory pattern recognition
- temporal aspects of audition, including:
    temporal resolution
    temporal masking
    temporal integration
    temporal ordering
- auditory performance with competing acoustic signals
- auditory performance with degraded acoustic signals

Readers should note that the above definition concerns itself specifically with the auditory system. **Memory, learning, attention, long-term phonological representation, and other higher-level neurocognitive processes are considered in the definition** *only as they relate to the processing of acoustic signals.*

This definition of central auditory processing has been criticized in the years since its proposal. Criticisms have included (1) the use of the term being defined (i.e., *processes*) in the definition of central auditory *processing*, (2) the lack of clarity and illumination afforded by the general phrase "auditory system mechanisms and processes," (3) the overly restrictive nature of the list of specific auditory behavioral phenomena provided in the definition with no acknowledgment of the possible interdependency of these behavioral abilities in auditory or spoken language processing and no mention of additional auditory abilities not included in the list, and (4) no elaboration of how "higher-level neurocognitive processes" relate to the "processing of acoustic signals."

Nevertheless, when viewed as a whole, several very important concepts and distinctions are implied by this definition:

- When talking about central auditory processing, we are referring to something that is fundamentally *auditory* in nature. That is, these are processes that take place in the auditory system and are, at their core, bottom-up or "input" factors related specifically to the representation of acoustic signals.
- Very basic auditory behavioral phenomena can be delineated that presumably underlie a wide variety of auditory perceptual events. For example, localization of a sound source is one of several important prerequisites for being able to attend to—and process—the signal coming from that sound source in a background of competing noise. Auditory discrimination certainly is a skill required for decoding and recognizing the sounds of a language and, thus, is one of many prerequisites for the ultimate comprehension of spoken language. Therefore, more complex auditory perceptual abilities can be decomposed into constituent auditory processes.
- It is possible, at least theoretically, to devise methods of assessing these constituent auditory processes for the purpose of identifying dysfunction in fundamental auditory input skills that may then lead to or be associated with difficulties in more complex auditory, language, and learning abilities.
- Higher-level neurocognitive processes (such as language, attention, and memory) will, in a top-down fashion, affect even these basic, fundamental auditory skills. Therefore, any consideration of central auditory processing and its disorders must, of necessity, include effects of these higher-order factors on auditory input processing.

A recent consensus conference—commonly referred to as the Bruton conference—on diagnosing central auditory processing disorders (CAPD) convened at the Callier Center in Dallas in April 2000 made these concepts somewhat clearer and more explicit (Jerger & Musiek, 2000). Along with recommendations for screening and diagnostic procedures, the consensus committee addressed several key issues that help to guide our conceptualization of this complex topic.

First, it was acknowledged that deficits in auditory processing are often associated with listening, comprehension, language, and learning difficulties; however, auditory processing disorders are, themselves, to be thought of as deficits that are specific to the auditory modality. When taken together with the previous (ASHA, 1996) definition, this may be thought of as a deficit in one or more of those fundamental, constituent auditory phenomena that underlie a wide variety of auditory perceptual and related skills—or a primarily "bottom-up," input disorder.

The emphasis on modality specificity in recent definitions of CAPD has led many to conclude, therefore, that a diagnosis of CAPD can be enabled only if it can be shown that a deficit exists that is specific to the auditory modality and *nowhere else*. Certainly, it is reasonable to insist that an auditory-specific deficit be demonstrated prior to applying the label of CAPD. However, when one considers the complexity of the central nervous system and the presence of multimodality association areas, inter- and intrahemispheric connections, and auditory responsive regions in "nonauditory" subcortical and cortical structures, some serious theoretical questions arise: Is it reasonable to expect that the auditory system, and the auditory system *alone*, will be affected by dysfunction at any level of the CANS above the brainstem? Or is it more reasonable to expect that dysfunction in certain subcortical or brain regions will give rise to deficits in fundamental auditory skills *that coexist with* deficits in other modalities or processes also subserved by the same anatomical regions or physiological mechanisms? And, if deficits in other modalities do exist, is the label *CAPD* truly appropriate, or would a more accurate label be "auditory manifestations of a central processing disorder"?

To illustrate this concept, let us consider the effects of corpus callosum dysfunction. It has been shown definitively that sectioning the corpus callosum can give rise to deficits in specific auditory processes, most notably dichotic listening and labeling of tonal patterns, which will be discussed later in this chapter. Certainly, the well-documented auditory findings in split-brain individuals would seem to support a diagnosis of CAPD. However, corpus callosum sectioning also results in specific deficits in tactile and visual modalities as well. Does the presence of these other, coexisting deficits then render the auditory findings insignificant? Would the label *CAPD* now no longer apply, even though auditory-specific deficits were demonstrated? Does the label even matter, or is it more important to focus our attention on addressing the auditory sequelae for management purposes?

It is my opinion that, when we are discussing central auditory processing and its disorders, we are, indeed, referring to those deficits that are specific to the auditory modality. However, **to expect that an auditory-specific deficit will exist in all cases of CAPD to the exclusion of deficits in any other sensory modality appears to be neurophysiologically untenable in light of our current knowledge of the incredible interconnectedness of nervous system function.** This is a hotly debated issue that is critical to appropriate conceptualization of central auditory processing and its disorders, and it will be explored further later in this chapter and in the chapters on central auditory diagnosis and interpretation.

A second topic emphasized in the proceedings from the Bruton conference was the need for investigating higher-order neurocognitive influences on auditory processing and controlling for "top-down" confounds such as attention, motivation, cooperation, and similar issues. Finally, in an effort to acknowledge the need for operational definitions and the vast complexity of the auditory system, including auditory-responsive areas that are outside the central auditory nervous system proper, it was recommended that the word *central* be dropped from the term, and that these disorders be referred to as "auditory processing disorders" (APD). This recommendation has met with some controversy since its proposal, and use of the term *APD* to describe these disorders is far from universal at the present time. Nevertheless, the term *APD* does seem to incorporate the important concept that the processing of acoustic input involves far more than just a step-by-step, hierarchical progression through the structures of the central auditory pathways. (*Note*: As discussed in the Preface, the previous term *CAPD* will be used throughout this text for the purposes of ensuring consistency in title and style with the previous edition.)

Dichotic Listening

The term *dichotic* **refers to auditory stimuli that are presented to both ears simultaneously, with the stimulus presented to each ear being different.** This term stands in contrast to *diotic* or *binaural*, which denote that the same, identical stimulus is presented to both ears simultaneously. Broadbent (1954) was the first to utilize a technique of presenting competing sets of digits to both ears simultaneously. Kimura (1961a, b) is generally credited with the introduction of dichotic speech tests into the field of central auditory assessment by adapting Broadbent's technique for assessing hemispheric asymmetry and unilateral lesion effects, and her research has served as the basis for much of the current theory regarding dichotic listening.

As discussed in Chapter 1, auditory input is represented both ipsi-

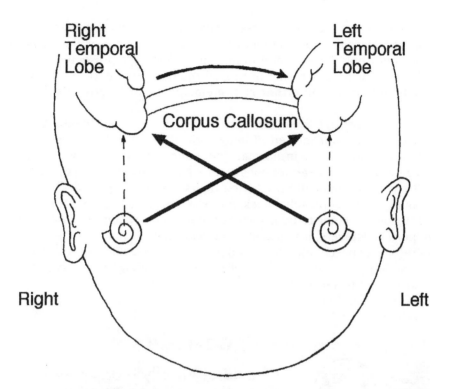

Figure 2-1. Kimura's theory of dichotic listening. Bold lines represent contralateral, dominant pathways; dotted lines represent ipsilateral pathways.

laterally and contralaterally throughout the CANS. Kimura theorized that **the contralateral pathways are stronger and more numerous than are the ipsilateral pathways** (Figure 2-1). When monotic or non-competing stimuli are introduced, either pathway is capable of transmitting the appropriate neural signal. However, **when dichotic (competing) auditory stimuli are presented, the ipsilateral pathways are suppressed by the stronger contralateral pathways.**

Because the language-dominant (usually left) hemisphere is required for the perception and verbal labeling of auditory linguistic stimuli, information presented to the left ear must traverse the right hemisphere and the corpus callosum in order to be perceived and labeled. Information presented to the right ear, on the other hand, is transmitted directly to the left hemisphere without the need for initial right-hemisphere or interhemispheric processing. Thus, processing and labeling of the information presented to both ears during dichotic listening paradigms are ultimately reliant on integrity of the left hemisphere. However, dysfunction in the right hemisphere or the corpus callosum would be expected to impact the message presented to the left ear only, as processing of the information presented to the right ear is not reliant on either right-hemisphere or interhemispheric integrity.

In the early 1960s, several researchers documented the existence of a cerebral dominance effect in dichotic listening, indicating a preexisting ear asymmetry in normal right-handed listeners in which the scores for the right ear are consistently higher than the scores for the left ear for dichotically presented digits (Bryden, 1963; Dirks, 1964; Kimura, 1961a; Satz, Achenback, Pattishall, & Fennell, 1965). This phenomenon has come to be known as the *right ear advantage (REA)* and, in normal listeners, it is usually apparent only upon dichotic stimulation (using speech stimuli) or other tasks that significantly challenge the auditory system (Kimura, 1961a). These findings have been considered as further evidence of the left hemisphere's dominance for speech perception.

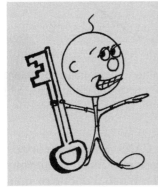

KEY CONCEPT

The REA typically is apparent only upon dichotic stimulation or other challenging auditory tasks.

It should be noted that some researchers have posited alternative theories regarding the mechanism of dichotic listening as it relates to speech perception (Sidtis, 1982; Speaks, Gray, Miller, & Rubens, 1975). One of the most compelling was set forth by Efron (1990), who suggested that left-right differences in dichotic tasks (or similar tasks in any modality) may be explained by the manner in which the brain prefers to scan the information presented rather than by the need for left-ear information to traverse additional pathways. For example, Efron demonstrated that, during presentation of visual stimuli to both visual hemifields, normal subjects tend to scan first the information presented to the right visual field, then move to the left visual field. Information presented within each hemifield tended to be scanned from left to right. Similar scanning effects were found for dichotically presented stimuli. Efron concluded that the brain has a tendency to scan information serially, which leads to one ear or visual hemifield having "superiority" over the other. He cautioned, therefore, that this directional bias should not be taken as evidence of the existence of hemispheric dominance for these tasks but, rather, evidence for serial processing in the brain. As such, Efron advised against inferring hemispheric specialization from dichotic (or similar) tasks.

Although Efron's arguments have merit, limited data exist to support his hypothesis. Furthermore, his caveat was directed solely toward the use of dichotic listening in the determination of hemispheric specialization. Finally, a substantial amount of evidence—both behavioral and electrophysiologic—exists to support Kimura's theory of dichotic listening.

Objective evidence in favor of Kimura's theory has come from studies of dichotic listening in subjects with surgical sectioning of the corpus callosum. Milner et al. (1968) and Sparks and Geschwind (1968) demonstrated complete left-ear suppression of dichotically presented stimuli following surgical sectioning of the corpus callosum. Musiek and colleagues, in a series of experiments delineating the neuroaudiological effects of surgical sectioning of the corpus callosum, have shown that surgical sectioning of the posterior, but not the anterior, portion of the corpus callosum results in a suppression of left-ear scores, whereas right-ear performance remains at preoperative levels (Baran, Musiek, & Reeves, 1990; Musiek, Kibbe, & Baran, 1984; Musiek & Reeves, 1990; Musiek et al., 1985).

Electrophysiologic evidence for Kimura's theory was provided by Aiello, Sotgiu, Sau, Manca, Conti, and Rosati (1995), who demonstrated that subjects with callosal agenesis, unlike normal subjects, exhibited more efficient transmission of monaural auditory stimuli through the ipsilateral, rather than contralateral, auditory pathways. In addition, Hugdahl and colleagues demonstrated via positron emission tomography (PET) that dichotically presented consonant-vowel (CV) syllables resulted in greater neural activation over the left temporal lobe whereas dichotically presented musical stimuli resulted in greater activation over the right hemisphere (Hugdahl et al., 1999). Similarly, Wioland, Rudolf, Metz-Lutz, Mutschler, and Marescaux (1999) demonstrated electrophysiologic correlates of perceptual asymmetries for dichotic tasks using tonal stimuli in subjects who demonstrated the expected REA for verbal dichotic stimuli. In their study, the authors found that normal subjects exhibited delayed latencies of the N2 and P3 auditory evoked potential components, along with prolonged reaction times for behavioral identification of targets, in response to dichotically presented stimuli, but not to binaurally presented stimuli. A clear left-ear advantage was observed in both the behavioral and electrophysiologic responses for dichotically presented tonal stimuli. The authors concluded that these findings strongly support Kimura's theory of dichotic listening, as well as confirming a right-hemisphere advantage for pitch discrimination.

Overall, these studies provide compelling evidence supporting the use of dichotic listening paradigms in the evaluation of right-hemisphere, left-hemisphere, and interhemispheric function. Therefore, Kimura's model of dichotic listening continues to be the one that is most widely accepted today.

Effects of Temporal Lobe Lesions on Dichotic Listening

In a study of twenty-eight left aphasic and twenty right nonaphasic lesioned adults, Sparks, Goodglass, and Nickel (1970) confirmed previous researchers' findings regarding temporal lobe lesions. They used double digits and familiar words (animal names) presented dichotically and concluded that, for subjects with right temporal lobe lesions, left-ear suppression/extinction occurs due to the contralateral effect previously discussed. Likewise, for subjects with left temporal lobe lesions, right-ear suppression/extinction occurs due to the contralateral effect. In addition, the authors explained that right-ear extinction does not occur with right temporal lobe lesions because the primary contralateral pathway to the left hemisphere remains intact; however, ipsilateral left-ear extinction can and does occur with left-hemisphere lesions due to the fact that the stimulus to the left ear must arrive at the right hemisphere, then cross to the left hemisphere by way of the corpus callosum. **Lesions affecting either the auditory areas of the left temporal lobe or the fibers of the corpus callosum would therefore interrupt the successful arrival of information at the speech-dominant left hemisphere** (Figure 2-2). The findings of Grote, Pierre-Louis, Smith, Roberts, and Varney (1995) supported this contention. In a study of forty-nine patients with seizures, the authors reported that, whereas right-ear impairment on dichotic listening tasks was always associated with left-hemisphere lesions, left-ear extinction occurred with lesions of either hemisphere.

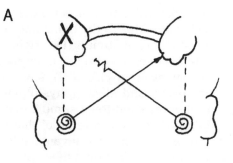

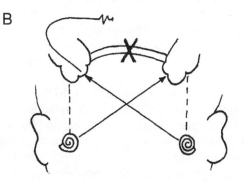

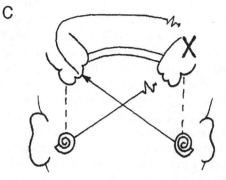

Figure 2-2. Effects of lesions of the CANS on dichotic listening showing pattern of interruption for (A) right temporal lobe lesion, (B) corpus callosum lesion, and (C) left temporal lobe lesion.

The authors also hypothesized that a reverse effect may be noted when using nonverbal stimuli due to the dominance of the right hemisphere for this type of acoustic stimuli (i.e., right-ear extinction of nonverbal dichotic stimuli in cases of right temporal lobe lesions). As previously mentioned, Wioland et al. (1999) demonstrated just such an effect both behaviorally and electrophysiologically. Therefore, when using dichotically presented tonal stimuli, one would expect to see a pattern of findings that is the reverse of that seen with speech stimuli, including presence of a left-ear advantage in normal listeners and bilateral suppression in cases of right-hemisphere dysfunction.

Damasio and Damasio (1979), studying patients with well-defined focal lesions, postulated further that seemingly "paradoxic" ear extinction (i.e., extinction of dichotically presented stimuli in the ear ipsilateral to the lesion) only occurs with deep suprasylvian lesions involving the pathway from the medial geniculate body of the thalamus to the cortex (thalamocortical pathway). Focal occipital and frontal lesions do not produce ear effects simply because no auditory areas are affected.

Berlin, Lowe-Bell, Jannetta, and Kline (1972) studied four temporal lobe lesioned patients using CV nonsense syllables presented simultaneously and with interaural lags of 15, 30, 60, and 90 msec. Their results also indicated depressed scores in the ear contralateral to the site of lesion, as well as ipsilateral ear extinction with lesions deep enough to interfere with the right-to-left interhemispheric transfer of information. In addition, the authors reported that **those subjects with posterior temporal lobe lesions exhibited greater auditory deficit,** which is consistent with placement of the primary and associative auditory areas in the more posterior aspect of the temporal lobe. In normal listeners, acoustic stimuli received at the right ear are generally reported more accurately, as shown by previous researchers, and the lagging message is better perceived when lags of 30–90 msec are utilized.

In conclusion, dysfunction in the non-language-dominant (usually right) temporal lobe can be expected to result in a left-ear suppression on dichotic speech testing. Dysfunction in the language-dominant (usually left) temporal lobe can be expected to result in bilateral suppression on dichotic speech testing. The opposite pattern may be found for dichotically presented nonspeech (or tonal) stimuli because of the reverse cerebral dominance for this type of auditory input. Finally, ipsilateral suppression or extinction typically occurs in isolation on dichotic speech testing only when the pathways from the thalamus to the cortex, or deep thalamocortical, suprasylvian pathways, are involved.

Effects of Corpus Callosum Lesions on Dichotic Listening

Milner, Taylor, and Sperry (1968) studied seven "split-brain" patients (i.e., they had undergone complete sectioning of the corpus callosum) and compared their results on a test of dichotically presented digit triads with normal listeners and cases of temporal lobectomies in which Heschl's gyrus was completely excised. Findings with normal listeners and temporal lobectomies agreed with the results of other studies: normal listeners exhibited a slight REA on dichotic tasks, left temporal lobectomy resulted in a bilateral deficit, and right temporal lobectomy resulted in an accentuation of right-ear superiority/contralateral left-ear deficit. With the split-brain patients, significant left-ear suppression or extinction resulted, even though monotic presentation of the digits to the left ear in these patients remained unaffected. The authors concluded that the left ipsilateral pathway can be utilized in cases of monaural stimulation; however, during the more challenging task of dichotic listening, the contralateral pathway is dominant.

In a similar study utilizing dichotically presented single digits and words, Sparks and Geschwind (1968) reported 100% left-ear extinction in patients with complete commissurotomies. When the listeners were instructed to attend closely to the left ear, performance for that ear improved but remained significantly depressed.

The authors also presented the verbal stimuli to the left ear along with contralateral white noise and babble masking to the right ear. They found that right masking did not affect left-ear performance significantly. The introduction of a distorted stimulus to the right ear impacted left-ear performance on dichotic tasks, depending on the degree of distortion. As the degree of right-ear distortion decreased, the degree of left-ear extinction increased. The authors concluded that the likelihood of left-ear extinction in split-brain patients increases when the stimuli delivered to both ears are very similar and that the localization and depth of the lesion significantly affect the degree of left-ear suppression/extinction.

Musiek, Reeves, and Baran (1985) investigated the effects of sectioning of the corpus callosum on a subject's performance on a variety of central tests. The subject was a patient undergoing a two-stage commissurotomy to control intractable epileptic seizures. The posterior portion of the corpus callosum was sectioned first, followed by anterior sectioning five months later. Following posterior sectioning of the corpus callosum, left-ear extinction on dichotic tasks occurred. In

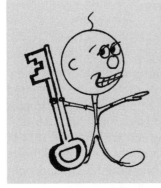

KEY CONCEPT

The degree of left-ear extinction in split-brain patients increases as stimuli delivered to the ears becomes more similar.

addition, right-ear performance was enhanced. The authors suggested that this finding was due to a release from competition: following posterior sectioning, the left hemisphere was required only to process information from the right ear. Subsequent anterior sectioning did not result in further auditory deficit.

In a related study, Baran et al. (1986) studied eight right-handed adults who underwent partial commissurotomies to control seizures. In all cases, the anterior portion of the corpus callosum was sectioned, leaving the posterior half intact. Results of the study indicated that, while complete commissurotomy results in a marked left-ear deficit on dichotic tasks, anterior sectioning alone does not. These findings led the authors to conclude that **the majority of auditory fibers travel interhemispherically in the posterior portion of the corpus callosum.**

In conclusion, interhemispheric dysfunction typically results in a left-ear suppression on dichotic speech tasks—a finding that is identical to that of right-hemisphere dysfunction. As a result, additional tests are indicated to diagnose right-hemisphere versus interhemispheric dysfunction differentially.

Effects of Other Pathological Conditions on Dichotic Listening

Roeser, Johns, and Price (1976) investigated the effect of bilaterally symmetrical sensorineural hearing loss on dichotic listening using digits and CV nonsense syllables as stimuli. Large ear advantages (right or left) were discovered in their subjects, suggesting that sensorineural hearing loss can significantly affect the size and direction of the ear advantage in dichotic listening tasks.

Table 2-1

Effects of Auditory System Pathology on Dichotic Listening

Site of Lesion	Effect(s) on Dichotic Listening
Right temporal lobe	Left-ear suppression/extinction
Posterior corpus callosum	Left-ear suppression/extinction, possible right-ear enhancement
Anterior corpus callosum	No effect on dichotic listening
Left temporal lobe	Bilateral suppression/extinction, may be more marked contralaterally
Cochlear	Depends on stimuli, CVs heavily confounded by cochlear hearing loss, digits relatively unaffected
Conductive	No effect at adequate presentation levels

Speaks, Niccum, and Van Tasell (1985) compared the performance of listeners with bilaterally symmetrical sensorineural hearing loss on three types of dichotic tests: digits, concrete noun words, and CV nonsense syllables. **As the difficulty of the test stimuli increased, the degree of ear advantage also increased. Digits appeared to be the least affected by sensorineural hearing loss.**

Conductive hearing loss does not appear to affect performance significantly on dichotic listening tasks as long as the stimuli are presented at an intensity of at least 12 dB above the monotic "knee" for the affected ear(s). The monotic knee represents that point in a performance-intensity function at which the listener reaches a 95% accuracy level for monotic presentation of the stimuli (Niccum, Speaks, Katsuki-Nakamura, & Van Tassell, 1987).

In cases of multiple sclerosis with cerebral involvement, left-ear suppression on dichotic tasks may be observed (Jacobson, Deppe, & Murray, 1983; Rubens, Froehling, Slater, & Anderson, 1985). It is possible that the existence of multiple sclerosis lesions in the deep white matter of the cerebral hemispheres results in an interruption of the auditory corpus callosal pathway, resulting in findings similar to that of split-brain patients (Rubens et al., 1985). The effects of pathology on dichotic listening are summarized in Table 2-1.

Temporal Processing

In this section, the term *temporal* **refers to time-related aspects of the acoustic signal.** Temporal processing is critical to a wide variety of everyday listening tasks, including speech perception and perception of music (Hirsh, 1959). For example, the perception of melody in music depends on the listener's ability to perceive the order of several musical notes or chords and to determine if the frequencies of the notes or chords are ascending or descending with respect to the adjacent chords or notes. In speech perception, temporal processing is one of the functions necessary for the discrimination of subtle cues such as voicing (e.g., voicing begins earlier in the word *dime* than in the word *time*) and the discrimination of similar words (e.g., discrimination between the words *boost* and *boots* depends in large part on discrimination of consonant duration and temporal ordering of the final two consonants of each word). These are just two examples of how the processing of time-related cues is used in everyday listening tasks.

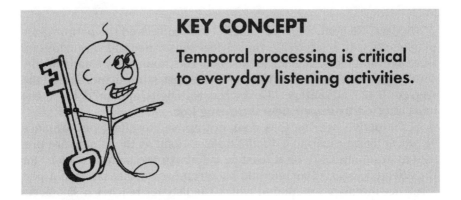

KEY CONCEPT

Temporal processing is critical to everyday listening activities.

Hirsh (1959) studied the effect of interstimulus intervals (ISI) on the perception of temporal order. Using a variety of acoustic stimuli, he determined that **an ISI of only 2 msec is required for the normal listener to perceive two sounds instead of only one; however, this ISI must be increased tenfold (or approximately 17 msec) for the listener to report which of the two sounds came first** with 75% accuracy. In addition, the judgment of temporal order appears to be independent of the acoustical nature of the sounds (e.g., the ISI necessary for the reporting of temporal order was approximately the same regardless of whether musical notes or clicks were used and whether certain variations in the acoustic characteristics of the stimuli were made). The author did note the existence of some minor exceptions to the above rule: although pitch had no effect, rise time and duration of click stimuli did have some minor effect on the perception of temporal order. In addition, when a burst of wide-band noise preceded a high-frequency, brief tone, the ISI necessary to perceive temporal order was slightly longer, possibly due to a forward masking effect. Hirsh concluded that the judgment of temporal order does not occur at the ear, but rather represents a central auditory function and that, **in cases in which a listener requires more than 15 or 20 msec to perceive the temporal order of two consecutive stimuli, the examiner should look to possible central involvement.**

In 1961, Hirsh and Sherrick explored the effect of sense modality on the perception of temporal order. They reported that an ISI of approximately 20 msec continues to be necessary to report temporal order with 75% accuracy, regardless of whether the stimuli are acoustic, visual, tactile, or a combination of modalities and despite the fact that the visual system requires a longer ISI to perceive a separation between two stimuli. Their results suggest that some type of time-organization system exists within the human brain that is independent of the peripheral and central modality-specific systems themselves. Similarly, it has been shown that some children with auditory, language, or reading disorders have difficulty processing rapidly occurring or short-duration stimuli, regardless of sensory modality (Farmer & Klein, 1995; Tallal, Miller, & Fitch, 1993). These "pansensory" disturbances provide further evidence of a non-modality-specific time organization system in the human brain.

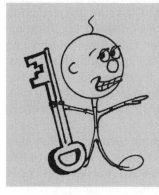

KEY CONCEPT

An ISI of about 20 msec is required to report temporal order of stimuli, regardless of modality.

Phillips (1999) and Phillips and Hall (2000) distinguished between *within-channel* and *between-channel* gap detection in temporal processing. In the typical gap detection paradigm, the stimulus preceding the gap is identical in spectrum and duration to the stimulus following the gap. That is, the typical gap detection paradigm involves the insertion of a silent period into the center of an ongoing auditory signal. As such, the auditory signal preceding the gap can be expected to stimulate the same neuronal pool that is stimulated following the gap. This is referred to as within-channel gap detection. As previously stated, studies have shown that the normal within-channel gap detection threshold is on the order of only 2 msec.

But gaps of only 2 msec do not typically occur during normal speech perception. For example, the perception of voice-onset time (VOT) necessary for discriminating between voiced and voiceless stop consonants is an excellent case of naturally occurring gap detection during running speech. Unlike the typical gap detection paradigms used in psychoacoustics laboratories, however, the spectral content and duration of the auditory signal preceding the gap in a voiced (or voiceless) consonant are quite different from those of the signal following the gap. As such, different neuronal pools can be expected to be stimulated before and after the gap. Indeed, as Phillips has shown, the normal gap detection threshold for stimuli in which the signal preceding the gap is different in spectrum and duration from the signal that follows the gap—a situation that is referred to as between-channel gap detection—is approximately 35 msec. It is perhaps not coincidental that this threshold of 35 msec also corresponds to the perceptual boundary between voiced and voiceless consonants. Therefore, **Phillips' findings suggest that between-channel gap detection paradigms may mimic temporal processing during normal speech perception more closely, and call into question the clinical utility and ecological validity of traditional within-channel gap detection techniques.** It should be noted that the same gap detection threshold of approximately 35 msec is also found when the stimulus preceding the gap is presented to one ear and the stimulus following the gap is presented to the opposite ear, even if both stimuli are identical in spectrum and duration. This would be expected, too, as the presentation of signals to opposite ears would stimulate different neuronal pools. Therefore, this, too, would be considered a between-channel gap detection paradigm.

Massaro (1972) posited a theory of auditory recognition in which auditory detection is distinguished from recognition and short-term memory storage. Using previous studies of forward (masking precedes stimulus) and backward (stimulus precedes masking) masking, Massaro suggested that auditory input results in the production of a preperceptual auditory image, or "echo," which preserves the characteristics of the stimulus and remains in storage for as long as 10 sec. Discrimination and recognition of the auditory input follows analysis of this preperceptual auditory image, rather than analysis of the initial input itself, which would require almost instantaneous perception—an impossible task. In addition, as contralateral masking does not appear to affect the detection of the stimulus but does interfere with recognition of the stimulus, Massaro suggested that the preperceptual auditory image is located centrally rather than peripherally. Finally, he hypothesized that, as the maximum duration of preperceptual auditory images is approximately 250 msec, **the first 100 to 250 msec of an auditory stimulus presentation are the most critical for stimulus recognition, which has significant implications for speech perception.** Moreover, recent research by Wright and colleagues (Wright et al., 1997) suggested that a deficit in auditory perception specifically related to backward masking and detection of very brief auditory stimuli may play a role in the language difficulties exhibited by some children.

Efron (1963) studied the effects of temporal lobe lesions on the perception of the temporal order of two consecutive visual or auditory stimuli. His subjects were inpatients, twelve of whom had documented lesions of the left hemisphere (eleven aphasics) and four of whom had documented lesions of the right hemisphere (no aphasics). The aphasic patients were considered to be the experimental group, the nonaphasics were used as controls.

Efron's results suggested that the lesions that resulted in disruption of temporal order perception of two consecutive stimuli all occurred in the left, or speech-dominant, hemisphere. The one patient who exhibited a left-hemisphere lesion but was nonaphasic exhibited temporal discrimination skills comparable to those of the controls. In addition, the expressive aphasics in Efron's study exhibited poorer performance on auditory sequencing, whereas the receptive aphasics performed worse on visual sequencing tasks. Finally, the patients with the most difficulty in understanding speech exhibited the least difficulty with auditory sequencing, and vice versa.

Based on his results, Efron suggested that, although unconscious temporal processing takes place at every synapse throughout the nervous system, **analysis of the temporal order of two stimuli takes place primarily in the dominant hemisphere, specifically in the temporal lobe and extending posteriorly to Wernicke's area and the angular gyrus.** The seemingly paradoxical finding that the most severe receptive aphasics exhibited the least difficulty with temporal sequencing is explained by the hypothesis that the functional deficit in speech understanding exhibited by the receptive aphasics occurs after the input is temporally sequenced. Thus, the receptive component of an expressive aphasic's difficulty may be at an earlier stage than the receptive component of a receptive aphasic, resulting in poorer temporal sequencing abilities in the expressive aphasic. Efron stressed that severity of cerebral damage cannot be correlated with results on a temporal sequencing task, as variability is high.

Efron also discussed the conscious perception of time as being mediated primarily in the dominant hemisphere. He set forth the theory that the conscious perception of an event occurs when the sensory data reach the left hemisphere. This theory helps to explain the existence of subjective time sense disturbances in patients with temporal lobe lesions. Efron also suggested that the phenomenon of *déjà vu*— the feeling that an individual has experienced an event previously— may occur because a lesion in the right temporal lobe delays the propagation of the sensory data to the left hemisphere. Thus, the patient "experiences" the sensory event twice: once directly, and once through delayed transmission from the right hemisphere, giving rise to the sensation of déjà vu.

In any case, early data concerning temporal processing suggest that, although temporal cues are processed throughout the CANS, the left temporal lobe is critical to the accurate perception of the temporal order of two stimuli. The perception and verbal report of the temporal order of more than two stimuli, or temporal patterning, appears to be more complex, however. Pinheiro and Ptacek (1971; Ptacek & Pinheiro, 1971) introduced a test of temporal processing involving triads of tone bursts. In each triad, two tone bursts are of the same frequency and a third is of a different frequency. The listener is required to report the order in which the bursts were heard (for example, high-high-low, low-high-low, etc.).

The mechanism underlying this Frequency Patterns task was described by Musiek, Pinheiro, and Wilson (1980) and is illustrated in Figure 2-3. Briefly, the perception and verbal labeling of the tonal pattern requires processing by both hemispheres of the brain (Pinheiro, 1976). The non-language-dominant (usually right) hemisphere of the brain subserves pitch perception (Jerger, 1997; Wioland et al., 1999), as well as recognition of the musical contour and gestalt pattern (Blumstein & Cooper, 1974; Nebes, 1971). The dominant (usually left) hemisphere, however, is required for verbalization of the response (e.g., Gazzaniga & Sperry, 1967). Therefore, verbal labeling of the tonal patterns used in this task requires, first, processing of the acoustic contour by the right hemisphere, then a transfer via the corpus callosum to the left hemisphere for the linguistic labeling component. When the linguistic labeling component is removed and the listener is asked to hum the pattern heard, only the right hemisphere is required. Thus, a comparison of performance in the linguistic labeling versus the humming condition provides an index of corpus callosum or left-hemisphere integrity, as right-hemisphere dysfunction will affect performance in both response conditions whereas corpus callo-

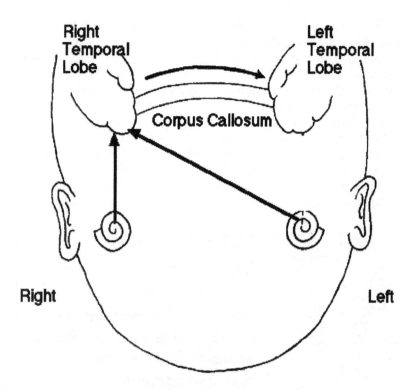

Figure 2-3. Mechanism underlying temporal patterning (i.e., Frequency Patterns) task.

sum or left-hemisphere dysfunction will affect performance in the linguistic labeling condition only.

Support for this model was provided by Musiek and colleagues in a series of experiments studying the effects of surgical sectioning of the corpus callosum on Frequency Patterns performance in the linguistic labeling and humming conditions (Baran, Musiek, & Reeves, 1986; Musiek, Kibbe, & Baran, 1984; Musiek & Reeves, 1990; Musiek, Wilson, & Pinheiro, 1979; Pinheiro, 1976). These studies demonstrated that, following surgical sectioning of the posterior portion of the corpus callosum, subjects were unable to label the tonal patterns verbally, despite preserved ability to hum or sing the patterns presented. Similarly, it has been shown that aphasic patients with documented lesions of the left hemisphere often retain the ability to sing or hum even when speech is problematic or impossible (e.g., Smith, 1966). Finally, the finding of left-ear (and right-hemisphere) advantages for the perception of tones or hummed patterns (King & Kimura, 1972; Zurif, 1974), when taken together with the research discussed above, provides further support for the theory that the acoustic pattern recognition is subserved by the right hemisphere whereas linguistic labeling of the pattern requires integrity of both hemispheres as well as the corpus callosum.

In conclusion, when a patterning test involving more than two successive auditory stimuli and linguistic labeling is involved, integrity of both hemispheres as well as the corpus callosum is necessary for normal performance. In cases of lesions involving the interhemispheric pathways, removing the linguistic labeling portion of the temporal patterning test results in performance closer to that of normal listeners.

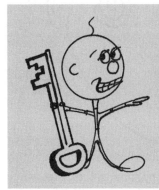

KEY CONCEPT

Integrity of both temporal lobes and the corpus callosum is necessary for the linguistic labeling of temporal patterns containing more than two successive stimuli.

Effects of Cerebral Pathology on Temporal Processing

Hughes (1946) discovered that, in normal listeners, **as the temporal duration of a brief tone decreases below 200 msec, the intensity required for threshold progressively increases.** This has been referred to as *temporal integration*, or *summation*. Results of studies investigating the effect of cerebral pathology on temporal integration have been somewhat variable (Cranford, 1984). In a study of a patient with bilateral temporal lobe lesions, Jerger, Lovering, and Wertz (1972) reported elevated temporal integration functions for both ears. Cranford, Stream, Rye, and Slade (1982) discovered that thresholds for brief tones may be elevated in the case of temporal lobe lesions, but that given a sufficient period of time following cerebral insult, the threshold functions may return to normal. However, the authors noted a significant increase in frequency difference limens (smallest detectable differences) for signals shorter than 50 msec in the ear contralateral to the temporal lobe lesion. They suggested that a cortical lesion may result in a dissociation between detection and discrimination of brief tones, indicating that the peripheral system is primarily responsible for detection of an auditory stimulus whereas the central system is the primary mediator for temporal analysis. The authors concluded that standard temporal integration tests may have little or no value in identifying cerebral lesions; however, frequency difference limens utilizing brief tones may have some utility.

Thompson and Abel (1992a, b) studied the effects of anatomical site of lesion on the processing of intensity, duration, and frequency cues. Using a two-alternative, forced-choice procedure, the authors obtained difference limens for the above three acoustic parameters from a subject group that included peripheral (cochlear) lesions, acoustic nerve lesions, and cortical lesions. Their findings indicated that the group with left temporal lesions exhibited the greatest deficits in processing all three acoustic parameters, and that the degree of deficit in duration processing was significantly correlated with consonant discrimination skills. Therefore, the authors concluded that tests of temporal processing may be good predictors of speech perception ability at the central level.

Carmon and Nachshon (1971) studied twenty-six patients with right-hemisphere lesions, twenty-one patients with left-hemisphere lesions, and forty-two controls without lesions and compared their performance on a task of temporal sequencing of auditory as well as visual stimuli. Although none of the subjects was overtly aphasic, the authors required a motor (pointing) response in case those patients with left-hemisphere lesions had subtle difficulties with verbalization. The authors found that those patients with left-hemisphere lesions demonstrated decreased performance on all sequencing tasks, whereas the patients with right-hemisphere lesions did not differ significantly from the control group. They concluded that **although temporal perception does not depend on speech, speech perception may well depend, at least in part, on the sequential analysis of temporal order.** This study also supported previous evidence that some types of temporal processing are mediated by the left hemisphere.

Swisher and Hirsh (1972) studied the effects of cerebral pathology on the ability to order two temporally successive stimuli. Using visual and auditory stimuli, the authors found that subjects with left-hemisphere lesions and fluent aphasia required the longest ISI to report the order of the two stimuli, especially when the stimuli were auditory in nature. Subjects with right-hemisphere lesions and no aphasia did not differ significantly from controls when both auditory stimuli were delivered to the same ear; however, they did require a longer ISI than controls to make temporal judgments when the stimuli were delivered to opposite ears. The authors concluded that the left hemisphere is particularly important for temporal ordering of events occurring at one place and that the right hemisphere also plays a part in the analysis of temporal order of tonal stimuli when one of the stimuli arrives at the left ear. This is consistent with Phillips' (1999) finding regarding larger gap detection thresholds when the stimulus preceding the gap is presented to one ear and the stimulus following the gap is presented to the other ear, discussed previously.

Lackner and Teuber (1973) utilized dichotic click stimuli varying in interaural ISI and asked subjects to hold up two fingers when two clicks were heard and one finger when the clicks fused and only one stimulus was heard. This activity was repeated in a bracketing paradigm in order to determine the subjects' threshold for click fusion/separation. The authors found that subjects with penetrative lesions of the posterior left hemisphere required a longer ISI in order to perceive a separation. Patients with right-hemisphere penetrative lesions did not differ from the normal control group in ability to perform the task. Therefore, temporal gap detection tasks also appear to rely on integrity of the left hemisphere.

In an ablation study using cats, Colavita, Szeligo, and Zimmer (1974) found that the ability to attend to a full pattern is successful only when the insular-temporal cortex is intact. Surgical ablation of the insular-temporal cortex in cats resulted in inability to order three stimuli, but did not affect the ability to order two stimuli. The authors suggested that the postablative deficit noted in their study may not be due to the inability to sequence temporally per se, but rather to a reduction in attention span so that triads of stimuli can no longer be processed. The authors concluded that, due to the predisposed tendency to attend to the full pattern in temporally ordering three or more consecutive stimuli, breaking down a complex message into its component parts may not be a useful strategy for individuals with brain damage.

Efron and his colleagues (Efron, 1985; Efron & Crandall, 1983; Efron, Crandall, Koss, Divenyi, & Yund, 1983; Efron, Dennis, & Yund, 1977; Efron, Yund, Nichols, & Crandall, 1977) conducted several studies to determine the effects of unilateral temporal lobe lesions on several auditory tasks, including gap detection and temporal ordering. Again, their findings suggested a clear pattern of deficit in the ears contralateral to posterior temporal lobe lesions. Interestingly, the authors also found contralateral deficits in patients with anterior temporal lobe lesions—an area previously thought to have no role in auditory processing. They suggested the possible existence of an efferent system responsible for enhancing the perception of auditory stimuli in the contralateral auditory space. Several other researchers have documented contralateral deficits in temporal ordering in cases of temporal lobe lesions (Belmont & Handler, 1971; Blaettner, Scherg, & Von Cramon, 1989; Karaseva, 1972).

As previously discussed, both corpus callosum and left temporal lobe lesions have been shown to interfere with the linguistic labeling, but not the perception (and humming) of acoustic patterns consisting of more than two stimuli (e.g., Musiek, Gollegly, & Baran, 1984). Subjects with temporal lobe lesions demonstrate significant bilateral deficits on Frequency Patterns tasks (Musiek et al., 1984; Musiek & Pinheiro, 1987). In addition, patients with lesions involving the left hemisphere or interhemispheric pathways exhibit great difficulty in verbally reporting patterns that differ in intensity and frequency, whereas, when asked to hum the patterns heard (thus removing the linguistic labeling component), these same subjects exhibit scores near the normal range (Musiek et al., 1980). Conversely, right temporal lobe lesions affect both the perception and linguistic labeling of auditory patterns.

In conclusion, temporal lobe lesions result in significant difficulty in the temporal ordering of two successive auditory stimuli in the ear contralateral to the lesion. Lesions of the dominant hemisphere result in deficits in traditional within-channel temporal gap detection; however, the effects of temporal lobe dysfunction on between-channel gap detection have yet to be studied. Although standard temporal integration tasks may not have much utility in the detection of cerebral lesions, evaluation of duration difference limens may differentiate peripheral from central pathology. Finally, lesions of the dominant (usually left) temporal lobe or the corpus callosum interfere with the ability to label linguistically (but not hum) a pattern consisting of more than two auditory stimuli, whereas lesions of the nondominant (usually right) temporal lobe disrupt auditory pattern perception altogether.

Effects of Other Pathological Conditions on Temporal Processing

The effect of brainstem lesions on subjects' ability to perform tasks of temporal ordering is variable and appears to depend on the site of lesion and the type of task (Musiek & Pinheiro, 1987). Cochlear lesions (peripheral hearing loss) do not appear to affect performance significantly on temporal patterning tests, provided that the stimuli are

Table 2-2

Effects of Auditory System Pathology on Temporal Processing

Site of Lesion	Effect(s) on Temporal Processing
Right temporal lobe	Bilateral deficit on temporal patterning tasks involving more than two stimuli when either verbal or humming response is required, poor performance on two-tone ordering tasks when signals are delivered to different ears, no effect on gap detection or two-tone ordering when both signals are delivered to the right ear
Left temporal lobe	Significant contralateral or bilateral effects, depending on type of task, bilateral deficit on temporal patterning tasks involving more than two stimuli when verbal report is required, poorer gap detection thresholds, poor performance on all two-tone sequencing tasks
Corpus callosum	Bilateral deficit on temporal patterning tasks involving more than two stimuli when verbal report is required
Brainstem	Variable, depends on site of lesion and type of task, temporal integration functions are less steep
Cochlear	Temporal integration functions are less steep, little or no effect on temporal patterning
Conductive	Little or no effect on temporal processing at adequate presentation levels

detectable (Musiek, Baran, & Pinheiro, 1990; Musiek & Pinheiro, 1987). In addition, Papsin and Abel (1988) found that subjects with VIIIth nerve pathology exhibited flat temporal integration functions, a finding that was supported by Thompson and Abel (1992b), who reported relatively little effect of stimulus duration on the ability of patients with acoustic neuromas to detect acoustic stimuli. Therefore, **it appears that tests of temporal processing may not be as sensitive to VIIIth nerve or brainstem pathology as they are to cerebral lesions.**

Cranford (1984) reported that temporal integration was affected by cochlear site of lesion, resulting in a significantly less steep integration function similar to those of subjects with brainstem lesions; however, the author was unable to correlate the slope of the temporal integration function with recruitment or etiology of sensorineural hearing loss.

Finally, conductive hearing loss appears to have little effect on temporal integration (Cranford, 1984) or temporal patterning. Therefore, it appears that some tests of temporal processing may have promise for use in evaluating central auditory processing in children and adults with hearing impairment. The effects of CANS lesions on temporal processing are reviewed in Table 2-2.

Binaural Interaction

The term *binaural interaction* refers simply to the way in which the two ears work together. Functions that rely on binaural interaction include but are not limited to localization and lateralization of auditory stimuli, binaural release from masking, detection of signals in noise, and binaural fusion (Durlach, Thompson, & Colburn, 1981; Noffsinger, Schaefer, & Martinez, 1984). As will be shown below, it is believed that auditory structures within the brainstem are most important for binaural interaction to occur, although the actual perception of the auditory event appears to occur in the cortex. As discussed in Chapter 1, **the superior olivary complex in the pons is the most caudal structure in the CANS to receive binaural input, which implicates the low brainstem as being particularly critical to binaural interaction.**

Localization and Lateralization

Studies of localization (determining direction of the source) and lateralization (place perception in the head) of auditory stimuli date back to the late 1920s (Greene, 1929). Several investigators have studied the mechanisms of localization and lateralization and the effects of various lesions upon listeners' ability to localize or lateralize auditory stimuli (Abel, Bert, & McLean, 1978; Bergman, 1957; Matzker, 1959; Norlund, 1964; Pinheiro & Tobin, 1969; Sanchez-Longo & Forster, 1958; Sanchez-Longo et al., 1957; Viehweg & Campbell, 1960; Walsh, 1957).

Bergman (1957) found that, in cases of unilateral middle ear surgery, the ability of listeners to localize was poor if the auditory stimulus was presented at a level below the threshold of the poorer ear; however, localization ability rapidly improved at suprathreshold levels and reached normal performance at 10 dB sensation level (SL) (re: poorer ear threshold). Nordlund (1964), in a study of subjects with a variety of lesions, discovered that lesions of the vestibular system had the least effect on localization ability whereas lesions of the auditory nerve and low brainstem and unilateral deafness had the greatest impact on listeners' ability to localize.

These two studies combined with the findings of the other researchers suggest that **although unilateral deafness and asymmet-**

rical hearing sensitivity degrades localization performance, auditory nerve and low brainstem lesions have a much greater impact upon localization and lateralization of an auditory stimulus. In addition, localization and lateralization ability is not easily predicted on the basis of the listener's audiometric configuration (Durlach et al., 1981). Therefore, it would appear that while peripheral considerations must be taken into account, a large portion of localization and lateralization involves at least the auditory nerve and low brainstem. In addition, Sanchez-Longo and Forster (1958) and Pinheiro and Tobin (1969) showed degraded performance on tasks related to localization in subjects with temporal lobe lesions. This finding indicates that although critical processing of localization and lateralization information occurs in the brainstem, the actual perception of sound location occurs in the cortex (Pickles, 1985).

Binaural Release from Masking

Licklider (1948) investigated the effects of interaural phase on the intelligibility of binaurally presented speech stimuli. He presented speech and white noise to both ears at the same time while systematically varying the phase relationship between the two ears. He found that when both speech and noise were in phase or out of phase (homophasic condition), the intelligibility of the speech was lower for normal listeners than when the speech was out of phase and the noise was in phase or when the speech was in phase and the noise was out of phase (antiphasic condition). In addition, speech intelligibility was found to be better for binaural antiphasic conditions than for monaural presentation alone. Conversely, speech and noise presented binaurally in a homophasic condition resulted in lower intelligibility than did monaural presentation. Therefore, he concluded that interaural inhibition (or the decrease in binaural performance over monaural performance in some conditions) may well be linked to interaural phase.

In a related study, Hirsh (1948) utilized a similar paradigm to investigate the effects of interaural phase, pure-tone frequency, and stimulus intensity on interaural summation and inhibition. The following six experimental conditions were utilized: (1) tone monaural/noise binaural and in phase (SNø); (2) tone monaural, noise binaural, and 180° out of phase (SNπ); (3) tone and noise binaural and in phase (SøNø homophasic condition); (4) tone and noise binaural and out of phase (SπNπ homophasic condition); (5) tone binaural and in phase/noise binaural and out of phase (SøNπ antiphasic condition); and (6) tone

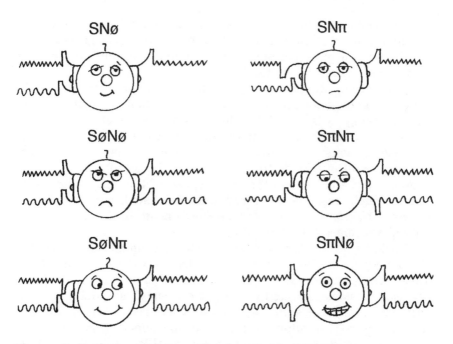

Figure 2-4. Phase conditions utilized in Hirsh's (1948) study.

binaural and out of phase/noise binaural and in phase (SπNø antiphasic condition). These conditions are illustrated in Figure 2-4.

Hirsh found that noise presented 180° out of phase to the two ears resulted in the listener perceiving the noise to be located at the ears, whereas noise presented in a homophasic condition resulted in a perception of the noise as being located in the middle of the head (midline). Therefore, the monaural pure-tone threshold was better when the noise was in phase since the noise was perceived at midline and the tone was perceived at the ear. Similarly, binaural pure-tone thresholds were much better for the antiphasic conditions since the pure tone was heard more easily when it was located at midline and the noise was located at the ears or vice versa, a phenomenon that has come to be known as "release from masking." An additional finding was the effect of stimulus frequency on binaural summation and inhibition: as the pure-tone frequency increased, localization on the basis of phase became more difficult. Thus, **the difference in binaural thresholds between homophasic and antiphasic conditions (otherwise known as the *masking level difference*, or *MLD*) decreased as the stimulus frequency increased.** The author added that the fact that the monaural pure-tone thresholds masked by noise in the same ear shifted when noise was added to the opposite ear suggests that masking is not merely a peripheral phenomenon but must involve some degree of central interaction.

A variety of stimulus variables affects the size of the MLD. The choice of a continuous masking stimulus will result in greater release from masking—a larger MLD—than will a masking stimulus that is designed to match the cycle of the pure tone (Green, 1966). An increase in stimulus intensity has been shown to result in a decrease in the amount of release from masking in the antiphasic condition (Townsend & Goldstein, 1972). Finally, **use of the antiphasic condition in which the signal delivered to the two ears is out of phase and the masking noise is in phase (SπNø) will result in the largest MLDs** (Olsen, Noffsinger, & Carhart, 1976).

That the mechanism of binaural release from masking occurs at the low brainstem level is evidenced by the work of Lynn, Gilroy, Taylor, and Leiser (1981), who found that whereas patients with low brainstem lesions exhibited very small or nonexistent MLDs, patients with cortical lesions exhibited release from masking comparable to normal controls. In addition, lesions of the upper brainstem corresponding to auditory brainstem response (ABR) waves IV and V do not affect the size of the MLD (Noffsinger, Schaefer, & Martinez, 1984).

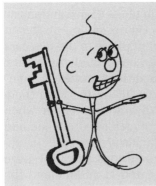

KEY CONCEPT

The MLD is not affected by cortical or high brainstem lesions, but is abnormally small in patients with lesions of the low brainstem.

Detection of Signals in Noise

The ability of a listener to detect a signal in a background of noise is critically related to the interaural relationship between the target signal and the masking signal (Durlach et al., 1981). Therefore, localization and lateralization play a crucial role in this ability.

It is generally known that two ears are better than one and that listeners with unilateral or asymmetrical hearing loss exhibit difficulty detecting signals in noise. However, **this "binaural advantage" is dependent not only upon the hearing sensitivity of the listener but also on the angle or direction of the noise as it relates to the target signal** (Nordlund & Fritzel, 1963). The binaural advantage, or improvement in masked threshold in the binaural condition over the monaural condition, is most evident when the speech and noise are separated by 90° and is essentially nonexistent when the speech and noise arise from the same angle or are separated by 180° (Dirks & Wilson, 1969; Tonning, 1971).

In essence, this dependence of the masked threshold on the angles of the signal and noise in sound field is analogous to the binaural release from masking (MLD) exhibited under headphones (Durlach et al., 1981). It is apparent from the literature that the ability to detect a signal in a background of noise can be affected by a variety of factors, including peripheral hearing sensitivity, localization/lateralization ability, and binaural release from masking. **Thus, we can infer that, for the listener with normal hearing sensitivity, similar processing mechanisms are engaged for speech-in-noise skills as for localization/lateralization and the MLD, which would implicate the low brainstem as being particularly important in the extraction of signals from noise.**

It is important to emphasize that binaural interaction skills, including localization and lateralization, are not the only prerequisites for detecting signals in a background of noise. Speech-in-noise abilities are complex, and are influenced by subcortical, cortical, corpus callosum, efferent auditory system, and attentional factors. Therefore, one cannot ascribe difficulties hearing in noise to a deficit in binaural interaction or, indeed, to any auditory-specific processing disorder as this is a general skill that is influenced by many auditory and nonauditory factors.

Binaural Fusion

Several investigators have studied the mechanism of binaural fusion (Lynn & Gilroy, 1975; Matzker, 1959; Smith & Resnick, 1972; Tobin, 1985; Willeford, 1976). Each of these studies has utilized the simultaneous presentation of high-pass filtered stimuli to one ear and low-pass filtered stimuli to the opposite ear in order to assess the listener's ability to fuse the two disparate inputs into one perceptual event.

In all studies, for normal listeners, the presentation of either band pass alone resulted in poor recognition scores; however, the binaural presentation of low-pass stimuli to one ear and high-pass to the other resulted in a significant improvement in recognition performance. Matzker (1959) found that the performance of subjects with cortical lesions was comparable to that of normal listeners whereas subjects with brainstem lesions had difficulty with the fusion task. The findings of Smith and Resnick (1972) and Lynn and Gilroy (1975) also indicated abnormal fusion performance in subjects with brainstem pathology, suggesting that **the mechanism of binaural fusion is also mediated primarily in the brainstem.**

Effects of Cerebral Pathology on Binaural Interaction

As mentioned previously, the mechanism of binaural interaction is mediated primarily in the low brainstem. Therefore, it would be expected that cerebral pathology would have little effect upon binaural processing. Indeed, Lynn et al. (1981) found that subjects with cerebral pathology demonstrated essentially normal MLDs. However, because the perception of the auditory event occurs in the cortex, lesions of the cerebral hemispheres also result in disrupted binaural perception. For example, binaural functions such as tracking moving auditory signals across the midline of the body, development of a concept of "auditory space," and even speech-in-noise skills are dependent on the integrity of cortical structures.

Sanchez-Longo et al. (1957) and Sanchez-Longo and Forster (1958) investigated localization ability in subjects with temporal lobe lesions. The authors found that subjects with lesions of the temporal lobe demonstrated impaired sound localization ability in the auditory field contralateral to the lesion.

Pinheiro and Tobin (1969, 1971) studied the amount of interaural intensity difference (IID) required for subjects to lateralize auditory stimuli. Whereas normal listeners required an IID of approximately 4 dB for lateralization, subjects with central lesions required a greater IID in the ear ipsilateral to the lesion in order to lateralize auditory stimuli successfully. Of the subjects in this study, those who exhibited neurological symptoms characteristic of temporal or parietal pathology demonstrated elevated IIDs, whereas those with symptoms of occipital or frontal lesions exhibited IIDs comparable to those of normal subjects. The corpus callosum also appears to play a significant role in binaural hearing. For example, the perception of midline fusion and tracking of auditory signals across the midline has been shown to be affected by corpus callosum dysfunction (Lepore et al., 1994; Lepore, Ptito, & Guillemot, 1986). Similarly, tasks involving speech-in-noise (or auditory figure-ground) skills, commonly considered to reflect binaural hearing ability, rely at least in part on corpus callosum integrity (Hoptman & Davidson, 1994; Jerger, 1997).

Based on these findings, it is clear that the auditory cortex and corpus callosum are extremely important in the development of the concept of auditory space as well as in the perception of the location of a sound source. Therefore, **although the preliminary groundwork for binaural abilities such as localization of sound sources occurs in the brainstem, higher-level structures play a critical role in binaural processing.**

Effects of Brainstem Pathology on Binaural Interaction

In addition to transmission of sound and reflexive action as seen in the acoustic reflex, the brainstem auditory pathways are responsible for reception and processing of binaural input (Noffsinger et al., 1984). Therefore, auditory functions involving binaural interaction are likely to be affected by brainstem lesions. The MLD paradigm represents the brainstem's ability to extract a signal from background noise and is the most sensitive behavioral procedure for assessing auditory brainstem integrity (Noffsinger et al., 1984). Specifically, lesions involving the pontomedullary junction are particularly likely to result in abnormal MLDs (Lynn et al., 1981; Noffsinger et al., 1984; Olsen & Noffsinger, 1976).

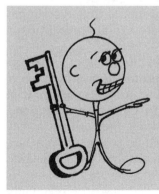

KEY CONCEPT

The MLD is the most sensitive *behavioral* technique for assessing brainstem integrity.

Multiple sclerosis has been shown to slow transmission time throughout the brainstem auditory pathways (Chiappa, 1980). Several researchers have studied the effects of multiple sclerosis on binaural interaction (Hendler, Squires, & Emmerich, 1990; Levine et al. 1993a, b; Noffsinger et al., 1972; Noffsinger et al., 1984; Olsen & Noffsinger, 1976; Quine, Regan, & Murray, 1983).

Olsen and Noffsinger (1976) studied a variety of subjects with cochlear and brainstem lesions using MLDs for tones and spondaic words. They reported that subjects with multiple sclerosis exhibited reduced MLDs for both tones and speech and concluded that this finding was most likely due to a disruption of brainstem integration of binaural input.

Quine et al. (1983) conducted a study in which the interaural delay of tones presented to one ear was varied relative to a fixed 1000 Hz tone in the other ear. Subjects were required to indicate which ear received the tone first. Responses were analyzed to determine the smallest interaural delay necessary for judgment, similar to temporal ordering tasks but involving both ears. The authors reported that the majority of subjects with multiple sclerosis exhibited significantly longer interaural delays than did control subjects. In addition, the authors found that this delay could be present at one, two, or all three of the frequencies tested (500, 1000, and 2000 Hz). Therefore, it appears that delays can occur for specific frequencies and not others, a finding that may be explained by the presence of local plaques of demyelination occurring at those anatomical sites responsible for the affected frequency or frequencies.

In a similar study investigating the ability of subjects with multiple sclerosis to process changes in interaural intensity, Noffsinger et al. (1972) found that 12 of 60 subjects were unable to experience a single fused midline image when tones presented to both ears were of equal intensity. Hausler and Levine (1980) reported that, of 29 patients with multiple sclerosis, 13 exhibited degraded interaural time discrimination abilities, and these findings were related to abnormalities in brainstem auditory evoked potentials.

Levine et al. (1993a, b) cautioned that **because multiple sclerosis may cause focal lesions anywhere throughout the auditory pathways, the performance of multiple sclerosis patients on various tests of central auditory processing is likely to be quite varied, depending on the site of lesion.** In their two-part study, the authors investigated the performance of subjects with multiple sclerosis on behavioral tests involving discrimination of interaural time and frequency. The findings on the behavioral tests were then compared to results of brainstem auditory evoked potential testing and magnetic resonance imaging (MRI) to determine site of lesion. The stimuli utilized were noise bursts that were either high-pass filtered (4000 to 2000 Hz) or low-pass filtered (20 to 1000 Hz). The authors' objective was to determine the just noticeable difference (jnd) in interaural time and interaural intensity required for subjects to perceive a displacement of sound from one ear to the other.

The authors' findings indicated that the majority of subjects exhibited abnormal time jnds for high-pass stimuli. Abnormal performance on any of the other tests was always associated with abnormal time jnds for high-pass stimuli. The least sensitive measures were the jnds for interaural intensity. In addition, the authors found that there were no "silent" multiple sclerosis lesions. Every subject with documented lesions of the brainstem auditory pathways exhibited some abnormality in tests that required microsecond accuracy in neural timing. Specifically, a disruption in interaural discrimination for high-frequency sounds was correlated with unilateral lesions between the cochlear nucleus (CN) and superior olivary complex (SOC). The authors suggested that **the processing of high-frequency sounds requires a greater amount of neural synchrony than does processing of low-frequency sounds and, thus, is most likely to be affected by lesions involving transmission of sound through the brainstem auditory pathways.**

In conclusion, pathological conditions involving the brainstem auditory pathways are likely to result in some disturbance of binaural interaction.

Effects of Cochlear Pathology on Binaural Interaction

Olsen and Noffsinger (1976) reported that subjects with unilateral Meniere's disease exhibited reduced MLDs for 500 Hz tones and spondaic words compared to normal controls. In addition, subjects with noise-induced cochlear hearing loss also exhibited reduced MLDs for speech, although MLDs for 500 Hz tones were within normal limits. They concluded that **binaural release from masking is affected by cochlear pathology when spondaic word stimuli are used** and that this finding may provide an explanation for why individuals with noise-induced hearing loss often report difficulty understanding speech in the presence of background noise.

Several other studies have shown that the MLD is often abnormally reduced in subjects with cochlear pathology (Hall, Tyler, & Fernandez, 1984; Jerger, Brown, & Smith, 1984; Quaranta & Cervellera,

1974; Schoeny & Carhart, 1971; Staffel, Hall, Grose, & Pillsbury, 1990). The abnormalities found in the MLD are likely to be more apparent with increasing severity of loss and interaural asymmetry in hearing sensitivity.

Regarding localization and lateralization abilities in subjects with cochlear hearing loss, it appears that cochlear lesions have a much lesser effect than lesions involving other parts of the auditory system and CANS (Nordlund, 1964; Roser, 1966; Pinheiro & Tobin, 1971). In addition, although subjects with asymmetrical hearing loss tend to do worse on these tasks, **unilateral deafness does not always destroy localization performance** (Gatehouse, 1976; Jongkees & Van der Veer, 1957; Tonning, 1971, 1975). The degree of difficulty in performing localization and lateralization tasks is difficult to predict on the basis of the degree of hearing loss or audiometric configuration (Nordlund, 1964; Tonning, 1971). The fact that some individuals with cochlear hearing loss report significant difficulty in activities such as understanding a speaker in a noisy situation and others do not may be explained, at least in part, by this variability found in binaural interaction skills in patients with cochlear pathology.

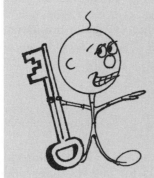

KEY CONCEPT

The degree of difficulty in localization and lateralization cannot easily be predicted on the basis of the audiogram.

Effects of Middle Ear Pathology on Binaural Interaction

Some of the most interesting research in the area of binaural interaction has concerned the effect of otitis media and other middle ear disorders on MLDs, particularly in children. **The MLD at 500 Hz is generally reduced in children as compared to adults and increases as a function of age, reaching adult values at approximately 5 to 6 years of age** (Hall & Grose, 1990). In addition, adults show a greater release from masking for time-compressed speech than do children of 8 to 9 years of age (Bornstein, 1994). Finally, children with a history of chronic otitis media have been shown to have difficulty recognizing words presented in a competing speech background (Jerger, Jerger, Alford, & Abrams, 1983).

Pillsbury, Grose, and Hall (1991) studied the MLD for 500 Hz tones in a group of children with a history of chronic otitis media with effusion (OME) and hearing loss. The children, ages 5 to 13 years, were tested just prior to the insertion of pressure equalizing (PE) tubes and one month following surgery. Several of the children also returned for additional testing three months postoperatively. Findings from this group were compared to those from a group of children with no history of otitis. The authors found that the children with a history of otitis media demonstrated significantly reduced MLDs and greater variability than did the control children. This MLD abnormality continued to be present for 64% of the children three months after the insertion of PE tubes.

The authors drew several conclusions from their study. Most important, **the extent of hearing disability associated with otitis media with effusion may be severely underestimated on the basis of pure-tone audiograms,** as many children may continue to have difficulty extracting signals from a background of noise even in light of essentially normal postoperative hearing sensitivity. Several possible explanations for the observed deficit in MLDs were posited. One focused on abnormal development of brainstem auditory structures responsible for binaural processing, a finding that would be consistent with the results of several animal studies in which asymmetrical conductive hearing loss resulted in abnormal development of auditory brainstem structures (Clopton & Silverman, 1978; Knudsen, 1983; Moore, Hutchings, King, & Kowalchuk, 1989; Moore & Irvine, 1981). Other possible explanations included inaccurate mapping of stimulus frequency onto cochlear place and reduced ability of the CANS to process cues for signal detection and extract the signal from the noise. Whatever the cause, it does appear from the authors' data that children having a significant history of chronic otitis media with effusion may exhibit long-term difficulty in binaural interaction, possibly due to sensory deprivation.

To explore further the relationship between abnormal MLDs and possible abnormal brainstem function in children with a history of otitis media with effusion, Hall and Grose (1993) studied a group of fourteen children, ages 5 to 9, all of whom had a significant otologic history and were tested approximately one month following the insertion of PE tubes. The authors compared MLD results with those of brainstem auditory evoked potential testing. Results of this study indicated modest correlation between abnormal MLDs and interaural asymmetry for interpeak interval values. There was no correlation noted between abnormal MLDs and absolute latency prolongation or interpeak intervals. The authors concluded that the degree of interpeak interval abnormality in one ear may be related to the degree of auditory deprivation in that ear relative to the other ear. In addition, the results suggested that reduced MLDs in children having otitis media with effusion may indeed be related to abnormal brainstem processing as opposed to more centrally located factors.

Hall, Grose, and Pillsbury (1995), in a longitudinal study of the effects of OME on MLD performance, reported that the above mentioned abnormalities in the MLD continued to be present up to two years following medical intervention. By three years postsurgery, a small proportion of children continued to exhibit reduced MLDs; however, the OME group did not differ significantly from the control group in terms of MLD performance. These results suggested a slow recovery of binaural function over a long period of time in children having a history of chronic otitis media with effusion.

Finally, conductive hearing loss can degrade localization and lateralization abilities significantly (Hausler, Colburn, & Marr, 1983; Nordlund, 1964; Roser, 1966), and abnormalities in binaural processing have been found to persist for some time even after hearing thresholds are returned to normal by middle ear surgery (Hall & Derlacki, 1986, 1988; Hall, Grose, & Pillsbury, 1990; Pillsbury et al., 1991). Table 2-3 summarizes the effects of CANS pathology on binaural interaction.

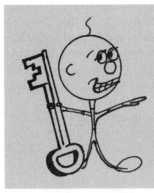

KEY CONCEPT

Even after chronic otitis media with effusion has subsided and hearing has returned to normal, auditory processing difficulties may continue indefinitely.

Table 2-3

Effects of Auditory System Pathology on Binaural Interaction

Site of Lesion	Effect(s) on Binaural Interaction
Temporal lobe	Impairment of localization in contralateral auditory field, greater IID required in ear ipsilateral to lesion for lateralization
Corpus callosum	Difficulty in tracking auditory sources across the midline, generalized localization and auditory figure-ground difficulties
High brainstem	No effect on MLD
Low brainstem	Deficit in all binaural interaction tasks
Cochlear	Variable, possible deficit in localization and lateralization, reduced MLD
Conductive	Reduced MLD, may exhibit ongoing deficit in binaural interaction tasks following resolution of conductive component

Speech-Sound Discrimination

The topic of speech-sound encoding at each level of the CANS was discussed extensively in Chapter 1, and that information will not be reiterated here. The precise mechanism whereby acoustic features of an auditory signal are put together to form what we perceive as a particular speech sound that is distinct from all other speech sounds is not yet completely understood—and, because of its complexity, it may never be. However, we do have some insight into those aspects of the speech signal itself that appear to be important for phonemic discrimination. We also know how dysfunction or damage to various levels of the CANS affect speech-sound discrimination abilities, as well as what role experience plays in our ability to discriminate sounds occurring in our own native languages.

Koch and colleagues suggested that speech can be characterized by a finite set of acoustic parameters that make up the fundamental sound structure of all languages of the world (Koch, McGee, Bradlow, & Kraus, 1999). Of primary importance to the discrimination of speech sounds are the frequency spectrum of the sounds, the way in which the spectrum changes over time, and the duration of the sound. These spectro-temporal and duration aspects of the speech signal are presumed to be encoded in various manners at each level of the CANS, as discussed in Chapter 1. Furthermore, running speech can be characterized by rapidly alternating amplitude peaks and troughs that correspond to vowels and consonants, respectively, as well as overall amplitude modulation corresponding to the syllabic structure of the ongoing speech message.

Virtually every level of the peripheral and central auditory systems plays a role in speech-sound encoding and, therefore, is important to phonemic discrimination. Certainly, we know that cochlear hearing loss can have a detrimental effect on the listener's ability to discriminate between similar-sounding phonemes, as well as on speech perception in noise and a variety of other auditory perceptual abilities. Similarly, pathologies that affect the auditory nerve and brainstem auditory pathways are notoriously destructive to speech-sound processing abilities. Disorders that diminish the auditory nerve fibers' ability to fire synchronously, such as auditory neuropathy or dyssynchrony, can eliminate speech perception skills altogether. Lesions such as acoustic tumors can result in asymmetrical findings on word recognition testing, with the speech perception abilities in the ear ipsilateral to the tumor being significantly poorer than those in the contralateral ear. Finally, speech sound representation and discrimination is ultimately reliant on the integrity of the thalamus and auditory cortex.

There is ample evidence to suggest that the auditory cortex is critical to the discrimination of speech sounds that contain rapid spectro-temporal changes, such as consonants, but that sounds with more slowly varying acoustic parameters (such as vowels) are not as reliant on cortical integrity (e.g., Kraus, McGee, King, Littman, & Nicol, 1994; Kraus, McGee, Littman, King, & Nicol, 1994; Phillips & Farmer, 1990). Moreover, integrity of the primary (left hemisphere) auditory cortex appears to be most critical for fine-grained acoustic discrimination of speech (especially consonant) stimuli (Phillips & Farmer, 1990). From these findings, we can conclude that the ability to discriminate between consonants that contain rapid spectro-temporal acoustic changes would be more vulnerable to subtle cortical disruption than would the ability to discriminate steady-state or slowly varying speech sounds, such as vowels or glides. Indeed, in cases of lesions of the primary auditory cortex, the ability to discriminate stop consonants is often affected, whereas vowel discrimination abilities are spared (Phillips & Farmer, 1990).

We should be cautious, however, in assuming that the acoustic-phonetic features of a speech signal will predict how a given person will *perceive* that speech signal. Although we can break phonemes down into their constituent spectral and temporal acoustic features, the ability of the listener to discriminate among those phonemes is highly dependent on many factors in addition to accurate acoustic encoding by the CANS. As will be discussed in the next section, these higher-level or top-down factors can affect the sensory percept even at its most basic level. Furthermore, these higher-level linguistic, cognitive, and related factors will also play a key role in determining how a deficit in the fundamental ability to discriminate between similar-sounding phonemes may relate to more generalized difficulties processing spoken language in a given individual.

Top-Down Factors in Auditory Processing

In the previous chapter, we provided a discussion and overview of the neuroanatomy and neurophysiology of the central auditory pathways, as well as acoustic signal encoding in the CANS, particularly relating to speech encoding. These bottom-up, or data-driven, factors are critical to the ultimate ability to perceive and understand speech; however, they are not in and of themselves sufficient. Indeed, even if basic sensory encoding unfolds perfectly at all levels of the ascending pathways, higher-order dysfunction or inadequate top-down, or concept-driven, factors can and will have a deleterious effect on the individual's ability to process, and ultimately comprehend, spoken language. Chief among these top-down factors are attention, memory, cognition, and language.

The purpose of this section is not to provide an in-depth tutorial of all of these complex areas. Indeed, an adequate treatment of any of these topics alone would fill volumes of text. An excellent overview of these topics can be found in Kolb and Whishaw (1996), Medin and Ross (1997), Restak (2001), or any of a number of other texts dealing with the subjects of cognitive psychology and the brain/mind connection. Instead, this section seeks to introduce readers to a few basic neuropsychological and psycholinguistic principles and to illustrate their applicability to the topic of auditory processing. It is not my intention to imply that deficits in the areas of language, attention, cognition, or other higher-order functions should fall under the umbrella of "auditory processing disorders." As previously discussed in this chapter, the modality specificity of CAPD has become a rather contentious topic of late, primarily due to the difficulty in demonstrating that a specific auditory deficit exists among children in whom CAPD is suspected or whether such a deficit may be an underlying cause for their learning difficulties (e.g., Watson & Miller, 1993; McFarland & Cacace, 1995; Cacace & McFarland, 1998). Nevertheless,

as our understanding of auditory processing and spoken language comprehension evolves, we find ourselves increasingly unable to ignore the vast body of evidence suggesting that the processing of auditory input involves far more than the sensory encoding of acoustic stimuli. Rather, we must acknowledge that the ultimate utility of basic acoustic encoding in the auditory system is inextricably intertwined with how the individual is able to use the information provided by such encoding in determining one's ability to process speech auditorily.

In our discussion of bottom-up factors in Chapter 1, we provided the admittedly extreme example of deaf individuals, in whom the lack of any sensory input would necessarily affect their ability to "process" auditory information. Let us take a look at another relatively extreme example at the other end of the processing continuum to see how higher-order functions factor into the processing equation. Consider, for example, children with significant attention deficit, for whom the task of merely attending to any stimulus long enough for it to be consciously perceived is nearly impossible. For these children, it may be irrelevant whether the central auditory system accurately encodes the stimulus, as their inability to be active listeners is impacted by the pervading attention deficit. As a result, their auditory processing skills may be as poor as those of deaf individuals, but for a vastly different reason.

At this point, many readers are undoubtedly thinking to themselves that neither hearing impairment nor attention deficit can or should be placed into the category of auditory processing disorders, notwithstanding their impact on the behavior of processing auditory information. This viewpoint would be entirely accurate. Indeed, the presence of either hearing impairment or attention deficit calls for specific interventions such as amplification or medical treatment, respectively. However, these examples are provided to illustrate the need for considering the entire system when attempting to determine why a given individual has difficulty listening to and comprehending spoken language. It may be that the difficulty is outside the realm of auditory processing per se, and that poor auditory processing skills are merely a by-product of a more pervasive dysfunction affecting abilities and skills across a wide variety of domains. Conversely, it may be that the problem is, indeed, auditory in nature, requiring auditory interventions. Or, it may be that a combination of auditory and higher-order factors are working together to impact auditory processing abilities in a given individual, and that intervention strategies should address listening skills across the continuum. Finally, it may be possible to employ higher-order strategies and to strengthen top-down factors and abilities to assist in compensating for an auditory processing deficit arising from poor sensory encoding. Whatever the case, it is necessary to consider all factors, be they auditory, cognitive, linguistic, or other, when assessing auditory processing abilities and determining methods for intervention and management.

Language Processing Versus Auditory Processing

I have stated that CAPD is primarily an "input" disorder, that is, it is a deficit specific to the processing of acoustic input. The behavioral manifestations of CAPD, however, often appear as language comprehension disorders. There does seem to be agreement among most in the scientific community that the terms *auditory processing* and *language processing* are not interchangeable. But the precise point at which auditory processing stops and language processing begins is unclear, and far from agreed upon.

Auerbach and colleagues distinguished between disorders that affect the perception of acoustic, or *prephonemic*, characteristics of speech sounds, giving rise to a secondary impairment in spoken word comprehension, and those that affect the identification of the speech sounds themselves, or *phonemic* deficits (Auerbach, Allard, Naeser, Alexander, & Albert, 1982). In this theory, phonemic deficits are those that occur after the basic sensory analysis of the spectro-temporal features, or waveform, of the acoustic signal is completed. The phonemic level of processing is the point at which categorical perception, or the ability to parse or categorize speech sounds into psychologically distinct percepts, occurs. Individuals with prephonemic deficits would have difficulty resolving the actual temporal and frequency aspects of the incoming acoustic signal, particularly those that change rapidly over time. Conversely, individuals with phonemic deficits would be able to resolve these features, but be unable to appreciate the fine boundaries between phonemes or to group sounds with different acoustic properties into instances of the same phoneme. This latter ability is important for spoken word comprehension, as *coarticulation* results in a given phoneme having different acoustic properties depending on the phonemes that immediately precede or follow it during running speech. A purely acoustic feature theory of auditory processing would state, then, that the point at which auditory processing becomes language processing is that point where prephonemic processing becomes phonemic.

This theory seems logical and, indeed, some conceptualizations of CAPD are based entirely on this premise. That is, a CAPD would be one in which one or more aspects of prephonemic processing are disrupted, leading to secondary phonemic and, therefore, word comprehension and related difficulties. Moreover, to support the validity of a diagnostic label of CAPD, it would need to be shown that (1) these types of prephonemic deficits, specific to the auditory modality, do exist; and (2) these prephonemic deficits then lead to difficulties in comprehending spoken language and additional communication and learning sequelae. As reviewed most eloquently by Cacace and McFarland (1998), there are only limited, if any, empirical data to support either of these points. In fact, it has been suggested that the rapid temporal processing deficits presumed by some to underlie reading and language difficulties in some children are not specific to the auditory modality, but are pan-sensory in nature (e.g., Farmer & Klein, 1995; Tallal, Miller, & Fitch, 1993). Studdert-Kennedy and Mody (1995) argued that some children exhibit difficulty with rapid perception that is, indeed, specific to speech stimuli and that is not apparent using rapid nonspeech stimuli, providing further evidence against the existence of a prephonemic deficit affecting resolution of the spectro-temporal aspects of the acoustic signal before the signal "becomes" phonemic in nature. Moreover, there is no compelling evidence to suggest that difficulties processing the prephonemic acoustic features of a speech signal lead to the types of language, communication, and learning effects ascribed to CAPD. Therefore, **if one views central auditory processing as involving only those auditory mechanisms that occur prior to phonemic processing in the auditory system, then there is no evidence at present to indicate that CAPD as a valid diagnostic construct actually exists at all.**

However, there are data to suggest that this line between pre-phonemic and phonemic processing is artificial, and does not reflect what actually occurs during normal speech perception in the real world. That is, there is no *ecological validity* to a theoretical construct that parses word comprehension into these specific, discrete stages. Instead, **there is increasing evidence supporting a global-to-local (or coarse-to-fine) hypothesis in real-world sensory perceptual processing.** That is, perceptual processing does not merely consist of the construction of global properties (e.g., phonemes, words, sentences) purely from an analysis and synthesis of lower-level local features (e.g., spectral and temporal acoustic characteristics of the signal) in a bottom-up fashion. Rather, early access to the global properties themselves (including familiarity with the speech sounds of the language and other higher-order aspects) influences and actually facilitates the processing of the finer, "lower-level" details (e.g., Goldstone, 1994). Thus, **any model that considers central auditory processes to be solely those mechanisms relating to the prephonemic processing of acoustic features would be inconsistent with the manner in which auditory perceptual processing occurs in the real world.**

Where, then, does the line between auditory processing and language processing really lie? There is no easy answer to this question. Certainly, individuals who exhibit entirely intact processing of auditory input—including good auditory discrimination abilities even during conditions of competing or degraded speech, intact phonological awareness and phonemic decoding abilities, good temporal processing abilities for speech and nonspeech signals, and related skills—yet who have difficulty comprehending the meaning of spoken and written communications in context would be considered to have a language processing disorder of some sort. Individuals who exhibit a deficit in the formulation of messages, either spoken or written, despite intact comprehension abilities would also fall into the language-disordered end of the continuum. Similarly, those who exhibit comprehension deficits that are restricted to words that occur with low frequency in the language or those that occupy specific semantic categories certainly would be considered to have language, rather than auditory, processing disorders. However, it is more difficult to draw a fine line between audition and language in some individuals for whom the perception and comprehension of verbally presented speech is impaired, especially when one considers the manner in which top-down, concept-driven factors influence basic bottom-up, data-driven auditory perceptual events.

Psycholinguistic views of CAPD focus on how auditory perception influences spoken language comprehension, taking into account the complexity of both the speech signal and speech perception. In these views, phonemic processing is not dependent solely on the input from lower-level, acoustic feature encoding. Rather, phonemic processing is influenced by many factors, including exposure to and experience with the speech sounds of the language, short-term memory required for even very basic auditory discriminations, and coarticulation influences on categorical perception (e.g., Groenen, 1997). Simply put, we do not perceive isolated, invariant spectro-temporal acoustic events and then put them together to create a holistic percept of the message in an acoustic-phonemic-linguistic hierarchical fashion. Rather, higher-order influences will have a significant effect on what is perceived even at the phonemic level, with the result that **acoustic and phonemic processing cannot be cleanly separated from one another or from higher-order linguistic influences.**

The processing of the basic acoustic features of speech is, without question, important to processing of spoken language. But the linguistic competence and experience of the listener, context of the surrounding message and communicative event, and other higher-level cues serve to direct speech processing, even influencing the most basic sensory perceptual events (Salasoo & Pisoni, 1985). As a result, even if the input is identical, what one listener hears may be quite different from what another listener hears. For example, the well-documented difficulty of Japanese listeners to discriminate between /r/ and /l/ arises from the lack of experience they have with these phonemes that do not appear in their language. Yet, the /r/ and /l/ differ in their acoustic makeup, and native English speakers can discriminate between them quite easily. Further, Japanese listeners can, with training and experience, learn to "hear" the differences between these two phonemes, even though they sounded the same to them previously (e.g., Bradlow, Pisoni, Akahane-Yamada, & Tokhura, 1999). Moreoever, experience with the language facilitates spoken word recognition when very fine discriminations among speech sounds within words are required (Bradlow & Pisoni, 1999). As such, acoustic parameters of the input signal may be very salient and accessible to listeners familiar with the speech sounds used, but be essentially nonexistent to non-native listeners. That experience modulates speech-sound processing even at a basic sensory, acoustic level demonstrates that spoken language processing requires far more than just the bottom-up, sensory encoding of the spectro-temporal features of the speech signal.

Even when a listener is familiar with the language, other contextual and language-related cues will have a significant influence on what is perceived. These cues may include knowledge of the prosodic, semantic, and pragmatic aspects of the speech signal, vocabulary, familiarity with the subject matter, and word predictability (e.g., Cole & Rudnicky, 1983; Hirsch, Reynolds, & Joseph, 1954; Lewellen, Goldinger, Pisoni, & Greene, 1993; Luce & Pisoni, 1998; Pisoni, 2000). Further, the ability to fill in missing pieces of a message and achieve *auditory closure* is highly dependent on even very subtle contextual information (Elliott, 1995; Kalikow, Stevens, & Elliott, 1977). In some cases, the missing pieces of the signal can be "filled in" so successfully that the listener is unaware that they were missing in the first place. Studies of *phonemic restoration* have shown that phonemes and even entire syllables that have been experimentally excised from a speech signal can be perceptually restored when contextual cues are available, especially if the gaps in the message are filled with some type of acoustic stimulus, such as noise (e.g., Bashford, Reinger, & Warren, 1992; Miller & Licklider, 1950).

Finally, a central principle of speech perception is that the same phoneme is represented by very different acoustic features when it occurs in different contexts, yet we perceive it as being the same speech sound each time it occurs. Therefore, auditory processing and speech perception must, of necessity, be at least equally influenced by psycholinguistic parameters as they are by the encoding of specific segments of sound that bear little or no relationship to our perception of these segments when they occur in running speech (Liberman, 1996). For these reasons, **psycholinguistic approaches appear to provide more ecologically valid views of central auditory processing than do purely psychophysical or acoustic feature models.**

Other Top-Down Factors in Auditory Processing

Ultimately, processing of spoken language—or, indeed, processing of any type of sensory stimuli—is reliant on general arousal state and attention. As such, anything that interferes with the ability to attend to the signal will necessarily affect auditory processing. Low-level dysfunction of the reticular activating system, which mediates overall arousal of the organism, can render a listener unaware that a signal has even occurred. Higher-order attention-related deficits, including attention-deficit/hyperactivity disorder (AD/HD), can have a significant impact on a listener's ability to attend to and process auditory input. Thus, dysfunction in various areas of the brain, including parietal and frontal regions, can ultimately affect auditory processing, even when the integrity of acoustic signal encoding in auditory regions remains intact.

Similarly, auditory processing is also reliant on adequate executive functioning. **The term *executive function* is used to denote a general set of overall cognitive control processes that serve to coordinate adaptive behavioral responses to the environment.** Like a general directing his troops, executive functioning can be thought of as "overseeing" problem solving, learning, memory, attention, planning and decision making, and goal-directed behavior (including listening and acting upon what is heard). The central nervous system regions involved in executive function are vast, and include multiple subcortical and cortical areas such as the basal ganglia, thalamus, frontal lobe, temporal lobe, and parietal lobe (Goldenberg, Oder,

Spatt, & Podreka, 1992). Disruption in any of the regions can affect executive functioning and, ultimately, listening abilities.

There are yet other sensory modalities that play a role in auditory processing. The well-known *McGurk effect*, in which visual input modulates what is perceived auditorily, is an excellent example of multisensory integration at a basic auditory sensory encoding level. Sams and colleagues (Sams et al., 1991) demonstrated that when listeners were provided with the auditory syllable /pa/, presented along with a videotape of a speaker saying /ka/, listeners reported hearing either what was seen (/ka/) or a syllable somewhere between the auditory and the visual input (i.e., /ta/). In other words, the normally simple task of identifying a consonant-vowel syllable was confounded by the introduction of discordant visual information. Even more interesting, neuromagnetic responses recorded over the left hemisphere indicated that when the visual and auditory signal did not match, a specific waveform occurred in the region of the supratemporal auditory cortex that was not present when the visual and auditory inputs agreed. This finding indicated that visual information was encoded in auditory cortex, perhaps at the level of very basic sensory encoding of acoustic stimuli.

More recently, it has been shown through functional magnetic resonance imaging (*f*MRI) that visual input can influence speech perception even before speech sounds are categorized into distinct phonemes. In a study using the *f*MRI technique, Calvert and colleagues recorded whole-brain activity during silent lipreading (mouth movements unaccompanied by auditory input). They demonstrated clear activation of primary auditory cortex and auditory association cortex during lipreading of mouth movements that corresponded to words or pseudowords, or what they termed "linguistic facial gestures" (Calvert et al., 1997). Conversely, mouth movements that did not correspond with plausible speech, such as nonlinguistic closed-mouth movements, did not result in auditory cortex activation. In short, these findings demonstrate eloquently that even the primary auditory cortex cannot be considered to be modality-specific. **Input from other sensory modalities can and does have an effect on the sensory encoding and perception of even the most basic acoustic events.**

When all of this information is taken together, only one conclusion can be drawn: although we are able to decompose auditory processing into constituent, auditory-specific skills, and perhaps even to tap those skills through carefully selected auditory tasks, the act of auditory processing is not and cannot be considered to be modality-specific. As such, any view of auditory processing disorders must take into account the influence of higher-order, top-down factors on sensory perception as well as the possibility that deficits in other sensory modalities may coexist with auditory processing disorders. Therefore, **rather than insisting on a modality-specific definition of CAPD, we must mold our conceptualization of this disorder to fit what is known about the incredible interconnectedness of the central nervous system while, at the same time, retaining primary focus on the auditory manifestations of central nervous system dysfunction.**

Summary

Central auditory processing encompasses a variety of auditory system mechanisms and is influenced by a host of top-down, higher-order influences. This chapter has focused on the underlying mechanisms of selected auditory processes, including dichotic listening, temporal processing, binaural interaction, and speech-sound discrimination. With an understanding of the neurophysiological bases of and pathological effects on these processes, clinicians may be better able to interpret tests of central auditory processing and make appropriate recommendations for management.

Dichotic listening is the processing of auditory stimuli that are presented to both ears simultaneously, with the stimulus being different in each ear. Theory regarding the mechanism of dichotic listening suggests that although auditory input is represented both ipsilaterally and contralaterally throughout the CANS, the contralateral pathways are stronger than the ipsilateral pathways. Thus, when competing auditory stimuli are introduced, the weaker ipsilateral pathways are suppressed by the contralateral pathways.

Lesions of the right temporal lobe result in contralateral (left-ear) suppression or extinction of dichotically presented auditory stimuli. Left temporal lobe lesions often result in bilateral suppression, as auditory information from both ears is prevented from arriving at the speech-dominant left hemisphere. Complete sectioning of the corpus callosum results in left-ear extinction of dichotically presented stimuli due to the interruption in interhemispheric transfer of auditory information from the right hemisphere to the left. Individuals with cochlear hearing loss may exhibit a greater ear advantage than do normal listeners. Conductive hearing losses do not appear to affect dichotic listening significantly.

Temporal processing refers to the processing of time-related cues in the auditory signal and is critical for speech and music perception.

The processing of temporal cues takes place throughout the CANS; however, the primary and associative auditory cortices appear to be particularly important for the processing of the temporal order of two consecutive stimuli. In addition, the corpus callosum is critical for the linguistic labeling of tonal patterns. Although VIIIth nerve and brainstem lesions may have some effect on temporal processing, lesions of the temporal lobe or corpus callosum are most likely to disrupt the processing of temporal cues.

Binaural interaction, or the way in which the two ears work together, is important for a variety of everyday listening activities, including localization and lateralization of auditory stimuli, binaural release from masking, detection of signals in a background of noise, and binaural fusion. The level of the pons in the low brainstem is implicated as being particularly crucial to the processing of binaural input, although the actual perception of the auditory event occurs in the cortex. Lesions of the low brainstem are most likely to disrupt binaural interaction. In addition, conductive hearing loss has been shown to have an effect upon binaural interaction, possibly due to abnormal development of brainstem auditory structures following sensory deprivation. Cochlear lesions may affect binaural interaction, depending on the extent of the pathology and the type of binaural interaction task. Finally, cortical structures, including the corpus callosum, are critical to a variety of binaural processes.

The mechanisms of speech-sound discrimination are not yet fully understood; however, it is known that the primary auditory cortex plays a critical role in the discrimination of phonemes that require precise spectro-temporal coding. As such, vowel discrimination is much less vulnerable to cortical dysfunction than is discrimination of stop consonants. However, as discussed in Chapter 1, virtually every level of the CANS as well as the peripheral auditory system are important to speech-sound encoding and perception.

Finally, it has been shown that higher-level influences such as language, cognition, attention, and executive function will influence the ability to listen and to process auditory input. Moreover, the fact that other sensory modalities influence auditory perception even at the most basic, prephonemic encoding level, combined with the finding of auditory-responsive areas in "nonauditory" regions of the brain, suggests that any definition of auditory processing and its disorders that insists upon modality specificity is neurophysiologically untenable. Therefore, our conceptualization of CAPD must, of necessity, be made consistent with our current knowledge regarding how information processing occurs.

Review Questions

1. Define the term *central auditory processes*.

2. Distinguish between dichotic and diotic listening.

3. Describe Kimura's theory of dichotic listening.

4. Define the term *right ear advantage*.

5. Describe the effects of pathology of the following structures on dichotic listening:

   right temporal lobe   left temporal lobe
   corpus callosum   cochlea
   middle ear

6. Define temporal processing.

7. Identify examples of listening tasks that rely on processing of temporal cues.

8. Describe the effects of pathology of the following structures on temporal processing:

   temporal lobe   corpus callosum
   brainstem   cochlea
   middle ear

9. Define binaural interaction.

10. Identify examples of auditory functions that rely on binaural interaction.

11. Describe the phenomenon of binaural release from masking (masking level difference) and define the following four stimulus conditions:

    SπN$\varnothing$ SπN$\varnothing$
    SπN$\varnothing$ S$\varnothing$Nπ

12. Which of the above four stimulus conditions will result in the largest MLDs in the normal listener, and why?

13. Describe the effects of pathology of the following structures on binaural interaction:

    temporal lobe   corpus callosum
    brainstem   cochlea
    middle ear

14. How does multiple sclerosis affect binaural interaction?

15. What types of speech sounds are most vulnerable to disruption by auditory cortex dysfunction, and why?

16. How do top-down influences such as language, attention, and executive function affect auditory processing? What implications does this have for the development of definitions and theories of central auditory processing disorders?

CHAPTER

THREE

Neuromaturation and Neuroplasticity of the Auditory System

Any discussion of central auditory processing in children must take into account the effects of maturation upon auditory function. Age-dependent morphological changes within the brain will determine in large part the child's ability to perform certain auditory tasks. Clinicians engaged in central auditory assessment must be familiar with normal variations in CNS development in order to select the most appropriate assessment tools, interpret test results in the context of age-appropriate normative data, and develop management plans based on the stage of neuroaudiological development. In addition, neuromaturation, or lack thereof, may remain a factor in the evaluation and remediation of a given child for several years following the initial assessment. Therefore, attempts to determine the efficacy of remediation must take into consideration those improvements in auditory function that may be attributed to CNS development over time as opposed to direct results of rehabilitative techniques.

   The term *functional plasticity* refers to the nervous system's ability to reorganize and adapt in response to internal and external

changes. Two familiar examples of neuroplasticity are the organizational rearrangement of neural pathways after a stroke or other pathology and the functional and morphological changes that occur as a result of sensory deprivation. The ability of the CNS to adapt to internal and external changes has important implications for learning. Because neuroplasticity is greatest in the early years and diminishes with age, early exposure to sensory stimuli is critical to the normal development of CNS structures and pathways. Likewise, early identification of pathological conditions will increase the chance of (re)habilitative success.

This chapter provides an overview of how age affects auditory function, including the normal course of development and maturation within the auditory system and implications for valid, age-appropriate assessment and interpretation. In addition, current research regarding neuroplasticity of the auditory system and its implications for remediation of CAPD will be discussed.

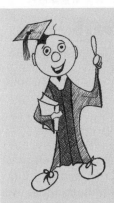

Learning Objectives

After studying this chapter, the reader should be able to:

1. Describe the prenatal development of the auditory system.
2. Describe the normal course of myelination and synapse formation in the maturing auditory system.
3. Discuss auditory behavioral correlates to neuromaturation of the auditory system.
4. Discuss neuroplasticity and its potential significance in remediation of central auditory processing disorders.

Prenatal Development of the Auditory System

It is not even remotely within the scope of this text to provide readers with a comprehensive discussion of human embryological development. Indeed, what is currently known about prenatal development of the auditory and central nervous systems would fill volumes of text. Therefore, the purpose of this section is to give readers a brief overview of the development of the auditory system, focusing in particular on the development of central auditory structures.

Prenatal Development of the Brain

First, it is important to note that the human brain is not fully developed at birth. Although the production of neurons through cell division is completed by approximately sixteen to twenty weeks after conception, **the development of new and more efficient synaptic connections continues at least into adulthood** (Kalil, 1989; Restak, 1986). In fact, the brain actually contains many more neurons than are needed at birth. During childhood, unused neurons are pruned away, and stronger connections are built among those CNS sites that are stimulated. This sculpting process forms the basis of neural plasticity, a subject that we will discuss later in this chapter. In addition, although it was once thought that we are born with our full repertoire of brain cells, new research in the area of cell regeneration and *neurogenesis* (creation of new neural tissue) suggests that new cells may be added even in adulthood, particularly in areas of the brain associated with memory and learning. For example, stem cells—cells that form the basis for all tissue in the fetus and, thus, are able to differentiate into any tissue in the body—have now been found to be present in human adult hippocampus and related regions throughout the life span. Moreover, it is possible that, under the right conditions, these stem cells, once thought only to create glia (or neural support tissue) can actually create new neurons in the adult (Palmer, Markakis, Willhoite, Safar, & Gage, 1999). As such, the human hippocampus may retain its ability to create new neurons throughout life (Eriksson et al., 1998).

Perhaps even more exciting is the finding that stem cells can be transplanted into brain regions that do not naturally contain these neural precursors and new neurons will be formed, neurons that will even create appropriate synaptic connections in areas that had previously degenerated (Magavi, Leavitt, & Macklis, 2000). Recent studies challenge our previously held notions that, at birth, we have all of the brain cells we will ever have and that lost brain cells can neither be repaired nor replaced.

Development of the brain and spinal cord begins during the third week after conception (gestational age, GA) with the appearance of the *neural plate*, a hollow tube approximately 3 mm in length. As the brain of a newborn baby contains more than 100 billion neurons, the developing brain must grow at the remarkable rate of about 250,000 nerve cells per minute throughout the course of pregnancy (Ackerman, 1992).

By 4 weeks GA, the main divisions of the brain can be seen: the *forebrain,* which will give rise to the cerebral hemispheres, *midbrain, hindbrain*, and *spinal cord.* Within another week, swellings appear that mark the future site of the cerebral hemispheres and other structures, becoming identifiable by 8 weeks GA. By 18 weeks GA, the primary grooves on the surface of the hemispheres have appeared, but the surface itself remains smooth. Finally, by 28 weeks GA, the primary lobes of the brain are clearly formed as is the lateral (Sylvian) fissure. From this point, the brain continues to grow in size and complexity of synaptic pathways, reaching an average weight of 8,400 g at birth.

Cell Differentiation and Migration in the Developing Embryo

At the earliest stages of development, all cells within the human embryo have the potential to develop into any cell of the body. However, at fifteen to sixteen days after fertilization, differentiation begins, with cells assuming specific "identities." The cells differentiate into three cellular layers, termed *germ layers*: the *ectoderm*, which will give rise to outer skin layers, the nervous system, and sense organs; the *mesoderm*, which is associated with skeletal, circulatory, and reproductive organs; and the *endoderm*, from which the digestive and respiratory organs will arise.

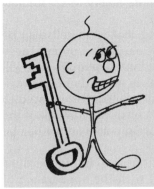

KEY CONCEPT

Although the brain is fully formed at birth, improvement in synaptic efficiency and development of new synapses continues into the teen years and beyond.

Following the appearance of the germ layers, a massive migration of cells begins wherein cells continually divide and travel to their final predetermined destinations. Upon arrival, each cell seeks out and recognizes others like itself, aggregating in groups in distinct regions and forming synapses. The exact mechanism through which this clustering and finely tuned differentiation occurs is not fully understood at this time; however, it is likely that both genetic programming and distinctive cellular secretions play a role (Restak, 1986).

Prenatal Development of the Auditory System

The outer ear, inner ear, and CANS structures arise from ectodermal tissues, which is why abnormalities of the outer ear may coincide with sensory or neural abnormalities. In contrast, the bony structures of the middle ear develop from the mesodermal germ plate. This section will focus on the prenatal development of the inner ear and CANS.

The inner ear is the first of the three anatomical divisions of the ear to appear embryologically, beginning with the appearance of the *otic placodes*—slight thickenings on the lateral aspect of the neural plate—at approximately 20 days GA. The otic placode consists of a small island of neural tissue that is similar to brain-wall ectoderm. In a short period of time, the otic placode sinks into the surrounding tissue and forms the otic pit, which subsequently deepens and forms a vesicle—the otocyst. By the end of the 5th week GA, the otocyst has divided into two lobes, which will ultimately become the organs of hearing and the vestibular system. **By the end of the 5th month GA, all of the structures necessary for inner ear function are present and adult-like in structure and size**. In fact, the youngest human fetus reported to have responded to acoustic stimuli was 26 weeks GA, a period that coincides with the completion of inner ear development (Wedenberg, 1965).

This is not the case with the structures of the CANS. As previously discussed, the human brain continues to change throughout life. Likewise, CANS structures, although present and functioning at birth, continue to form new synaptic connections and to increase synaptic efficiency until adolescence and possibly early adulthood. With further aging in the adult, we see additional structural and functional changes in the CANS, consisting of *reduced* neural density, synaptic efficiency (including myelination), and cross-sectional size of some structures. These structural changes often are accompanied by concomitant functional deficits in central auditory processes in the aging adult. Therefore, unlike the structures of the peripheral auditory system, the CANS remains a work-in-progress long after an infant is born.

Little is known about the prenatal development of the central auditory pathways. It is known that cells of the cochlear ganglion begin to migrate toward the brainstem during the 6th week GA and that the cochlear nerve appears abruptly at approximately 7 weeks GA, with its appearance occurring in all parts of the nerve's course simultaneously (Streeter, 1906). It is likely that the fibers of the auditory brainstem structures develop at the same time as the nerve fibers of the otic vesicle; however, there are no empirical data to determine the timing of their maturation definitively (Maue-Dickson, 1981). **That the brainstem auditory pathways are structurally complete by 30 weeks GA is evidenced by the ability to obtain brainstem auditory evoked potentials from infants as young as 10 weeks premature** (Cervette, 1984; Despland & Galambos, 1980; Galambos, Wilson, & Silva, 1994; Starr, Amlie, Martin, & Sanders, 1977). **However, the synaptic efficiency of auditory brainstem fibers continues to improve until approximately 3 years of age** (Cox, 1985; Salamy, 1984; Salamy, Mendelson, Tooley, & Chaplin, 1980). The information presented here regarding prenatal development of the auditory system is summarized in Table 3-1.

Neuromaturation of the Auditory System

It is a well-accepted fact that normal human infants, just minutes after birth, can hear. Newborns startle to loud sound and even turn, to the degree that their immature musculature will allow, toward an off-center sound (Kelly, 1986; Wertheimer, 1961). This behavioral orienting response, basic to hearing, has been shown to be affected by the type of stimulus used. Very brief stimuli appear to be unsuccessful in eliciting a response in newborns (Butterworth & Castillo, 1976; McGurk, Turnure, & Creighton, 1977), but high-frequency, longer duration stimuli such as rattle sounds and human speech are extremely effective in eliciting head turns (Brazelton, 1973; Muir & Clifton, 1985; Weiss, Zelazo, & Swain, 1988).

In addition, evidence suggests that newborns exhibit definite preferences not only to certain types of sounds, but even to content of linguistic stimuli. A study was undertaken at the University of North Carolina in which pregnant mothers were asked to read a children's book (*The Cat in the Hat* by Dr. Seuss) twice every day during the final

Table 3-1

Overview of Prenatal Development of the Brain and Auditory System

Gestational Age	Developmental Characteristics
15–16 days	Differentiation of cells into three neural germ layers
3rd week	Appearance of neural plate
20 days	Appearance of otic placodes
4 weeks	Main divisions of the brain can be seen
5th week	Division of otocyst into lobes that will give rise to organs of hearing and balance
6th week	Cells of cochlear ganglion begin to migrate toward brainstem
7 weeks	Cochlear nerve appears abruptly
18 weeks	Primary grooves have appeared on brain surface
5 months	Structures of inner ear are present and adult-like in structure and size
28 weeks	Primary lobes of brain and lateral fissure are fully formed
30 weeks	Brainstem auditory pathways structurally complete; auditory brainstem response can be obtained
Birth	Brain weighs approximately 8,400g

six months of their pregnancy. Shortly after birth, the newborn infants were attached to a device that monitored sucking activity. The infants learned immediately to alter their sucking patterns to produce a tape-recorded rendition of the mother reading the familiar book; however, taped renditions of the mother reading another children's book with similar intonation failed to elicit the sucking response (Kolata, 1984). Although it is not clear which auditory cues were most influential in the infants' preferences, **these findings suggest that the ability of infants to perceive differences in the linguistic content of auditory stimuli is present to some degree at birth, and may even be present prior to birth while still in the womb.**

Although newborn infants exhibit surprisingly sophisticated auditory abilities, there is no question that the auditory system of the infant and child is not like that of the adult. **In the infant and small child, masked thresholds are higher** (Schneider, Trehub, Morrongiello, & Thorpe, 1989), and **discrimination of intensity, frequency, and temporal cues is poorer** (Hall & Grose, 1994; Irwin, Ball, Kay, Stillman, & Bosser, 1985; Jensen, Neff, & Callaghan, 1987;

Wightman, Allen, Dolan, Kistler, & Jamieson, 1989). As will be discussed more extensively later in this chapter, **the right-ear advantage on linguistically loaded dichotic listening tasks is more pronounced** (Keith, 1984; Willeford & Burleigh, 1994), and changes occur in a variety of other auditory capabilities as well. What accounts for these marked differences between the auditory perceptual abilities of children and adults? The answer, simply, is neuromaturation. While the auditory system of the newborn may be structurally intact from a gross anatomical and physiological perspective, the efficiency of the system continues to develop and improve for several years following birth (Aoki & Siekevitz, 1988).

Age-Dependent Morphological Changes of the Central Auditory Nervous System

A variety of age-dependent morphological changes occur in the brain and influence auditory behavior, the most prominent of which is degree of myelination (Romand, 1983). Myelin is the white matter of the brain, a multilayered sheath that insulates and protects the nerve fiber. The speed of transmission of nerve impulses depends on the diameter of the nerve fiber and its degree of myelination. Some areas of the brain are heavily myelinated; others (gray matter) are unmyelinated.

The formation of myelin begins during fetal development and continues until maturity. Therefore, the time span of myelination is directly related to the development of sensorimotor and cognitive development (Lecours, 1975; Lenneberg, 1967). **Myelination proceeds in a caudal to rostral direction, with those structures of the brainstem necessary for survival completed before the first year of age whereas cortical communication areas may not be fully myelinated until early adulthood** (Yakovlev & Lecours, 1967). Myelination of the corpus callosum, critical for interhemispheric transfer of information, continues through adolescence (Salamy, 1978). Recent research using MRI technology indicates that although myelination can be observed in the brainstem by 29 weeks GA and in the cerebellum as early as the fifteenth day of life, initial deposits of myelin are not visible in the corpus callosum until approximately 5 to 6 months of age (Ballestros, Hansen, & Soila, 1993; Barkovich & Kios, 1988; Girard, Raybaud, & DuLac, 1991). In addition, although some researchers have contended that the corpus callosum becomes adult-like by age 10 to 12 (e.g., Hayakawa et al., 1989), others have found evidence of corpus callosum growth and increased efficiency into the early adult years (Johnson, Farnsworth, Pinkston, Bigler, & Blatter, 1994; Pujol, Vendrell, Junque, Marti-Vilalta, & Capdevila, 1993). Moreover, Pujol et al. (1993) demon-_____ that the growth and refinement of integrative brain areas, _____ the corpus callosum, parallels the attainment of maximum _____ efficiency in cognitive processing, which also reaches _____ n the mid-20s. Thus, the corpus callosum and related _____ re among the latest maturing and highest-order networks

_____ t different areas of the brain undergo myelination and _____ different times has profound implications for auditory _____ hose processes that depend upon brainstem function will develop much earlier than will those that rely upon efficient inter- and intrahemispheric communication. Furthermore, additional age-related changes in the adult brain will also have a direct impact on auditory processing. Although brainstem auditory structures, once developed, remain relatively stable throughout life, cortical communication areas demonstrate significant changes. For example, the corpus callosum, among the last structures to fully develop, is also one of the first to show age-related structural changes, demonstrating a decrease in size of some regions as early as age 20 in men, but not until the mid-50s in women (Cowell, Allen, Zaltimo, & Dennenberg, 1992). These structural changes are accompanied by functional deficits in auditory processing that arise earlier for men than for women (Bellis & Wilber, 2001). When taken together, the available evidence suggests that the time course of structural changes in the CANS resulting either from development or from aging will be accompanied by functional changes in auditory processing abilities that rely on the affected CANS structures. Therefore, once again, knowledge of the underlying neurophysiology of specific auditory processes, as well as of how maturation and

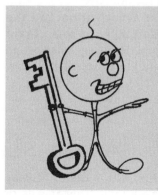

KEY CONCEPT

Those processes dependent upon brainstem integrity will mature much earlier than will those that rely upon integrity of the corpus callosum.

aging affect specific areas of the CANS, is critical for clinicians engaged in diagnosis and management of central auditory processing disorders.

Another factor that affects degree of neuromaturation is *arborization,* or *dendritic branching.* Dendrites are extensions of the nerve cell body that transmit information to the cell body from other, adjacent cells. As the organism develops, the dendrites branch out in various directions, thus increasing the surface area available for synapses with the axons of other nerve cells. As a result, additional connections are made for the transfer of more information.

In addition to developmental effects on dendritic branching, the extent and precision of arborization is also due in large part to degree of stimulation—or how much the particular pathways are being used. Animal studies have indicated that lack of stimulation results in a disruption of normal patterns and density of afferent innervation in the auditory brainstem which, in turn, impacts proper sound representation in auditory brainstem structures (e.g., Gabriele, Brunso-Bechtold, & Henkel, 2000; Gold & Knudsen, 2000). Auditory experience appears to affect even very basic, neurochemical characteristics of the CANS as well. Futai and colleagues (Futai, Okada, Matsuyama, & Takahashi, 2001) have shown that auditory stimulation results in a downregulation (or decrease) in the amount of NMDA excitatory neurotransmitter receptor protein at auditory synapses which, in turn, allows for faster and more precise neural firing. This is necessary for high-fidelity transmission of high-frequency auditory input in the CANS. Without stimulation, however, the NMDA downregulation does not occur, and high-frequency signals cannot be transmitted accurately. Therefore, it is difficult to separate cleanly the effects of neuromaturation alone from the effects of stimulation that occur with exposure to and experience with auditory stimuli in the environment. Both work hand-in-hand to shape the ultimate functioning of the CANS.

There is some evidence to suggest that arborization and the development of new synapses continue indefinitely in some brain systems. In fact, those systems responsible for learning must retain some ability to alter neural "wiring" throughout life; otherwise, no new learning could take place (Kalil, 1989).

Electrophysiological Indicators of Auditory Neuromaturation

The caudal to rostral course of neuromaturation within the CANS may be illustrated through the use of electrophysiological measures of

CANS function, in which the speed of transmission appears to be directly related to the degree of myelination (Musiek, Verkest, & Gollegly, 1988).

The Auditory Brainstem Response

The auditory brainstem response (ABR), first described by Jewitt and Williston (1971), is an electrical, far-field recording of synchronous activity in the auditory nerve and brainstem and is characterized by five to seven waveforms which occur within 10 msec following presentation of auditory stimuli (clicks or tone pips). A typical adult ABR is illustrated in Figure 3-1. The ABR is most often analyzed according to absolute wave latencies of waves I, III, and V; interwave intervals; and interaural latency differences, as well as interwave amplitude ratios in order to obtain information regarding hearing sensitivity and neurological brainstem integrity (Jacobson, 1985).

Although absolute generators of the ABR have been in dispute for a number of years, it is generally agreed that **wave I represents the action potential within the acoustic nerve and wave II arises from the VIII nerve.** Wave III appears to receive most of its activity from the region of the cochlear nucleus. Waves IV and V represent the sum of synchronized neural activity from multiple generator sites; therefore, they cannot be attributed to activity in single generator sites. Wave IV

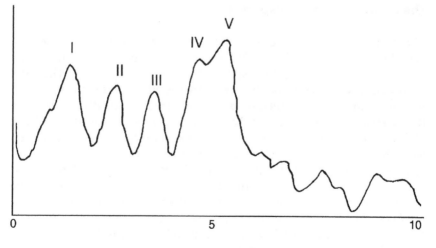

Latency (msec)

Figure 3-1. Typical auditory brainstem response (ABR).

possibly represents activity in the region of the superior olivary complex, cochlear nucleus, and lateral lemniscus. Wave V appears to be related to activity in the lateral lemniscus and inferior colliculus (Chiappa, 1983; Hood, 1998; Moller, Janetta, & Moller, 1981).

Studies of the effects of age on the ABR provide us with valuable information regarding neuromaturation of the brainstem. As previously mentioned, waves I, III, and V of the ABR may be obtained by 30 to 32 weeks GA. However, absolute wave latencies, interwave intervals, and amplitude ratios continue to change as a function of age, with **waves III and V continuing to change until age 2 or 3 even though absolute latency of wave I reaches adult values by 3 months of age** (Cox, 1985; Salamy et al., 1980). The caudal-to-rostral maturation of the brainstem is evident in the time course of auditory brainstem response maturation which reflects, in part, speed of transmission through the brainstem auditory pathways. Because the brainstem auditory pathways are not fully myelinated at birth, absolute wave latencies are prolonged. Following wave I, wave III attains adult absolute latency values next. Wave V is the last to reach adult latency values. As a result, interpeak intervals are, likewise, prolonged in infants and toddlers, with the I–V and III–V interpeak intervals being the last to normalize. It is important for clinicians employing auditory brainstem response measures in infants and toddlers to use age-specific normative values for both absolute and interpeak latencies so that responses can be interpreted appropriately.

The Middle Latency Response

The middle latency response (MLR) was first described by Geisler, Frishkopf, and Rosenblith (1958). Like the ABR, the MLR can be recorded from the scalp in response to tone pips or clicks. **The MLR follows the ABR, occurring between 10 and 90 msec following stimulus onset and is characterized by waves Na, Pa, and Pb** (Figure 3-2). **Brain structures thought to be involved in the generation of the MLR include auditory-specific structures as well as structures outside the CANS.** Presumed generators include the temporal lobe or thalamocortical projections (Kileny, Paccioretti, & Wilson, 1987; Kraus, Ozdamar, Hier, & Stein, 1982; Ozdamar & Kraus, 1983), the reticular formation in the midbrain and thalamus (Buchwald, Hinman, Norman, Huang, & Brown, 1981; McGee, Kraus, Comperatore, & Nicol, 1991; Osterhammel, Shallop, & Terkildsen, 1987), the inferior colliculus (Caird & Klinke, 1987; Fischer, Bognar, Turjman, & Lapras, 1995; Hashimoto, Ishiyama, Yoshimoto, & Nemoto, 1981; McGee et al., 1991), and the medial geniculate body in the thalamus (Fischer et al., 1995).

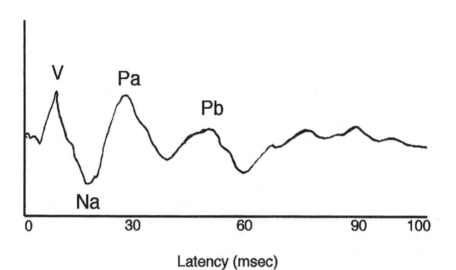

Latency (msec)

Figure 3-2. Typical middle latency response (MLR). Wave V of the ABR can be visualized.

It has been reported that **MLRs obtained from infants and young children show longer latencies, poorer waveform morphology, and greater variability than those from adults** (Suzuki, Hirabayashi, & Kobayashi, 1983). This finding has resulted in limited clinical usage of the MLR in the pediatric population. However, it should be noted that the variability of the MLR in children is related to sleep, particularly depth of sleep stage. Specifically, peak Pa of the MLR is virtually always identifiable in children when they are awake or during stage 1 (light) sleep. Similarly, the response is most often present in children during rapid-eye-movement (REM) sleep. However, during deep sleep, particularly stage 4, the MLR is frequently absent (Kraus, McGee, & Comperatore, 1989). Sleep affects the MLR in adults in a similar fashion, with response amplitudes being significantly smaller in deep sleep stages 3 and 4 as compared to wakefulness, stage 1, and REM sleep (Bellis, 1985; Osterhammel, Shallop, & Terkildson, 1985). However, the effects of sleep on the MLR are much more pronounced in children, and the detectability of the response in deep sleep increases with increasing age from birth to adolescence (Kraus, Smith, McGee, Stein, & Cartee, 1987).

The reason for the differential effect of sleep on the MLR in children and adults appears to lie in the neural generators for the response and in the time course of maturation of those generators.

Remember that both the reticular formation—responsible for arousal in the organism—and the thalamocortical auditory pathways contribute to the MLR. It has been suggested that the thalamocortical contributions to the MLR provide a stabilizing influence, allowing the response to be detected even during alterations in subject state (Kraus, Smith, & McGee, 1988). Because the thalamocortical pathways are not fully myelinated until puberty or later, the MLR in younger children is dominated by the reticular formation, rendering it much more susceptible to subject state. As such, the increased detectability of the MLR with age may be directly related to maturation of the thalamus and cortical generators of the response.

Although these findings may suggest that the MLR is so variable in children that it cannot be used clinically, my own experience suggests otherwise. In very small children who are unable to sit still for testing and who, therefore, must be evaluated during sleep, it is possible to obtain robust MLRs if sleep stage is monitored via analysis of ongoing electroencephalographic (EEG) activity and records are collected only during favorable sleep stages (i.e., stages 1, 2, and REM). Because infants spend so much of their time in deep sleep stages, this can be time-consuming, and it requires special knowledge regarding EEG characteristics of the sleep stages when evaluating all children during sleep. For older toddlers and children who are able to sit quietly and watch a video of their choice, testing can be accomplished during wakefulness when the MLR is best identified. Therefore, **the MLR, when performed and interpreted appropriately, can be a clinically useful tool for central auditory assessment even in very young children.**

The Late Event-Related Potentials

The ABR and the MLR are considered to be primarily *exogenous* potentials; that is, they occur in response to external events (although subject state does have an effect upon the MLR, as discussed above). Portions of the late event-related potentials (LEPs), conversely, are *endogenous* potentials, occurring in response to internally generated events related to attention to the stimulus (Squires & Hecox, 1983). As such, **the generators of the LEPs are those that involve the integrative and attentional functions of the brain including the limbic system and the auditory cortex itself** (Perrault & Picton, 1984; Ritter, Simson, Vaughan, & Macht, 1982; Scherg, Vasjar, & Picton, 1989; Vaughan & Ritter, 1970).

The typical LEP consists of the P1, N1, P2, N2, and P3 waves which occur at 100, 200, and 300 msec poststimulus, respectively (Picton, Woods, Baribeau-Braun, & Healey, 1977) (Figure 3-3). Whereas the N1 and P2 can be elicited simply by presentation of tonal, click, or speech stimuli to an awake, passive individual, the P3 requires conscious attention to and discrimination of stimulus differences (Sutton, Braren, Zubin, & John, 1965). In addition, speech stimuli may be used to elicit these potentials (e.g., Bellis, Kraus, & Nicol, 2000; Rugg, 1984a, b) as can visual and somatosensory stimuli (Davis, 1939).

It is important to recognize that these are not the only event-related potentials to auditory stimuli that can be recorded. Indeed, neural responses can be recorded to virtually any auditory stimulus, including sentences involving semantic anomalies and signals requiring auditory-visual integration. However, the responses discussed here are those that are in clinical use most commonly because of equipment availability and familiarity on the part of the clinical community.

Presumed generators of the LEP include multiple subcortical and cortical structures. Therefore, these late responses represent the sum of neural activity across several generator sites (Naatanen & Picton, 1987). Specifically, peak P1, which is considered by some to be a component of the MLR, appears to receive its major contribution from the associative auditory cortex and the (mostly nonprimary) thalamocortical projections to it (Liegeois-Chauvel, Musolino, Badier, Marquis, & Chauvel, 1994). N1 consists of contributions from both primary auditory cortex and associative (including non-modality-specific) cortical

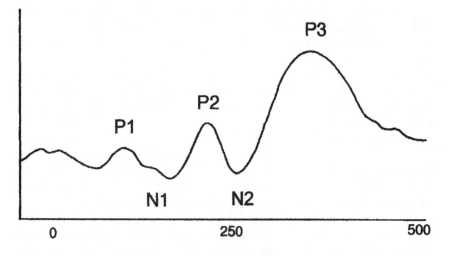

Figure 3-3. Typical adult late event-related potentials (LEP), including P300 response to deviant stimuli.

regions (Makela & McEvoy, 1996; Naatanen & Picton, 1987). When taken together, the P1–N1 complex appears to reflect basic sensory encoding of acoustic stimuli (Eberling, Bak, Kofoed, Lebech, & Saermark, 1982; Pantev, Ross, Berg, Elbert, & Rockstroh, 1998). They are often referred to as "obligatory responses" in that they do not require any conscious attention on the part of the listener. Instead, the subject must merely be awake and alert, but can be attending to something else during stimulus presentation.

In contrast, P2 does not appear to be generated in the auditory cortex but, rather, reflects in large part activity of the non-modality-specific reticular formation, making it particularly susceptible to subject state (Naatanen & Picton, 1987; Yingling & Skinner, 1997). Similarly, N2 is also affected significantly by attention as well as a variety of stimulus characteristics (Perrault & Picton, 1984). Therefore, the P2 and N2 responses do not appear to reflect basic sensory encoding. Instead, they appear to arise from some as yet unspecified higher-order processes that occur after basic sensory encoding and, possibly, stimulus evaluation and analysis.

Finally, the P300 is elicited by an "oddball paradigm" in which a random, unexpected stimulus occurs in a series of standard, expected stimuli (Sutton, Braren, Zubin, & John, 1965). The P300 can be obtained using auditory, visual, or tactile stimulation. Unlike the P1 and N1, the P300 requires that the listener actively attend to the stimulus contrasts. Therefore, the P300 appears to reflect aspects of attention, discrimination, and memory (Picton & Hillyard, 1988).

The maturational time course of the LEP is different for each of the components, reflecting the developmental time course of the underlying generators. As such, the effects of maturation on these potentials are complex and have only recently begun to be fully delineated. P1 and N1 responses demonstrate a gradual decrease in latency with increasing age from age 5 or 6 until age 15 or 16; however, amplitude of these responses exhibits a rather abrupt change at approximately age 10, when synaptic density of cortical neurons decreases rapidly (Huttenlocher & Dabholkar, 1997; Ponton, Eggermont, Kwong, & Don, 2000). Like latency, amplitude of the P1 and N1 responses attains adult-like values by age 15 or 16 (Ponton et al., 2000).

In contrast to the P1 and N1 obligatory responses, P2 demonstrates little, if any, latency changes as a function of age from age 6 through adulthood, although amplitude of the response does decrease with increasing age, reaching asymptote by approximately age 18. Absolute latency of N2 is shorter in children than in adults, and increases at approximately age 19 or 20. N2 amplitude reaches adult-like values by approximately age 17; however, the effect of age on N2 amplitude differs depending on the scalp recording site (Ponton et al., 2000). Finally, the P300 response appears to reach its shortest latency values in the early to mid teenage years (Courchesne, 1978; Davis & Onishi, 1969; Goodin, Squires, Henderson, & Starr, 1978; Polich, Howard, & Starr, 1985). The fact that the different components of the LEP follow markedly different maturational time courses provides further support to the theory that different, independent neural generating systems are responsible for each component.

The significant maturational changes that occur in the LEP during childhood, combined with the fact that some of the components may not be identifiable in very young children, have led some clinicians to assert that LEPs cannot be recorded in the pediatric population. However, as with the MLR, recording, analyzing, and interpreting LEPs in even toddlers and very young children is possible as long as the clinician is knowledgeable about the characteristics of these responses.

First, it is important to note that **the LEPs recorded from young children do not look like those of adults.** Whereas the adult response is frequently dominated by a very small P1 followed by a very large N1 component, the young child's response is dominated by a large P1 response (Sharma, Kraus, McGee, & Nicol, 1997). The P1 may be followed either by a broad negativity, or by two negativities (referred to as N1a and N1b, also characteristic of the adult response). The emergence of the distinct dual-negativity, N1a and N1b, increases with increasing age (Sharma et al., 1997). Finally, later components such as the P2 and N2 may not be evident in very young children. Similarly, because the P300 requires conscious attention to stimulus differences, it too may be absent in very young children. A typical LEP recorded from a 4-year-old child is illustrated in Figure 3-4.

Finally, attention must be given to recording conditions in the pediatric population. Because of the extreme lability of LEPs to subject state, they cannot be obtained during sleep. Therefore, even the obligatory responses require that the child be awake and alert, although attention to the stimuli is not required. As such, it has been my experience that these responses can be reliably obtained from small children as long as they are able to sit still and remain awake— an ability that typically occurs in normal children during the preschool years. A useful method of accomplishing this goal is to have the child watch a video or look at a favorite book during testing. The youngest child I have been able to record both MLRs and LEPs from using this method is 2½ years.

Before we end this section, we should mention an additional auditory event-related response that has received a good deal of attention in the literature in recent years. The *mismatch negativity* (MMN) is a

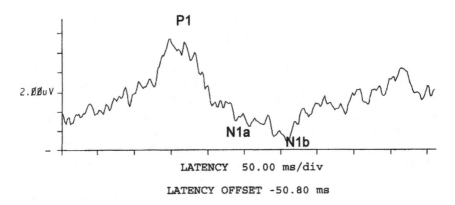

Figure 3-4. Late event-related potential recorded from a 4-year-old child. Note the dominance of the P1 response, followed by a dual-peaked N1 negativity. High-frequency activity is present due to the use of wide filter settings during recording.

preattentive response elicited by stimulus change using an oddball paradigm, and can be obtained to much smaller differences in stimuli than that required for the P300 (Sams, Paavilainen, Alho, & Naatanen, 1985). As such, the MMN appears to reflect basic sensory discrimination of auditory stimuli even before conscious perception of stimulus differences occurs. The MMN consists of a prolonged negativity in the 150–275 ms range, and is presumed to arise from sources in the non-primary thalamus and auditory cortex (Kraus, McGee, Littman, Nicol, & King, 1994; Scherg, Vajsar, & Picton, 1989). A typical MMN is illustrated in Figure 3-5.

Because the MMN can be elicited from infants and young children, demonstrates no age-related maturational effects during childhood, does not require attention or conscious perception of stimulus differences, yet appears to reflect basic sensory encoding of those differences, much excitement has arisen regarding use of this paradigm in the evaluation of central auditory processing disorders. Adding to this excitement is the finding that, for some children with auditory-based learning disorders, difficulty discriminating small differences in phonemic stimuli (e.g., /da-ga/) is accompanied by absence of the MMN to the stimuli whereas other phonemic contrasts (e.g., /ba-wa/) that the same children are able to discriminate psychophysically also elicit the MMN (Kraus et al., 1996). Moreover, when listeners are trained to discriminate new speech-sound contrasts that they previously were unable to differentiate, emergence of the MMN precedes behavioral discrimination ability, demonstrating early physiologic

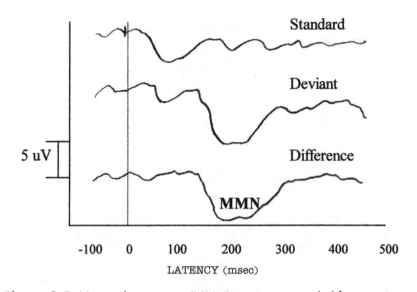

Figure 3-5. Mismatch negativity (MMN) response recorded from an 8-year-old child in response to synthetic /ba-wa/ stimuli.

effects of auditory training even before such effects can be measured psychophysically (Kraus et al., 1995; Tremblay, Kraus, & McGee, 1998; Tremblay, Kraus, Carrell, & McGee, 1997). Thus, the MMN has been heralded as an objective measure of fine-grained auditory discrimination ability, a contention that is very attractive from a clinical standpoint.

However, concern has arisen over the individual reliability of the MMN. Although it has been shown to be robust when responses from several listeners are averaged together and group data are presented, it has often been reported that the response is difficult to identify in individual listeners (Dalebout & Fox, 2000; Kurtzberg, Vaughan, Kreuzer, & Fliegler, 1995). Moreover, the MMN may be obtained on one occasion and not on another, and may not always be present in listeners who are, nevertheless, easily able to discriminate behaviorally the stimulus contrast used to elicit the response (Dalebout & Fox, 2000). Even when it is obtained from the same listener on more than one occasion, its reliability may be quite poor when identifiability and replicability are considered (Dalebout & Fox, 2001).

These concerns are not trivial ones. My own experience with the MMN is that it can be a very time-consuming procedure. Further, absence of a response is difficult to interpret unless it is robustly present to other, more perceptually salient contrasts (e.g., /ba-wa/) and the pattern of absence versus presence of response can be correlated with behavioral discrimination ability and can be replicated over two or more test sessions. Conversely, the fact that the response may be present in listeners who are *unable* to discriminate the stimulus contrasts behaviorally (Tremblay et al., 1998) leads one to question the ecological validity of the MMN, as our ultimate goal is to determine how the listener functions in the real world.

At present, it appears that further investigation into the clinical utility of the MMN is needed before it can be embraced as a valuable addition to the central auditory assessment battery. Of primary importance is the development of techniques to quantify what constitutes a response, as well as methods of improving individual subject reliability and enhancing detectability. Although some gains have been made in these areas (e.g., McGee, Kraus, & Nicol, 1997; Ponton, Don, Eggermont, & Kwong, 1997), it is my opinion that **much work still needs to be done before the MMN can be recommended for general clinical use.**

In conclusion, examination of the available data regarding maturation of auditory electrophysiology measures reveals a **caudal-to-rostral progression of maturation with auditory brainstem potentials reaching adult values by age 3, followed by middle latency potentials and, finally, late potentials, which may not reach adult values until the teen years.** Furthermore, recent findings indicate that the late components undergo additional changes with aging in the adult, particularly relating to left- versus right-hemisphere asymmetry of response amplitudes (Bellis, Nicol, & Kraus, 2000). These findings are consistent with those regarding maturation and age-related morphologic changes in the CANS.

Developmental Psychoacoustics

Given the fact that neuromaturation of the CANS continues for several years following birth, it would be expected that those behavioral auditory phenomena and processes that rely upon auditory system integrity would follow a maturational course consistent with the physiological neuromaturation of the system. Indeed, when psychophysical data regarding the effect of age on the ability of children to perform certain auditory tasks are studied, this does appear to be the case. Following is a discussion of maturational effects upon the auditory processes and behaviors described in Chapter 2.

Maturation and Dichotic Listening

The effect of age on dichotic listening may be different depending on the type of stimuli used. As discussed in Chapter 2, dichotic listening requires communication between cerebral hemispheres as well as functional integrity of both temporal lobes. A review of the literature on dichotic listening and children suggests that **the more linguistically loaded the stimuli presented are, the more pronounced the maturational effects are likely to be.**

Berlin, Hughes, Lowe-Bell, and Berlin (1973) studied the performance of normally hearing children between ages 5 and 13 on a test of dichotic, consonant-vowel (CV) nonsense words. Their results showed a right-ear advantage (REA) that remained relatively constant throughout the age range. However, the number of incidences in which stimuli presented to both the left and the right ear were reported correctly increased significantly as a function of age. The authors suggested that this improved performance reflected an increase in the brain's ability to process two-channel stimuli as a function of age.

In contrast, when dichotically presented sentences are used, right-ear scores reach adult values by age 5 while the left ear exhibits poor performance which improves with age, resulting in a decrease in the size of the REA with increasing age (Willeford & Burleigh, 1994). Age-related normative data from our own clinic show the same general trend. The REA for dichotically presented digits declines from approximately 15% at age 7 years to approximately 2% by age 11. However, our normative data using dichotic sentence stimuli indicate that 7-year-olds exhibit an REA on the order of nearly 50% which rapidly decreases as a function of increasing age, reaching adult values by age 10 to 11. Right-ear performance of younger children using dichotic sentences is not significantly different from that of adults (Figure 3-6). It should be noted that, in our clinic, normative data for children younger than age 7 are not available due to the high variability found in these children on central tests.

A possible explanation for these findings lies in the degree of complexity of the stimuli utilized. CV nonsense syllables (as well as digits) are less linguistically complex than sentences. As such they may place fewer or less complex processing demands on the two hemispheres and the interhemispheric connections. In contrast, dichotic sentences are more heavily linguistically loaded. As discussed in Chapter 2, processing of dichotic speech stimuli requires adequate interhemispheric communication via the corpus callosum as well as integrity of both temporal lobes. **Poor left-ear performance on dichotic sentence tasks**

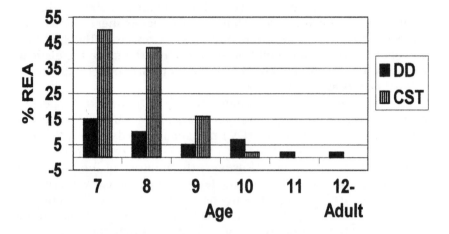

Figure 3-6. Comparison of the size of the REA for Dichotic Digits (DD) and Competing Sentences (CS) as a function of age from 7 years to adult.

in children may reflect a decreased ability of the corpus callosum to transfer complex stimuli from the right hemisphere to the left hemisphere. As the child becomes older and myelination of the corpus callosum is completed, interhemispheric transfer of information improves and left-ear scores approach those found in adults (Musiek, Gollegly, & Baran, 1984).

Maturation and Temporal Processing

Like dichotic listening, there appear to be definite effects of age on temporal processing. Werner, Marean, Halpin, Spetner, and Gillenwater (1992) studied the ability of 3-, 6-, and 12-month-old infants to perform gap detection tasks. The infants were conditioned to respond when a gap occurred in the presentation of broadband noise, but not when the noise was continuous. In addition, the effect of masker frequency on gap detection was investigated. High-pass, continuous maskers with cutoff frequencies of 500, 2000, and 8000 Hz were added that would allow the listener to use only those frequencies below the masker cutoff to detect gaps in the broadband noise stimulus. The authors found that although the infants' ability to perform the gap detection task was quite poor as compared to adults, the general effect of masker frequency on gap detection was the same for infants as for adults, with improvement in gap detection as masker frequency increased. In other words, **infants performed qualitatively**

KEY CONCEPT

The more linguistically loaded the dichotic task, the more pronounced the REA will be in children.

like adults, suggesting that the poor temporal resolution in the younger population was due to the primary effect of age.

Studies of temporal resolution in older children have exhibited the same general finding. Irwin et al. (1985) found that gap detection ability improved in subjects from age 6 up until approximately ages 8 to 10. Morrongiello and Trehub (1987) reported a progressive increase in duration discrimination from infancy to adulthood. Wightman et al. (1989) found that, for subjects in their study, gap detection improved from age 3 to 5, but was not significantly different from adults by age 6. However, the authors reported that the within- and across-subject variability in their population was very high, with some very young children at times performing comparably to adults. The authors suggested that memory or attention may have played a role in these findings, although a very real age effect on temporal resolution did appear to be present. Trehub and colleagues (1995) also investigated the effects of maturation on gap detection abilities. Their results indicated that even 6.5-month-old infants exhibit some gap detection abilities. The authors also demonstrated a significant difference in gap detection ability between 5-year-old children and adults. The authors concluded, therefore, that gap detection abilities exhibit a rather prolonged maturational time course. Although, on the surface, this conclusion may appear somewhat contradictory to that of previous studies, a topic that was addressed by the authors, Trehub and colleagues did not investigate gap detection in subjects age 6 year (the age at which gap detection had previously been found to become adult-like). When considered in this light, the finding of significant differences in gap detection abilities between age 5 and 21 does not appear to conflict with previous findings after all.

More recently, Keith (2000) collected normative data for gap detection performance on the Random Gap Detection Test (a revision of the Auditory Fusion Test—Revised; McCroskey & Keith, 1996). This test uses a standard gap detection paradigm, requires listeners to hold up one or two fingers corresponding to the number of stimuli heard, and includes tonal stimuli of octave frequencies 500 to 4000 Hz. Similar to the findings of Wightman et al. (1989), Keith found very little if any difference in gap detection performance between ages 5–7 and 10–11. Children younger than age 5 were not, however, evaluated. It should also be noted that this test is considered a *within-channel* gap detection test, as discussed in Chapter 2. The effects of maturation on *between-channel* gap detection have yet to be investigated. Finally, Grose, Hall, and Gibbs (1993) found that the temporal resolution in their subjects improved as a function of age to 7 to 10 years of age.

As discussed in Chapter 2, temporal encoding occurs in the peripheral auditory system and is represented at various levels throughout the CANS. However, extraction and analysis of temporal cues in an auditory stimulus appear to be primarily a central function. In a study of eighteen listeners ages 4 years to adult utilizing a temporal modulation task, Hall and Grose (1994) found that **the peripheral mechanism responsible for encoding temporal aspects of the acoustic signal appeared to be well developed in young listeners. However, the ability of the CANS to extract and process temporal cues appeared to improve as a function of age.**

The effect of age on tests of temporal patterning may be inferred from studies of patients with corpus callosal involvement (Musiek et al., 1980; Musiek, Kibbe, & Baran, 1984). **Performance on temporal patterning tasks involving linguistic labeling of nonspeech stimuli would not be expected to reach adult values until neuromaturation of the neural structures critical to the task, particularly the corpus callosum, is complete.** Indeed, our own clinic norms, in which adult values on the Frequency Pattern and Duration Pattern tests are not attained until age 11 to 12, support this hypothesis.

To summarize, **the development of temporal processing abilities appears to follow the course of neuromaturation, with skills improving as a function of age until approximately age 12.** In addition, the effect of age upon temporal processing will depend on the task selected and, to some degree, on attentional factors.

Maturation and Binaural Interaction

As previously mentioned, a newborn will turn toward an off-center sound, indicating that at least a portion of those brainstem structures necessary for basic localization are developed by birth (Kelly, 1986; Wertheimer, 1961). However, stimulus frequency and stimulus duration have a significant effect on the newborn's ability to localize. High-frequency stimuli appear to be most effective in eliciting head turns in the newborn, as do stimuli at least 1 sec in duration. Stimuli less than 500 msec in duration result in nonresponsiveness (Clarkson, Clifton, & Morrongiello, 1985; Clarkson, Clifton, Swain, & Perris, 1989; Morongiello & Clifton, 1984).

Interestingly, when infants reach approximately 6 to 8 weeks of age, they stop turning toward a sound source (Field, Muir, Pilon, Sinclair, & Dodwell, 1980; Muir, Abraham, Forbes, & Harris, 1979). Muir and Clifton (1985) suggested that this change in behavior does not reflect infants' sudden inability to process interaural cues but, rather, the maturational shift from a subcortical to a cortical site of processing control. Whereas the head turn of a newborn toward a sound source may be almost a reflexive action, **the reappearance of the head-turning behavior at approximately 4 months of age, accompanied by visual searching, may signal the onset of conscious perception of auditory space.**

Although infants age 4 months and older demonstrate repeatable orienting responses toward sound, the precision and accuracy of their ability to localize when the sound is presented at decreasing angles from midline continues to improve until approximately age 5 (Litovsky, 1991). Again, it appears that factors other than simply binaural sensitivity are at work in the developing infant. Rather, this developmental change in localization acuity may well be attributed to the integration of binaural cues with head movement and changing head size (Ashmead, Davis, Whalen, & Odom, 1991; Knudsen, Esterly, & Knudsen, 1984).

Results of studies of the effect of age on the masking level difference (MLD), described in Chapter 2, have been somewhat contradictory. Nozza (1987) reported that the MLD for 500 Hz tones was significantly smaller in infants than in adult subjects. In a related study, Nozza, Wagner, and Crandall (1988) concluded that although significant differences appear to exist between the size of the MLD for infants and adults, those of preschool children do not differ significantly from those of adults when sensation level of masking presentation is taken into account. Likewise, other studies have suggested that the MLD of 4- to 6-year-old children does not differ significantly from that of adults (Roush & Tait, 1984; Sweetow & Reddell, 1978).

In a study of twenty-six children ages 3.9 to 9.5, Hall and Grose (1990) found that the MLD for a pure tone presented in a wide-band (300 Hz) masker progressively increased up to approximately age 5 or 6. In addition, MLDs presented in narrow-band (40 Hz) maskers were smaller for 6-year-old subjects than for adults. The authors concluded that **these developmental changes observed in the MLD of children younger than age 6 are most likely related to central auditory processing rather than to sensitivity to interaural timing cues.**

A review of the data regarding brainstem neuromaturation supports this hypothesis. As previously discussed, the ABR reaches adult values by age 3, indicating that the brainstem structures necessary for the detection of interaural cues are essentially intact at this age. However, the higher-level pathways responsible for integration and processing of binaural cues continue to mature beyond this age. Therefore, the time span of neuromaturation in the developing auditory system may be correlated with the development of localization acuity and binaural release from masking in the infant and child. **Overall, it appears that binaural interaction abilities continue to improve from infancy until at least age 6.**

Maturation and Speech-Sound Discrimination

Babies are born with the ability to discriminate all of the speech sounds that occur in any language of the world. In fact, speech-sound discrimination-related MMN electrophysiologic responses have been recorded from healthy premature infants ages 30 to 35 weeks GA (Cheour-Luhtanen et al., 1996). This finding indicates that the human brain is able to discriminate among speech sounds even at preterm ages.

What is fascinating about maturation and speech-sound discrimination, however, is not what the infant is able to do at birth but, rather, what the infant becomes *unable* to do during the first year of life. Maturation of speech-sound discrimination is characterized less by improvement in skills and more by the gradual loss of discrimination abilities that are unnecessary for particular infants to process their native languages.

Specifically, infants are born with a generalized auditory processing mechanism that allows for the detection of differences between phonetic units. At first, this mechanism is non-language-specific, and appears to be related primarily to the acoustic features of the speech (or nonspeech) signal. As such, infants are able to discriminate contrasts that form phonetic categories in all languages, an ability that is shared by animals as well (Kuhl, 1979; Kuhl & Miller, 1978). However, by age 12 months, these same infants are unable to discriminate phonetic contrasts that do not occur in their native languages (Werker & Tees, 1999).

One theory to explain this alteration in discrimination abilities during the first year of life is the Native Language Magnet model. For an excellent review of this model, readers are referred to Kuhl (2000). Briefly, this model suggests that experience with a particular language, through hearing it daily, creates a "map" onto which those phonetic characteristics and contrasts that occur regularly are drawn. In a sense, this map serves as a kind of language filter that alters the acoustic input, rendering those acoustic events that are characteristic of the infant's native language more perceptually salient and those that do not occur in the native language less salient. As a result, what one person hears (or perceives) is not the same as what another person hears, even if the acoustic input is identical. For example, as previously discussed in Chapter 2, native Japanese speakers have extreme difficulty producing the /l/ phoneme because it does not occur in the Japanese language. Instead, they substitute the closest native phoneme, the /r/. It is also true that native Japanese listeners are unable to discriminate between the /r/ and /l/ because, to them, the two phonemes sound the same, despite the fact that they differ significantly in their acoustic makeup. Yet a native English listener hears the exact same stimuli as being quite different. Therefore, perception does not always reflect reality, and our perceptions of phonetic contrasts are largely formed during the first year of life.

It is important to note that this perceptual mapping, or "tuning," of the auditory perceptual mechanism to those sounds that occur in the native language appears to occur *prior to* word learning and, indeed, assists in the learning of the native language (Kuhl, 2000). Moreover, the formation of this language-specific acoustic filter appears to occur between 6 and 12 months of age.

At age 6 months, infants respond equally well to contrasts in native and non-native languages. Similarly, they are able to recognize when the same phoneme occurs in different contexts or in different positions in a syllable or a word, or when spoken by different speakers (Kuhl, 1979). Physiologically, 6-month-old infants also exhibit MMN responses to both native and non-native phonetic contrasts. Similarly, 6-month-old infants do not exhibit a preference for prosodic (or stress- and intonation-related) patterns that occur in their native language. However, by 9 months of age, the same infants will begin to respond preferentially to syllabic stress patterns that occur in the native language (Jusczyk, Cutler, & Redanz, 1993). They will also respond preferentially to those phonetic combinations or sequences that are "legal" in their native language, but not to those that are not permissible (such as /vl/, a combination that occurs in Norwegian languages, but not in English). Finally, by one year of age, infants only "hear" those phonetic contrasts and combinations that occur in their native language, and basic speech-sound discrimination abilities appear to be developed fully (Kuhl, 2000; Werker & Tees, 1999). Therefore, in many ways, our auditory perception is influenced less by the acoustic properties of the phonemes themselves than by our early experience with the use of those same acoustic phonemes in language. Perception is altered by—and cannot be separated from—experience.

That these phonetic maps have distinct physiologic underpinnings is illustrated by the findings of Naatanen et al. (1997), who demonstrated through whole-head magnetic recordings that phonemes occurring in a listener's native language are represented primarily in the auditory cortex of the left hemisphere. Similarly, studies using fMRI to investigate early and late second-language acquisition indicate that, when a second language is learned early in life, the cortical regions activated overlap those used for the native language. When, however, second-language acquisition occurs later, after perceptual "mapping," different cortical areas are recruited for representation of the second language (Naatanen & Alho, 1997). It is as if the neural circuitry is committed to the mapping of the primary language, and the learning of a second language with additional phonetic contrasts requires the creation of a new "map," one that must rely on circuits that are not already in use (Kuhl, 2000). In contrast, when both languages are learned early enough, the maps for each language can share the same neural substrates.

The previous discussion has centered primarily on the overall ability to discriminate phonetic contrasts. Children become more accurate at behaviorally discriminating fine-grained acoustic/phonetic differences between speech stimuli up to approximately age 8; however, older children do not differ from young adults in this ability (Bellis, Kraus, & Nicol, 2000; Kraus, Koch, McGee, Nicol, & Cunningham, 1999). In fact, this type of speech discrimination ability does not seem to change until older age, when adults begin to demonstrate poor discrimination abilities for phonetic contrasts that contain rapid spectro-temporal acoustic changes even when peripheral hearing sensitivity is normal. Furthermore, the typical left-hemisphere dominance for speech-sound encoding that is seen in the child and young adult is not evident in older adults, providing physiologic evidence of age-related alterations in the cortical representation of speech stimuli (Bellis et al., 2000).

The fact that speech-sound discrimination abilities appear to be developed at relatively young ages should not be taken to mean that other mechanisms related to speech processing do not exhibit longer maturational time courses. For example, the ability to recognize degraded speech or speech in backgrounds of noise does not reach adult values until adolescence (Elliott, 1979; Marshall, Brandt, Marston, & Ruder, 1979; Palva & Jokinen, 1975). It is likely that these abilities rely on efficient functioning of those auditory pathways that mature later, particularly thalamocortical, cortical, and interhemispheric communication areas. It is also likely that, as will be discussed in the next section, development and maturation of higher-order, top-down language, attention, and related skills serve to facilitate more complex auditory discrimination tasks that exhibit prolonged maturational time courses.

Maturation and Top-Down Factors in Auditory Processing

A complete discussion of maturation of cognitive, language, attention, and other top-down factors that, as presented in Chapter 2, will have an enormous impact on the processing of spoken language is not within the scope of this book. However, it is important to know that many executive function abilities, such as generalized attention, decision-making and problem-solving skills, organization and planning of responses, social judgment, and similar abilities are reliant on efficient functioning of prefrontal cortical regions, among others. These areas of the brain are among the last to mature and, indeed, a multitude of anatomical, neurochemical, and hormonal changes will impact the functioning of the prefrontal regions up to adolescence and beyond. Just as occurs early in life, a proliferation in synaptic connections occurs during puberty and is followed by pruning away of unused connections through experience and learning during the teenage years (Durston et al., 2001). Functional changes that accompany this structural development can have an impact on a child's ability to attend and respond appropriately to sensory, including auditory, stimuli.

Furthermore, as previously discussed, inter- and intrahemispheric communication structures, such as the corpus callosum, also continue to develop well beyond the childhood years. So, too, will experience with more complex linguistic forms and concepts, exposure to new topics and ideas, and simply the ongoing act of experiencing life in all its richness mold and shape the functioning of our higher-order brain centers and, in turn, our ability to process information. In a sense, although discrete auditory processing skills may show finite developmental time courses, we should always remember that the overall ability to process auditory information is a function of many brain regions working in concert. As such, changes in auditory processing abilities can be expected to occur throughout the life span.

To conclude, auditory behaviors reflect a developmental course that can be explained in large part by neuromaturation of the auditory system. The implications for clinicians involved in the assessment of central auditory processing abilities in children are obvious. **Assessment must be undertaken with an awareness of maturational effects upon the test protocols utilized, and age-related normative data must be obtained up through age 11 to 12, at which time performance on the majority of central tests will have reached adult values.** Consideration should also be given to the development of separate normative values for adult males and females, as auditory processing abilities—particularly those that rely on efficient interhemispheric communication—have been shown to be affected by both aging and gender (e.g., Bellis & Wilber, 2001). **The assessment of children under age 7 must be undertaken with caution due to the high degree of variability in performance seen on many of the commonly used tests in this younger population.** The information presented in this section is summarized in Table 3-2.

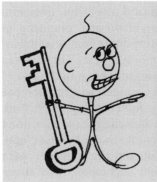

KEY CONCEPT

Although speech-sound discrimination abilities are present at birth, they will continue to be shaped by linguistic experience and other bottom-up and top-down factors.

Neuroplasticity of the Auditory System

The term *neuroplasticity* refers to the nervous system's ability to undergo organizational changes in response to internal and external

Table 3-2

Effects of Neuromaturation on Selected Auditory Processes.

Process	Neuromaturational Effects
Dichotic listening	Right-ear advantage reaches adult values by age 10 to 11
	Neuromaturational effects on REA more pronounced for linguistically loaded stimuli
	Overall performance improves until age 12 or 13
Temporal processing	Temporal resolution abilities improve until age 8 to 10
	Gap detection abilities appear to be adult-like by age 6 or 7
	Performance on temporal patterning tasks reaches adult values by approximately age 12
Binaural interaction	Gross localization abilities are present at birth
	Conscious perception of auditory space occurs at 4 months of age
	Precision and accuracy of localization abilities improve until approximately age 5
	MLD reaches adult values at approximately age 6
Speech-sound discrimination	Ability to discriminate among all phonemes in all languages of the world present at birth
	By 9 months of age, preferential responses are seen to phonemic sequences, contrasts, and prosodic patterns of the native language
	By 12 months of age, discrimination abilities are restricted to phonemic constructs that occur in the native language only
	Accuracy of speech-sound discrimination improves until approximately age 8
Top-down factors	Maturation of attention, problem-solving, memory, and related executive abilities continues through puberty and beyond
	Ongoing linguistic, cognitive, and experiential changes occur throughout the life span

factors. In 1949, D.O. Hebb suggested that synaptic changes occur in response to synaptic activity in the CNS and that these synaptic changes are critical to learning and memory. While it was once thought that CNS representation of sensory events was predetermined and unchangeable, it is now understood that the CNS can and does alter its neural wiring to at least some degree throughout life. Neuromaturation, as discussed in the previous section, is one example of the nervous system's ability to form new connections as the organism grows and changes and as the tasks placed upon it become more and more challenging.

The majority of research conducted in the area of neuroplasticity has examined the effects of sensory deprivation upon the CNS. Studies of the effects of sensory deprivation on the visual system of cats indicate that the blocking of action potentials at any time during the critical two-month period following birth results in abnormal development of the visual nervous system, indicating that visual stimulation is crucial to the normal development of the visual system in cats (Kalil, 1989; Kalil, Dubin, Scott, & Stark, 1986; Stryker & Harris, 1986).

The reorganization of the somatosensory cortex following peripheral nerve injury has been demonstrated in a variety of mammals. For example, sectioning the median nerve in the wrist of adult monkeys results in reorganization of the somatosensory cortex over time, with those areas of the brain responsive to the adjacent, intact digits expanding to occupy the deprived area (Merzenich & Haas, 1982). The fact that these organizational changes were observed in adult monkeys suggests that **plasticity is not simply confined to the immature or developing mammal.**

Studies of the barn owl have shown that neurological mapping of information related to spatial hearing occurs very early in life and is influenced by both auditory and visual experience (Knudsen & Knudsen, 1985; Knudsen et al., 1984). When one ear of the barn owl is plugged, a disruption in localization ability occurs (Knudsen, 1987). These effects of early auditory deprivation appear to occur in humans as well.

It is currently accepted that an early history of chronic otitis media with effusion (OME) is associated with a higher incidence of learning difficulties, language deficits, and attention disorders (Haggard & Hughes, 1991). Pillsbury et al. (1991) have shown that children with a history of OME often exhibit abnormally reduced MLDs, and that this reduction continues even after the placement of PE tubes, resulting in a reduced ability to extract signals from noise in these children. In addition, ABR interwave intervals were found to be abnormal in the affected ear(s) of many of these children, suggesting a physiological correlate to early auditory deprivation (Hall & Grose, 1993). Furthermore, **deprivation need not occur solely during the developmental years in order to have an impact on brainstem auditory processing. Similar results have been seen in adults in whom**

hearing was repaired following several years of otosclerosis (Hall & Derlacki, 1986; Hall, Grose, & Pillsbury, 1990).

The effect of sensory deprivation upon the auditory cortex may be examined through the use of electrical recording of cortical activity before and after inducing auditory deprivation in animals. Studies have demonstrated reorganization of the topographic representation of the auditory cortex following induced cochlear lesions (Irvine, Rajan, Wize, & Heil, 1991; Robertson & Irvine, 1989). Similar reorganization has been observed in auditory brainstem structures following sensory deprivation (Gabriele et al., 2000; Gold & Knudsen, 2000) and includes both structural and neurochemical alterations (Futai et al., 2001). It has been suggested that **the ability of the auditory cortex to reorganize continues throughout life and reflects the ability to acquire new skills and behaviors** (Kalil, 1989; Merzenich, Rencanzone, Jenkins, Allard, & Nudo, 1988).

If auditory deprivation results in morphological changes in the CANS and the nervous system retains the ability to reorganize throughout its lifetime, then it may be hypothesized that an increase in auditory stimulation may also result in morphological alterations within the CANS. Indeed, studies have shown that frequency response characteristics of single neurons can be altered by behavioral auditory conditioning (Disterhoft & Stuart, 1976; Kitzes, Farley, & Starr, 1978; Olds, Disterhoft, Segal, Kornblith, & Hirsh, 1972; Ryugo & Weinberger, 1978). In addition, Rencanzone, Schreiner, and Merzenich (1993) have shown that changes in the cortical tonotopic representations of monkeys following auditory training are correlated with improvements in discrimination ability. In other words, **auditory deprivation may result in morphological changes within the CANS that correlate with decreased auditory processing ability, but auditory stimulation and training have been shown to facilitate improvement in auditory processing abilities.** Stimulation and experience activates and strengthens neural pathways whereas unstimulated pathways atrophy (Aoki & Siekevitz, 1988; Rauschecker & Marler, 1987).

One of the mechanisms thought to be responsible for this improvement in processing abilities is **long-term potentiation (LTP). LTP is the increase in synaptic activity and efficacy following strong and repeated stimulation of a sensory system** (Bliss & Lomo, 1973; Gustafsson & Wigstrom, 1988). Although it is not clear whether all brain systems exhibit LTP in the same manner or whether the changes in synaptic activity observed are permanent, there have been reports of morphological and structural alterations within nerve cells, including increases in size and postsynaptic density, accompanying LTP (Gustafsson & Wigstrom, 1988).

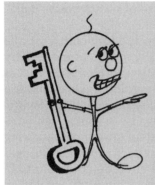

KEY CONCEPT

Auditory stimulation may result in structural, morphological, and functional changes in the CANS, and this potential for change may extend throughout an individual's lifetime.

The implications of these findings are monumental when one considers the potential for remediation of children with auditory processing disorders. **Auditory stimulation of inefficient CANS pathways may result in morphological and functional alterations, culminating in improvement in auditory processing abilities.** For example, Jirsa (1992) demonstrated a significant decrease in P3 latency and an increase in P3 amplitude in the evoked potentials obtained from children with CAPD following an intensive therapeutic intervention program. The children in the experimental group also exhibited improvement on selected auditory tasks and positive changes in overall school performance as reported by parents and teachers. Age-matched controls of individuals with and without CAPD demonstrated no such change, suggesting that the therapeutic intervention utilized was, at least in part, responsible for the changes observed in the experimental group. It should be noted that Jirsa (1992) did not describe the specific auditory stimulation activities utilized in his study but, rather, stated that the activities focused on intensive listening exercises emphasizing auditory memory and language comprehension.

In recent years, the literature has abounded with articles relating principles of neuroplasticity to stimulation via auditory training. Merzenich et al. (1996) and Tallal et al. (1996) demonstrated that intensive, computer-based auditory training can alter the language abilities of some children with language learning impairments. The authors contended that their intervention resulted in neural reorganization and a concomitant improvement in the ability to process rapidly changing auditory input. Specifically, the authors suggested that intensive stimulation and training results in greater coherence and synchrony in auditory cortical neuronal activity (Recanzone, Merzenich, & Schreiner, 1992). Neurophysiologic support for this theory comes from findings of increased amplitude of late event-related potentials elicited by speech sounds following discrimination training (Tremblay, Kraus, McGee, Ponton, & Otis, 2001). Additional neurophysiologic evidence of neuroplasticity following auditory training has been observed in animals (e.g., Recanzone, Schreiner, & Merzenich, 1993; Weinberger, 1993) and humans (e.g., Kraus, McGee, Carrell, et al., 1995; Naatanen, Schroger, Karakas, Tervanieme, & Paavilainen, 1993). Moreover, recent findings indicate that alterations in the neural representation of speech contrasts may precede behavioral demonstration of improved discrimination abilities following speech-sound training (Tremblay, Kraus, & McGee, 1998). Finally, the fact that the neurophysiologic and behavioral effects of speech discrimination training can generalize to other, similar phonetic contrasts, even when those contrasts were not specifically trained, provides great support for auditory training as a therapy tool in ameliorating auditory processing deficits (Tremblay, Kraus, Carrell, & McGee, 1997).

Although the results of studies regarding auditory neuroplasticity appear promising, it must be recognized that data regarding specific treatment efficacy are scarce. **Therefore, a comprehensive approach to management of CAPD, including compensatory strategies and environmental modifications as well as therapeutic intervention, should be undertaken. In addition, because auditory neuromaturation and neural plasticity depend upon auditory stimulation, aggressive management of CAPD should begin as early as possible** (Chermak & Musiek, 1995). For more information regarding deficit-specific management of CAPD, readers are referred to Chapters 8 and 9.

Summary

Neuromaturation and neuroplasticity of the auditory system have important implications for the assessment and remediation of children with CAPD. **As neuromaturation of some portions of the auditory system may not be complete until age 12 or later, age-appropriate normative data should be obtained for any assessment tools utilized clinically. In addition, due to the high degree of variability in children under age 7, many central tests may not be appropriate for use with this young population.**

Recent findings regarding auditory neuroplasticity suggest great promise for therapeutic intervention with children exhibiting CAPD. Further research is needed in the area of specific treatment efficacy; however, management of CAPD in children should be undertaken as early and aggressively as possible.

Review Questions

1. At what gestational age do the brain and spinal cord begin to develop?

2. At what gestational age are the primary lobes of the brain clearly formed?

3. Identify the anatomical structures which arise from the following three embryonic cell layers:

    ectoderm   mesoderm
    endoderm

4. By what gestational age are the structures necessary for hearing, including the brainstem auditory pathways, structurally complete?

5. Define myelination and discuss the course of myelination within the nervous system.

6. Define dendritic branching.

7. Briefly describe the following electrophysiological measures and discuss the maturation of each:

    ABR   MLR
    LEP

8. Discuss the effects of maturation on dichotic listening.

9. Differentiate the effects of maturation on linguistically loaded versus nonlinguistically loaded dichotic listening tasks.

10. Discuss the effects of maturation on temporal processing.

11. Discuss the effects of maturation on binaural interaction.

12. Discuss the effects of maturation on speech-sound discrimination and top-down factors in auditory processing.

13. By what age do children's performance on tests of central auditory function reach that of an adults?

14. Why is it important to obtain age-appropriate normative data on tests of central auditory processing?

15. Define neuroplasticity.

16. Discuss the effects of auditory deprivation on auditory processing.

17. Define long-term potentiation.

18. Discuss the implications of neuroplasticity in the remediation of children with CAPD.

PART

TWO

Central Auditory Screening and Assessment Procedures

CHAPTER

FOUR

Screening: A Multidisciplinary Approach

I n response to the topic of screening children for auditory processing disorders, many questions spring to the minds of administrators, clinicians, and special education professionals. Chief among these are: *What is the purpose of CAPD screening? Who should be responsible for CAPD screening? What will occur after a child is identified through the screening process?* The task of providing a plan for the development of a CAPD screening program and associated follow-up services often falls to the audiologist or speech-language pathologist in the school setting.

The intent of this chapter is to assist readers in developing a CAPD screening program using a multidisciplinary team approach that will efficaciously identify children in need of comprehensive diagnostic central auditory processing assessment with a minimum amount of money and time investment on the part of the already taxed school or clinical system. The rationale behind the need for such a program is similar to that found for other screening programs, not the least of which is a reduction in the number of inappropriate referrals of children with learning disabilities who are erroneously suspected of having CAPD. **By**

143

effectively selecting the most appropriate population for comprehensive central auditory assessment, overall costs are reduced and efficiency of identification and rehabilitation is improved.

It should be emphasized that, in this context, the term *screening* is used somewhat differently than it is in many audiology- and speech/language-related arenas. That is, in many areas of our work, screening techniques are employed with large numbers of individuals for the purposes of separating those who do not exhibit a given disorder from those who might. Indeed, when one considers the advent of universal newborn hearing screening and school-based hearing screening, the picture that comes immediately to mind is that of a specific process that is both time- and cost-effective and that will be used for virtually every child in the system, regardless of whether specific concerns have been raised.

In this chapter, the term *screening* refers to a method by which the determination of need for further testing can be made for children *who are already exhibiting some type of learning or communicative difficulty and for whom the issue of CAPD has already been raised.* In other words, screening for CAPD in this context may be thought of as comparable to using a high-risk registry for hearing impairment. Those children who will undergo the CAPD screening process are those who exhibit behavioral symptoms, sequelae, and difficulties that *may* be indicative of CAPD. Therefore, the implication is *not* that CAPD screening should be included in routine hearing screening practices and programs for school-age children, but rather that CAPD screening should be a first step in determining the need for and appropriateness of further central auditory assessment.

The rationale behind the need for a screening procedure for CAPD is clear. In recent years, with the advent of greater public and professional awareness of CAPD and increased accessibility to information regarding general indicators of possible CAPD, we have witnessed an explosion in the number of referrals for central auditory assessment services. Because CAPD, from a behavioral checklist standpoint, may look like many other disorders, virtually any child who demonstrates difficulty listening, attending, spelling, or a host of other symptoms has become a possible referral for auditory processing assessment. In my experience, the topic of CAPD frequently arises even before the nature of the child's language, cognitive, and academic difficulties has been explored adequately. This situation renders a diagnosis of CAPD difficult at best, and of questionable utility when one is attempting to determine the degree to which a given auditory-based deficit may be contributing to a child's overall behavioral and academic difficulties.

Finally, it is sometimes the case that a child is referred for central auditory assessment who clearly does not exhibit symptoms of CAPD (beyond general "listening" or "comprehension" difficulties) and for whom such assessment is not indicated. The ruling-out of CAPD occasionally is included as part of an overall "shotgun" approach to determining what is underlying a child's presenting difficulties. Although this practice is not necessarily inappropriate in and of itself, when a clinic or school is dealing with hundreds of such requests per year, and when each comprehensive evaluation is both time- and cost-intensive, it is important to attempt to ensure that time and resources are spent wisely. One method of doing this is to make every attempt to verify the appropriateness of each referral for comprehensive assessment. That, in particular, is the overall aim of the screening guidelines set forth in this chapter.

The focus of this chapter will be on how clinicians may use the results of the multidisciplinary team assessment of cognitive, psychoeducational, and speech/language functions, along with audiologic information and behavioral checklists, to answer four primary questions: **(1) Are the current evaluations that have already been completed sufficient in nature and scope to provide a picture of the child's strengths and weaknesses across cognitive, academic, and speech/language domains prior to addressing the issue of CAPD? (2) Is there sufficient evidence to support the likelihood that a CAPD is present that would necessitate further comprehensive auditory processing assessment? (3) Is the child capable of participating in comprehensive central auditory assessment, or will age, cognitive status, or other factors interfere with our ability to obtain reliable central auditory assessment results? (4) Would results of comprehensive central auditory assessment add information that is likely to affect the overall assessment and management of the child's learning and communication difficulties, or are current intervention strategies already sufficient to address the child's areas of need?**

Finally, the overall philosophy of the screening approach advocated in this chapter is based on the fundamental premise that, if a child is exhibiting significant language, learning, or communication difficulties in school, then **possible CAPD should not be a starting point in the assessment process.** Instead, it is important for all involved to ensure that a good picture of the child's overall functional strengths and weaknesses across a wide variety of domains be obtained prior to determining the need for specialized testing that focuses on only one aspect of the child. It is for this reason that the screening process requires that general measures of cognitive, psychoeducational, language, and associated abilities be obtained as part of the multidisciplinary team assessment process *prior* to initiating a referral for CAPD services, and that the whole child is considered throughout the process. Although the question of whether school districts resist such an approach is a common one, it has been my experience that, once the rationale behind this specific approach to screening is explained, resistance is rarely, if ever, encountered. Indeed, the focus on children in their entirety, and the inclusion of the multidisciplinary team in the screening process, typically is perceived as not only logical, but most efficacious. Furthermore, by its very nature, this approach to screening for CAPD fosters interaction and consultation among the various individuals involved, which is beneficial for all who work with children with disabilities of any nature. Thus, this chapter emphasizes a process in which we begin with the whole child, with all of his or her strengths and weaknesses, and only then do we begin to decompose his or her abilities into underlying contributing deficits. As will be seen in the chapters on management, this process is then reversed so that the functional strengths and weaknesses of the whole child are, once again, considered and made use of when planning management and intervention strategies.

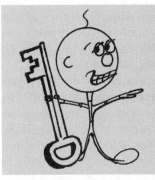

KEY CONCEPT

Evaluation for CAPD should be considered ONLY after measures of cognition, learning, speech, and language have been obtained.

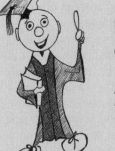

Learning Objectives

After studying this chapter, the reader should be able to:

1. Discuss the rationale for a CAPD screening program.
2. Identify categories and types of test tools and measurements that should be included in the screening process.

3. Develop a CAPD screening program for use in the educational setting.
4. Determine the need for referral for comprehensive central auditory evaluation on the basis of screening results.

Rationale for Central Auditory Processing Disorders Screening

Lessler (1972) stated that the purpose of screening is to acquire preliminary information about individuals' characteristics, particularly those that may have significant impacts on their health, education, or well-being. In addition, the author emphasized that the screening process should be economical in terms of money, time, and resources, because screening, by definition, will deal with larger numbers of people than will comprehensive assessment.

The justification for a CAPD screening program should comply with the above-stated factors, and should take into account concerns regarding the need, cost, design, and outcomes of the program. To this end, we will attempt to deal with some of the questions that may be posed by administrators and others in the special education profession regarding the need for a CAPD screening program. In this manner, clinicians should be able to justify the screening program's development, implementation, and maintenance.

Do central auditory processing disorders exist? Are tests available that can diagnose these disorders and provide information to assist in the remediation process? Are effective intervention strategies available? Although these questions may seem irrelevant to some, the fact is that many professionals in the educational setting have, over time, come to disallow the existence or effective treatment of CAPD. Citing a lack of valid diagnostic tools and effective therapeutic interventions, these professionals prefer either to ignore the existence of CAPD as a whole or to label it as a kind of learning disorder that is best addressed through the use of a generic list of compensatory strategies appropriate for "all" children affected by the disorder. Therefore, a screening program, as the first step in the overall diagnosis of CAPD in a given educational population, may not be seen as a priority in many educational arenas.

A second factor interfering with the justification of need for a screening program for CAPD is the existence of several test tools that purport to assess central auditory function and are currently administered by psychologists, educational diagnosticians, and speech-language pathologists. These tools, which will be reviewed later in this chapter, often include "auditory perceptual" subtests that presumably provide descriptive information regarding a wide range of auditory abilities, from auditory memory and sequencing to auditory discrimination and attention. Given the fact that many of these test tools have been in use for several years within the educational setting, the question arises as to the need for additional testing that, on the surface, adds little or nothing to the overall picture.

Finally, it seems that the term *central auditory processing disorder* has become a catch-all phrase used, often inappropriately, to explain a wide variety of learning and attention problems. In my experience, in many instances, if a child exhibits difficulty with verbal information processing or storage, the child automatically earns the label of CAPD, regardless of whether valid central auditory tests have been performed. In recent months, I have had the experience of hearing the term *CAPD* linked automatically or used interchangeably with learning disabilities, dyslexia, attention-deficit/hyperactivity disorder (AD/HD), and receptive language disorders by professionals within the fields of psychology, neurology, speech-language pathology, and even audiology. Although, as emphasized in Part One of this book, difficulty with the processing of auditory information and generally poor listening abilities frequently accompany many of these disorders, it is important that we make every effort to either differentiate CAPD from these disorders or, in the case of comorbidity of disorders, determine to what degree a child's difficulties may be due to a deficit in auditory processing specifically.

All of this creates a formidable task for clinicians devoted to developing state-of-the-art assessment and management programs for CAPD in the educational setting. To obtain administrative support and funding for these projects, clinicians must be able to show that (a) central auditory processing disorders do, in fact, exist as distinct entities and significantly impact children's ability to learn; (b) current measurement tools used by psychologists, speech/language pathologists, educational diagnosticians, and other professionals may suffice for screening purposes; however, comprehensive central auditory testing remains essential for defining the disorder and providing direction for management; and (c) remediation techniques are available that can assist in managing the disorder. Finally, **the first, vital step in this process is a multidisciplinary screening program that will serve to identify those students for whom a comprehensive central auditory evaluation appears warranted while, at the same time, reducing the number of inappropriate referrals.**

The subsequent chapters in this book address the topics of defining CAPD, administering and interpreting a comprehensive CAPD assessment, and developing a management program. The current chapter is concerned primarily with the need for a screening program that will provide preliminary information needed to determine if further evaluation is warranted. **Therefore, the first question that must be addressed is the basic one of "Why screen?"**

Musiek, Gollegly, Lamb, and Lamb (1990) listed several reasons why a screening program for CAPD is necessary. Included in their rationale were that accurate screening and identification of CAPD would:

- help to identify conditions that may require medical attention
- foster increased educators' and parents' awareness of CAPD
- reduce the shopping around associated with attempts to determine the cause of a particular child's listening and learning difficulties
- minimize psychological factors on the part of the child arising from anxiety, stress, and fear of the unknown
- allow for insightful educational planning based upon the individual child's auditory strengths and weaknesses

Finally, the authors stated that it cannot be overlooked that audiologists have a basic responsibility to evaluate the entire auditory system. **Although traditional audiological evaluation procedures have focused primarily on the peripheral auditory system, the central auditory system cannot be ignored.**

I would add to this list that screening for CAPD also would reduce time and cost investments on the part of the special education team by reducing the number of overreferrals for comprehensive CAPD evaluation and other diagnostic assessments, and by helping to provide direction to special educators, speech-language pathologists, rehabilitative audiologists, and others entrusted with the task of developing a remediation program that will help to manage children's disorders in the most efficient way possible.

Finally, a factor that must be taken into account in the justification of any screening program is the number of children potentially affected by the disorder. If, for example, only a very few children are likely to exhibit the disorder in question, it may not be cost-effective to develop a program designed to identify the disorder. If, however, the given disorder is likely to affect a large portion of the population, then the cost, in terms of time and money, of developing and implementing a screening and identification program becomes much easier to justify.

Lewis (1986) estimated that **3% to 7% of all school-age children exhibit some form of learning disability. Although it is true that, due to the lack of adequate identification procedures to date, the number of children with CAPD within this population cannot be stated with certainty, it is likely to be quite high** (Hurley & Singer, 1989). Therefore, if a program designed to identify the presence of CAPD is not in place, a good number of children exhibiting the disorder will be missed altogether or remain unidentified until long after effective management strategies might have been undertaken.

In conclusion, **the need for a CAPD screening program is justified when one considers the large numbers of school-age children who are likely to be affected by the disorder, combined with the need for a reduction in the number of inappropriate referrals for central auditory evaluation or additional diagnostic tests.** Appropriate identification of children with CAPD can assist in the development of effective management and educational strategies, and may also serve to reduce or eliminate the amount of shopping around and anxiety on the part of children and parents that occurs when the underlying reason for learning difficulties is not clearly understood. Finally, a CAPD screening program may help to identify those children in need of medical follow-up who might otherwise have gone undetected. The information discussed in this section is summarized in Table 4-1.

The Central Auditory Processing (CAP) Team

The main purpose of assembling a multidisciplinary CAP team is to allow its members to gather sufficient information about children in question so that a preliminary understanding of their abilities across a wide variety of functional domains may be obtained. **A team approach to CAPD screening allows for the gathering of information regarding educational, social, speech/language, cognitive, and medical characteristics, and helps to reduce the time demand placed upon any one individual.** Finally, a team approach in which a multitude of data is collected allows for a more insightful answer to the question of whether additional testing is indicated to define a specific child's learning difficulties more fully. Bellis and Ferre (1996) emphasized that, regardless of whether audition, language, and learning are approached from a "bottom-up" or "top-down" perspective, it is important to realize that a good deal of interdependency exists. Therefore, when attempting to determine the contribution of CAPD to learning and language difficulties in the educational setting, the whole

Table 4–1

Rationale for CAP Screening

Why Screen for CAPD?

- Many children are likely affected by the disorder.
- Screening will reduce the number of inappropriate referrals for comprehensive central auditory testing, thereby reducing long-term time and cost investment.
- Screening will help to identify children in need of medical intervention.
- Psychological effects of CAPD can be minimized.
- Appropriate identification of children with CAPD will allow for insightful educational planning.
- A screening program will help to foster awareness on the part of educational professionals and parents regarding CAPD.

child must be taken into account, and the identification process must reflect this interdependency.

To this end, a multidisciplinary team approach to CAPD identification should be implemented. A brief discussion of the relative contribution of various team members follows (Table 4-2).

Table 4-2

The CAP Team

Member	Responsibilities
Audiologist	Manages and coordinates CAP effort; performs audiological evaluation to rule out peripheral hearing loss
Speech-language pathologist	Defines child's receptive and expressive language skills, as well as written language and associated abilities
Educator	Provides information regarding child's listening and learning behavior in the classroom
Psychologist	Determines child's cognitive skills and capacity for learning
Social worker	Serves as primary liaison between school and family
Parents	Provide information regarding developmental milestones, auditory behavior in the home, and medical and academic history
Physician	Rules out presence of pathology that may affect learning abilities

The Audiologist

Typically, **the audiologist will be responsible for managing and coordinating the CAPD screening effort,** as it will fall to this professional to perform comprehensive central auditory assessment if the need for such is determined. Therefore, the audiologist should gather information from the other team members, evaluate and discuss the results of findings with the team, and aid in determining the need for comprehensive central auditory evaluation. In addition, the audiologist should perform standard audiological evaluations on children suspected of CAPD in order to rule out peripheral hearing loss as a possible contributing factor to listening or learning difficulties. Finally, the audiologist should be alert for signs that would indicate the need for special tests of auditory and neurophysiologic function such as otoacoustic emissions or electrophysiologic testing and, if these tests are not available on site, should be aware of resources in the community to whom children can be referred.

The Speech-Language Pathologist

The speech-language pathologist is instrumental in defining children's receptive and expressive language abilities. Using test protocols that are within their domain, these professionals can provide valuable information regarding relative strengths and weaknesses in children's oral and written language abilities. Also, as will be discussed later, many of the speech-language test tools that are currently in use contain auditory perceptual subtests that help identify specific areas of functional auditory difficulty.

The Educator

The special education and classroom teachers are the primary source of descriptive information regarding children's listening and learning behavior within the learning environment. Information that may be obtained from these professionals includes, but is not limited to, identification of specific subjects in which children exhibit the greatest amount of difficulty, daily listening behaviors in group and individual learning situations, reading and writing competencies, comprehension of instructions, general problem-solving skills, and overall attitudinal and behavioral characteristics. In addition, the educator (or educational diagnostician) may administer basic skills testing that will serve to illuminate relative areas of academic strengths and weaknesses as well as cognitive functioning.

The Psychologist

The psychologist is the professional qualified to administer and interpret cognitive assessments that provide information concerning children's cognitive skills and capacity for learning. Information regarding the possibility of attention-related disorders or emotional disturbances that may interfere with the learning process may also be provided by the psychologist. In addition, portions of various psychological tests, like those of the speech-language pathologist, tap general auditory behaviors. Finally, as discussed in Part One, children should have a mental age of 7 or 8 years before many tests of central auditory function can be administered. Results of psychological testing may help to establish cognitive or mental age.

The Social Worker

The social worker is often the primary link between school and family. As such, social workers are invaluable members of the multidisciplinary team because of their input regarding family dynamics, socioeconomic factors that might affect the ability to assess or manage children's auditory deficits, and impact of the children's difficulties on socialization and related activities. In addition, the social worker frequently is the person who works as a liaison between the school district and the family, helping to ensure that legal and practical matters are understood and agreed upon and facilitating the teamwork that is so important when children have a disorder or disability.

The Parents

Valuable information regarding developmental milestones, auditory behaviors and difficulties encountered in the home environment, medical history, and academic sequelae can be obtained only by including the parents in the screening process. The parents can provide valuable insight regarding the impact of the learning difficulties experienced on the overall well-being of their children as well as an analysis of family history of hearing or learning disorders, early history of otitis media or head injury, and other valuable information. Furthermore, similarities and discrepancies between parental and school-based reports of a specific child's difficulties may serve to illuminate possible contributing factors and provide directions for intervention both at home and at school.

The Physician

Medical doctors and school nurses are key players in ruling out the presence of pathological conditions that may cause learning difficulties in children. In many cases, referral to a physician may be indicated for diagnosis and treatment of otologic and neurologic disorders that threaten the health and well-being of the child.

The individuals discussed above may be considered the core members of the CAP team; however, in certain cases, additional persons or professionals significant in a child's life may be included. The inclusion of these individuals in the screening process allows for the efficient gathering of a wide variety of data so that a picture of the whole child begins to emerge. What would, in fact, be an overwhelming task for just the audiologist can be managed much more easily and effectively via a team approach. In all but a few situations, the requirements for screening on the part of the team members would coincide with the duties they already perform as part of an initial or triennial evaluation in gathering information for special education consideration.

Screening Test Tool Considerations

A key factor in considering tools for screening is the time involved in administration. As a general rule of thumb, **the time involved in gathering preliminary information, with respect to any team member, should not exceed the time needed for comprehensive central auditory assessment.** Fortunately, many of the tests recommended as screening tools either will have been administered already, or will be in the process of being administered, as part of a multidisciplinary evaluation resulting from a special education referral. Therefore, much of the information necessary for the determination of need for comprehensive central auditory evaluation should already be available for review. If current test results are unavailable, certain tests may need to be updated to get a more accurate picture of a child's current level of functioning across domains.

Additionally, it should be noted that many of the test tools discussed herein are not specifically designed to gather information regarding auditory processing abilities, but rather are used diagnostically within each discipline to rule out speech, language, cognitive, or other disorders. For example, the information obtained from cognitive testing is designed to provide information regarding children's cognitive capacity, not auditory processing skills. However, the data gleaned from such tests may provide useful information in determining whether a central auditory processing disorder might be present, as well as in deciding whether a child possesses the cognitive ability to participate in central auditory assessment procedures.

Finally, although speech-language, psychoeducational, and cognitive tests exist that purport to assess auditory processing abilities, it should be recognized that most of these tests are confounded by language and other higher-level neurocognitive variables, do not provide for sufficient acoustic control, or have no documented validity in the identification of disorders of the central auditory nervous system. Therefore, **these tests should be considered as screening tools from an auditory processing perspective and should never be utilized for central auditory diagnostic purposes.** Validity and reliability of central auditory assessment materials will be discussed in subsequent chapters, and the information provided will help guide clinicians in determining the relative worth of any test that claims to assess central auditory processing abilities.

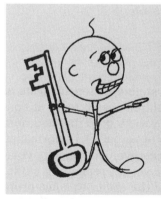

KEY CONCEPT

Most nonaudiological tests that purport to assess "auditory perceptual abilities" should not be considered diagnostic tools for CAPD, and should be used for *screening* purposes only.

It is recommended that, whenever possible, the decision regarding which test or tests to utilize in the screening process be left up to individual professionals' discretion within their specific disciplines. In other words, although measures of receptive and expressive language skills are important in the overall screening process, audiologists should not presume to tell speech-language pathologists which test(s) should be utilized in language assessment.

With that said, what follows is a general overview of some of the more commonly used tests within each discipline that may provide information regarding auditory perceptual abilities.

Tests of Cognitive Capacity and Psychoeducational Function

In my opinion, **few components of the multidisciplinary evaluation provide more qualitative information regarding children's functioning across domains that is useful in screening for CAPD than cognitive and psychoeducational assessment.** However, it should be emphasized that the information to be gleaned from this assessment will not be found in the overall IQ score or school grades. Rather, an analysis of a child's functioning within specific subcomponents of the assessment can be used to identify *patterns* of difficulty areas that may be suggestive of CAPD. Conversely, examination of levels of functioning across subtests may provide supportive evidence that a higher-order, more global dysfunction is the likely culprit in a child's listening and learning difficulties.

Although several test tools are available for cognitive and academic assessment in the school-age population, this section will review the two most commonly used measurement tools.

Weschsler Intelligence Scale for Children—Third Edition (WISC-III)

The WISC-III (Kaplan, 1995) is one of the most comprehensive tests of cognitive capacity available for use with children ages 6 to 16. It consists of several subtests that assess a wide variety of verbal and non-verbal abilities, leading to composite scores of verbal IQ, performance IQ, and full-scale IQ (verbal and performance cognitive capacity combined). Verbal capacity is an indicator of verbal reasoning skills, whereas performance capacity is an index of the ability to solve problems using nonverbal, visual-spatial information. The full-scale IQ is thought to represent the overall cognitive capacity; however, extremely poor performance on one or more subtest (i.e., significant scatter in skills) can lead to a skewing of the full-scale IQ score so that it does not, in some cases, accurately reflect actual overall cognitive ability. A significant discrepancy between verbal and performance scales may qualify a child for special education services under the classification of learning disabled, as may a significant discrepancy between indicators of cognitive capacity and actual academic proficiency or performance.

Each subtest of the WISC-III delivers a scaled score that ranges from 1 (lowest) to 19 (highest), with a score of 7 to 12 (mean: 10) being average. Percentile scores that indicate how the child performed relative to same-age peers are also provided. Composite scores of verbal, performance, and full-scale IQ are expressed in standard scores, with 100 being average. In addition, four additional "Index" scores may be derived from combinations of scores on various subtests. These Index scores consist of: (1) Verbal Comprehension, which provides an indication of the ability to understand verbal information and to use words to solve problems; (2) Perceptual Organization, or the ability to perceive, organize, and solve problems using visual-spatial information; (3) Freedom from Distractibility, which measures the ability to perform tasks that require sustained attention, concentration, and mental control; and (4) Processing Speed, which is an index of the ability to perform visual perceptual paper-and-pencil tasks with speed and accuracy. Of these Indexes, the one that usually holds the most interest for the purposes of CAPD screening is that of Verbal Comprehension.

Subtests within the Verbal scale of the WISC-III include:

- Information—fund of general knowledge
- Similarities—abstract verbal reasoning abilities
- Arithmetic—ability to solve verbal arithmetic problems, providing an index of numerical reasoning abilities along with attention and short-term memory for meaningful information
- Vocabulary—knowledge of word meanings
- Comprehension—ability to comprehend verbally presented information, particularly relating to social judgment
- Digit Span—short-term memory for orally presented non-meaningful information (i.e., strings of numbers)

Subtests within the Performance scale of the WISC-III include:

- Picture Completion—attention to visual detail and visual closure abilities
- Coding—visual-motor skills and processing speed

- Picture Arrangement—sequential reasoning abilities and attention to visual detail
- Block Design—visual abstract abilities
- Object Assembly—part-to-whole synthetic reasoning
- Mazes—graphomotor planning skills, visual-motor coordination, and visual-motor speed

Woodcock-Johnson III Tests of Achievement

The Woodcock-Johnson III Tests of Achievement (WJ III ACH; Woodcock, McGraw, & Mather, 2001) comprise the academic achievement portion of the Woodcock-Johnson Complete Test Battery, which is the latest edition of the Woodcock-Johnson Psycho-Educational Test Battery—Revised (WJ-R; Woodcock & Johnson, 1989). In addition to tests of academic achievement, the WJ III Complete Battery also has the Tests of Cognitive Ability (WJ III COG), which include tests of long- and short-term memory and retrieval, auditory- and visual-processing-related abilities, processing speed, crystallized and fluid intelligence, and similar tasks. The WJ III may be administered from age 24 months through adulthood. This discussion will focus primarily on the academic achievement tests of the WJ III.

The WJ-III ACH may be used to assess academic achievement and skills in the areas of reading, written language, mathematics, oral language, and academic knowledge. It is an extremely useful tool for providing a basis for comparison between cognitive capacity and actual achievement in a variety of areas. There are twelve tests in the Standard Battery, including:

- Letter-Word Identification
- Reading Fluency
- Story Recall
- Understanding Directions
- Calculation
- Math Fluency
- Spelling
- Writing Fluency
- Passage Comprehension
- Applied Problems
- Writing Samples
- Story Recall—Delayed

Various combinations of these twelve tests can be grouped to form twelve "cluster" scores designed to provide a profile of skills and abilities in four major academic areas: reading, oral language, math, and written language. Each cluster score focuses on a specific aspect of each academic area, allowing the interpreter to gain a better understanding of areas of difficulty underlying poor achievement in a given broad area.

In addition to the tests and clusters discussed above, the Extended Battery includes nine additional tests as well as nine additional clusters. Use of the extended battery allows for additional investigation into a given child's academic difficulties and more fine-grained analysis of underlying deficit areas.

The WJ III ACH provides an excellent overview of abilities across a wide variety of domains, especially when used together with the cognitive ability tests. It should be emphasized that **both the WJ-III and the WISC-III must be administered and interpreted by a professional trained and licensed or certified to provide such assessment.** Thus, these assessments usually are administered by psychologists or educational diagnosticians. Furthermore, it must be remembered that these tests are measures of higher-order cognitive abilities and, as such, are reliant on the ability to comprehend what is expected during the testing, ability to attend to the task, and a host of other factors. Therefore, in some instances, these tests may not be accurate representations of a child's actual abilities within some domains.

Although there are several additional test tools that can be employed to assess cognitive capacity and academic achievement, the WISC-III and WJ III are two of the most commonly used as well as being, in my opinion, the two that provide the most complete information for the purposes of auditory processing screening.

Subtest Analysis of Cognitive and Psychoeducational Measures

When reviewing the results of any cognitive and psychoeducational assessment tools for purposes of CAPD screening, our primary aim is to gain a qualitative understanding of the types of activities and tasks that present a problem for the individual child in question. In particular, we are interested in scatter across subtests that conveys a pattern or carries a common theme, which may indicate that a child has particular difficulty with specific types of tasks. Thus, we are *not* reinterpreting the tests for purposes of determining cognitive capacity or academic abilities. Rather, **we are looking for specific indicators that the child's difficulty indeed lies in "auditory" domains, or that there is a possibility that an auditory deficit may be affecting his or her performance on the battery.** Therefore, it is not the overall score that is important to us during CAPD screening, but the nature of the child's difficulties across academic and cognitive domains. I refer to this process as *subtest analysis*.

Perhaps a couple of examples will serve to illustrate this concept. At one extreme lies the child who exhibits relatively little scatter in skills, that is, who exhibits equal difficulty across subtests within cognitive and academic testing. Because many of these tests rely on abilities that cannot truly be considered to be taxing from an auditory perspective (e.g., tasks in the Performance scale of the WISC-III; Processing Speed, Visual Processing, and Math Calculation in the WJ III), difficulty across domains would be a more likely indicator of a higher-order cognitive deficit that is affecting processing in many modalities, including auditory, than it would be an indicator of a primary central auditory processing disorder.

At the other extreme lies the child who clearly exhibits difficulties only on those tasks that rely on auditory abilities. For example, there may be a clear discrepancy between verbal and performance scales on the WISC-III, with performance abilities significantly better than verbal ones. In addition, on the WJ III, the child may exhibit difficulty with any test component that requires auditory decoding or comprehension skills, including, but not limited to, tasks that require repetition of verbally presented material, "auditory processing" subtests, tests of overall comprehension or knowledge (due to the listening comprehension component inherent in these tasks), fluid reasoning tasks (specifically in the verbal analogies component), reading abilities (especially Letter-Word Identification and similar areas), Mathematics Reasoning (because of the auditory comprehension necessary for solving word problems), and Basic Writing Skills (particularly in taking dictation). Conversely, this child may do well on tasks that are less auditorily loaded, such as those that require basic mathematics calculation, visual-spatial processing, and the like. Certainly, this pattern of responses across subtests provides a clear indicator that the child has difficulty with any task that contains a significant auditory component. However, it should be emphasized that **the nature of the underlying auditory difficulty cannot be ascertained from subtest analysis of cognitive and psychoeducational measures.** Rather, these measures provide a qualitative indicator of the functional difficulties a child is experiencing that *might* be due to an underlying auditory deficit. This information is important in determining the possible functional impact of a given auditory processing deficit; however, it does not allow us to determine where our auditory intervention strategies should focus as we do not yet know what the nature of the auditory processing deficit is, or even whether a primary central auditory processing disorder exists at all. As such, this pattern of findings would certainly suggest that additional testing in the area of central auditory processing is indicated.

Unfortunately, not all children fall into one of these two extremes. In fact, in my clinical experience, the vast majority of children do not present as clear a pattern as the above two examples do. Therefore, when reviewing the results of these, or any, tests of cognitive and psychoeducational abilities, one must take into careful consideration the task demands of each individual subtest and determine whether the possibility of an auditory confound exists. At the end of this chapter, case studies will be provided that illustrate the use of subtest analysis of cognitive and psychoeducational tests, along with additional measures to be discussed subsequently, in the determination of the need for formal central auditory evaluation.

Finally, it should be remembered that an additional purpose of CAPD screening is to determine whether the child is capable of participating in comprehensive central auditory assessment. Clues pertaining to this issue may also be found in the results of the cognitive and psychoeducational battery. For example, if the child is unable to repeat four digits in quiet (WISC-III, Digit Span subtest) or to repeat simple sentences or two or more words in isolation (WJ III, Short-Term Memory cognitive test), then one must ask whether a valid indicator of this child's central auditory processing abilities may be obtained from an assessment that will require the child to repeat digits, words, and sentences *in dichotic, or competing, conditions*; or to remember, sequence, and verbally label tonal patterns. If the child is unable to perform these tasks in a relatively quiet, noncompeting auditory environment, it certainly is unreasonable to expect the child to perform them under conditions of auditory competition. Therefore, results of central auditory evaluation may be equivocal, as poor performance on central auditory tests may be due to the child's memory and sequencing difficulties in general, and not to central auditory deficit specifically.

Speech and Language Tests

Speech-language pathologists have a lengthy list of tests to draw from in the assessment of children's language abilities. It is not within the scope of this text to provide an overview of all the speech and language tools on the market, nor is such an overview necessary. Instead, I have attempted to identify some of the more commonly used test tools that either include subtests that help to describe auditory perceptual abilities, or that focus on auditory-related skills such as phonological awareness and auditory comprehension. It should be cautioned once again that these tests do not provide information regarding the underlying nature of a specific auditory deficit and, therefore, cannot be used diagnostically for central auditory assessment (Musiek, Gollegly, Lamb, & Lamb, 1990).

It is not my intention to imply that all of the following tests be included in the screening process, but rather to increase readers' awareness regarding test tools—both old and new—that are available commercially and to suggest that the addition of one or two of the following materials may help provide auditory-related data to the overall information-gathering process. It should be emphasized that the following is not a comprehensive list of all speech-language assessment tools that may provide information for auditory processing screening purposes. It is merely intended as a representative list of some commonly used measures that are presently available. For ease of reference, the tests discussed in this section are listed in Table 4-3.

Auditory Discrimination Test—Second Edition (ADT)

The ADT (Wepman & Reynolds, 1986) assesses the ability to detect subtle phonemic differences between word pairs. It is a quick and easy-to-administer test that requires listeners to determine whether

---

Table 4-3
Lists of Selected Cognitive, Psychoeducational, and Speech-Language Tests

- Weschler Intelligence Scale for Children—Third Edition (WISC-III)
- Woodcock-Johnson III Tests of Achievement (W-J III ACH) and Tests of Cognitive Ability (W-J III COG)
- Auditory Discrimination Test—Second Edition (ADT)
- Carrow Auditory-Visual Abilities Test (CAVAT)
- Clinical Evaluation of Language Fundamentals—Third Edition (CELF-3)
- Comprehensive Test of Phonological Processing (CTOPP)
- Goldman-Fristoe-Woodcock Test of Auditory Discrimination (G-F-W TAD)
- Lindamood Auditory Conceptualization Test, Revised Edition (LAC-R)
- The Listening Test
- Phonological Awareness Profile
- Phonological Awareness Test (PAT)
- Test for Auditory Comprehension of Language—Third Edition (TACL-3)
- Test of Auditory Perceptual Skills—Revised (TAPS-R)

two words are the same or different. The ADT was designed for children ages 4 through 8.

Carrow Auditory-Visual Abilities Test (CAVAT)

The CAVAT (Carrow-Woolfolk, 1981) contains several subtests that may be used to help identify children with language learning disabilities. Several auditory abilities are assessed, including general auditory memory for related and unrelated stimuli, auditory sequencing, short-term auditory memory, digit span repetition (forward and reversed), auditory discrimination, sentence and word repetition, and auditory blending. In addition, this test helps to describe auditory-visual integration and motor abilities. The CAVAT was designed for use with children who are 4 years to 10 years, 11 months, in age.

Clinical Evaluation of Language Fundamentals—Third Edition (CELF-3)

Although the CELF-3 (Semiel, Wiig, & Secord, 1995) is primarily a test of language, it provides valuable information regarding auditory comprehension and sentence recall abilities. Furthermore, because it assesses a wide range of language abilities, it is a good tool for exploring overall language-related difficulties. The CELF-3 was designed for ages 6 through 21.

Comprehensive Test of Phonological Processing (CTOPP)

The CTOPP (Wagner, Torgesen, & Rashotte, 1999) examines a variety of phonological awareness abilities and is separated into two versions based on age: Version 1 (children age 5 or 6), and Version 2 (individuals ages 7 through 24). Version 1 includes such tasks as phonological manipulation, rapid color and object naming, sound matching and blending in words, memory for digits, and nonsense word repetition. Version 2 includes additional tasks such as rapid letter naming, phoneme reversal, sound blending in nonwords, and phoneme segmentation in words and nonwords.

Goldman-Fristoe-Woodcock Test of Auditory Discrimination (G-F-W TAD)

The G-F-W TAD (Goldman, Fristoe, & Woodcock, 1970) was designed to assess the ability to discriminate speech sounds in quiet and noise. It can be used with children age 3 to adulthood, and uses a picture-pointing response in an effort to minimize spoken or written language confounds.

Lindamood Auditory Conceptualization Test, Revised Edition (LAC-R)

The LAC-R (Lindamood & Lindamood, 1979) measures auditory skills in the two primary areas of sound discrimination and sequencing of speech sounds in an attempt to relate auditory deficits in these areas to problems with spelling and reading as well as expressive speech. It may be used with children from kindergarten through high school.

The Listening Test

Because the ability to listen is so closely tied to overall communication and learning abilities, The Listening Test (Barrett, Huisingh, Zachman, Blagden, & Orman, 1992) was developed to assess children's ability to attend to, process, and respond to verbally presented information. The test was designed to measure elementary school-age children's listening skills in "real-life" situations such as those found in typical classrooms. The five tasks included in the test assess the ability to determine the main idea of a passage, answer questions relating to specific details, apply basic concept and vocabulary knowledge, draw inferences from verbally presented information, and comprehend a story. The Listening Test was designed for children age 6 years and older, with normative values established for children who are 6 years, 0 months, through 11 years, 11 months, in age.

Phonological Awareness Profile

Designed to evaluate both phonological processing and sound-symbol association, the Phonological Awareness Profile (Robertson & Salfer, 1997) includes tasks of rhyming, phoneme manipulation (including segmentation, isolation, deletion, substitution), sound blending, and phonological decoding. It is particularly valuable in determining outcome measures following therapy through the development of an overall performance profile. The Phonological Awareness Profile was designed for use with children ages 5 through 8.

Phonological Awareness Test (PAT)

A relatively recent addition to speech-language pathologists' armamentarium, the PAT (Robertson & Salfer, 1997) provides an indicator of the ability to perceive and manipulate speech sounds. The test consists of several subtests that measure a wide variety of phonological awareness abilities, including, but not limited to, rhyming, phoneme discrimination, speech-sound production, segmentation, sound blending, identification of speech sounds in various positions within words, and invented spelling (or word attack) skills. This tool provides excellent information about the nature of phonological awareness abilities, and frequently is found to be very useful in screening for CAPD and in selecting goals in planning for auditory intervention. When results of the PAT are viewed in combination with information from tests such as the reading subtests of academic achievement test batteries, discussed above, relationships between perceptual difficulties and spelling/reading difficulties may be illuminated. This test can be administered to children with developmental ages of 5 through 9.

Test for Auditory Comprehension of Language—Third Edition (TACL-3)

The TACL-3 (Carrow-Woolfolk, 1998) consists of three subtests that measure receptive language abilities, including comprehension of word classes and word relations; grammatical morphemes such as those that denote tense, possession, and plurals; and comprehension of complex sentence structures. In contrast to auditory comprehension subtests of cognitive and psychoeducational tests, such as the WISC-III and the Woodcock-Johnson, the TACL-3 does not require verbal responses, thus eliminating any expressive language confound. This test was designed for administration to children ages 3 through 9.

Test of Auditory Perceptual Skills—Revised (TAPS-R)

The TAPS-R (Gardner, 1996) measures auditory perceptual skills in areas such as digit span (forward and reversed), sentence memory, word memory, interpretation of directions, dictation, word discrimination, and reasoning. It was designed for use with children ages 4 through 13. An upper extension, the TAPS: Upper Level, is available for assessing these skills in children ages 12 through 18 (Gardner, 1994).

Tests of Written Language Ability

Tests of reading and written language can provide valuable information regarding phonemic representation, word attack skills, reading comprehension, and other abilities. Some speech-language assessment tools also include written language supplements. In addition, a multitude of oral reading, reading comprehension, written language, spelling, and related tests is available. I strongly suggest that information regarding reading and written language abilities be obtained for any child suspected of CAPD.

Audiological Tests

The only audiological test battery to date that has been designed specifically for the purpose of screening for CAPD is the SCAN: A Screening Test for Auditory Processing Disorders (Keith, 1986). A revised version was recently published (SCAN-C Test for Auditory Processing Disorders in Children—Revised; Keith, 2000a). The original version of the test consists of three subtests: Filtered Words, Auditory Figure-Ground, and Competing Words. It was designed to be administered easily and quickly using a portable cassette tape player with headphones and may be administered by virtually any individual on the screening team.

The SCAN-C includes the original three subtests as well as one additional subtest: Competing Sentences. Additional differences between the SCAN and the SCAN-C include the conversion from audiocassette to compact disc, the deletion of some items in the Competing Words subtest, new methods for calculating composite scores, and the rewording of the recorded instructions to render them easier to understand by young children. Both versions of the SCAN were designed for use with children from ages 3 to 11; however, children below age 5 may be unable to complete the tasks for a variety of reasons. Normative data for children who are 5 years, 0 months, to 11 years, 11 months, in age are now available for the SCAN-C (Keith, 2000b). Results of both the SCAN and the SCAN-C have been shown to correlate with findings on selected tests of auditory processing, and the test appears to demonstrate validity for the identification of learning disabilities.

The SCAN has been criticized for the absence of a measure of temporal processing and for the fact that there is no documented validity of the test with listeners having known lesions or disorders of the central auditory nervous system (Musiek, Gollegly, Lamb, & Lamb, 1990). In addition, the subtests within the SCAN have a limited number of items and may not allow for adequate investigation into the auditory functions that are assessed. Therefore, **results of the SCAN should be viewed in light of other data for determining if diagnostic evalua-**

tion is needed and should not stand alone as a diagnostic test of central auditory function. An upward extension of the SCAN designed to screen auditory processing abilities in the adolescent and adult population, the SCAN-A, is also available (Keith, 1994b).

Auditory Continuous Performance Test (ACPT)

The ACPT (Keith, 1994a) is an excellent test for looking at attention-related auditory abilities. This test, which is essentially a test of auditory vigilance, requires listeners to attend to strings of monosyllabic words, and to raise their thumbs whenever the word *dog* occurs. Both impulsivity and omission errors are scored, and performance at the beginning of the test is compared to performance at the end of the test to provide an indicator of auditory vigilance over time. I have found that the inclusion of this test in the screening process provides invaluable information regarding a child's ability to sustain attention to auditory stimuli. Further, the use of this test along with measures of visual vigilance may assist in the differential diagnosis of attention-related disorders.

Other Audiological Screening Tests for CAPD

A recent consensus conference convened at the University of Texas at Dallas reviewed the topic of screening for CAPD (Jerger & Musiek, 2000). **Of the many central auditory test tools on the market, one in particular was judged to be appropriate for screening as well as diagnostic purposes: the Dichotic Digits test (Musiek, 1983a). In addition, a measure of temporal processing, such as a gap detection test, was recommended.** Validity, administration, and scoring of both the Dichotic Digits test and gap detection tests will be discussed in subsequent chapters.

In addition to the possible administration of these screening tools, combined with serving as the CAP team leader, the greatest contribution to the screening process that audiologists can make is the assessment of peripheral hearing sensitivity to rule out peripheral hearing loss as a contributing factor to academic or listening difficulties. To this end, **all children suspected of CAPD should undergo complete audiological assessment of peripheral auditory system function prior to referral for comprehensive central auditory evaluation,** to include pure-tone air- and bone-conduction testing, speech reception threshold (SRT) and word recognition testing, immittance (tympanometry and acoustic reflex) testing, and otoacoustic emission testing, when indicated.

Behavioral Checklists and Questionnaires

Several behavioral checklists and questionnaires exist that are designed to provide qualitative information regarding function across environments and situations. Two of these, in particular, are useful for obtaining information regarding auditory function in children: the Children's Auditory Performance Scale (CHAPS; Smoski, Brunt, & Tannahill, 1998) and Fisher's Auditory Processing Checklist (Fisher, 1985).

The CHAPS consists of a rating scale of +1 to -5 to indicate the degree of difficulty children exhibit in relation to same-age peers in a variety of situations and listening conditions, with +1 indicating less difficulty and -5 indicating inability to function at all. Listening conditions included in the CHAPS include noise, quiet, ideal, with multiple inputs, conditions requiring memory sequencing, and conditions requiring sustained auditory attention. Situations include various auditory behaviors and requirements, such as "when paying (or not paying) attention," "when being given simple (or complex) instructions," "when immediate (or delayed) recall is required," and the like. Performance scores are derived that indicate the child's ability to function in each of the listening conditions and a graphic display of the data allows the evaluator to determine in which conditions the child is at risk for auditory difficulties. The CHAPS may be completed by classroom teachers, special education service providers, parents, or any other appropriate persons. Indeed, a comparison of CHAPS results across different environments (e.g., home versus classroom versus small-group therapy) can provide important information about discrepancies in function depending on the environment, which may help guide decisions for management and intervention.

The Fisher's Auditory Processing checklist is somewhat more restricted in scope than the CHAPS, but also provides good information regarding children's functional listening behaviors in the classroom. The checklist is designed to be completed by classroom teachers.

There are several other auditory-based checklists that may provide valuable information regarding listening skills in a variety of settings. These include the Screening Instrument for Targeting Educational Risk (S.I.F.T.E.R.; Anderson & Matkin, 1996), the Listening Inventory for Education (L.I.F.E.; Anderson & Smaldino, 1998), and the Children's Home Inventory of Listening Difficulties (CHILD; Anderson & Smaldino, 2000).

Other checklists that may be used to investigate children's psychological, attention-related, or other functional behavior in real-world situations include, but are not limited to, the Conners' Rating Scales—Revised (CRS-R; Conners, 1996), which looks at possible attention-related deficits; the Behavior Assessment System for Children (BASC; Reynolds & Kamphaus, 1998), which provides information regarding possible psychological status in clinical (problem behavior) and adaptive (appropriate behavior) areas and includes both parent and teacher versions; and the Child Autism Rating Scale (CARS; Schopler, Reichler, and Renner, 1988), which is designed to identify children at risk for autism.

Despite the availability of these and a myriad of other behavioral checklists and questionnaires, it should be emphasized that **the value of simple, old-fashioned behavioral observation in both classroom and nonclassroom environments should not be underestimated.** Questions to be asked include those such as: *Does the child participate in group discussion? When the child is unable to follow verbal directions, is he or she paying attention to the speaker at the time the directions are given? Does the child exhibit greater difficulty during group discussions or when excess noise is present? Can the child independently complete activities or tasks once he or she knows what is expected? Is the child able to comply with daily procedural expectations, such as putting away a coat, taking a seat, and similar activities? What is the acoustic environment like? Does the child exhibit greater difficulty in some environments or classes than others? What teacher-, acoustic-, or group-related characteristics are present in those environments that are not present in those in which the child demonstrates less difficulty?* Answers to questions like these can provide valuable information in determining whether an auditory processing deficit may be present, or whether attention, behavior, or other issues are interfering with the child's ability to comply with auditory demands and instructions and to understand verbally presented information.

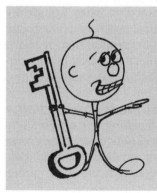

KEY CONCEPT

Behavioral observation in both classroom and nonclassroom environments provides invaluable information regarding listening behaviors.

Determining the Outcome of the CAPD Screening Process

The decision whether to refer a given child for comprehensive central auditory assessment should be a team one and should be based on information gathered during the screening process. At the beginning of this chapter, four primary questions to be answered by the screening process were listed. If the answer to all four questions is affirmative, then referral for comprehensive central auditory evaluation is warranted. Let us now see how a review of results from multidisciplinary assessments such as those listed above, along with findings from additional professionals such as occupational and physical therapists and medical professionals, may be used to answer these four questions.

Are the current evaluations that have already been completed sufficient in nature and scope to provide a picture of the child's strengths and weaknesses across domains? As emphasized previously in this chapter, it is critical that a good view of the child's functioning across cognitive, speech/language, academic, and other related domains be obtained prior to referral for central auditory assessment services. This practice not only fosters interdisciplinary interaction, but also helps in focusing on the whole child when the possible impact of CAPD and directions for management are being determined. Therefore, if basic, standardized assessments within these key areas have not yet been performed for children who are exhibiting language, learning, or communicative difficulty, it should be recommended that such information be obtained. Additional assessments, such as those relating to fine and gross motor skills, visual-motor integration, and similar multimodality functions may also be indicated prior to central auditory assessment referral. Finally, if possible medical conditions exist that may impact functioning (e.g., attention deficit with or without hyperactivity, seizure disorder, otitis media, neurologic disorder, psychiatric disorder), they should be addressed prior to initiating a referral for central auditory assessment, as conditions such as these either present an immediate danger to the health and well-being of the child or may impact processing and performance across modalities and affect reliability and validity of test results obtained.

Is there sufficient evidence to support the likelihood that a CAPD is present? Children with CAPD tend to exhibit certain common indicators of an auditory deficit. Often, they will behave as if they have a peripheral hearing loss, particularly in noisy or other low-redundancy listening situations, even though hearing sensitivity is within normal limits. This is frequently the initial symptom that causes referral for CAPD screening. Once the multidisciplinary assessment has been completed, the next step is to look for general trends and patterns across the information obtained that are characteristic, in general, of the CAPD population.

Audiologically, children with CAPD typically, but not always, exhibit normal hearing sensitivity. If a screening test such as the SCAN or SCAN-C is used, the child may fail one or more subtests; however, it has been my experience that many children with CAPD pass the SCAN. The reverse also is true. Therefore, **a passing score on audiologic screening tools such as the SCAN (or SCAN-C) should not be taken as evidence that further evaluation is unnecessary. Rather, it should be viewed in light of all other data obtained during the screening process.**

As previously discussed, children with CAPD will often demonstrate significant scatter across subtests within the domains assessed. For example, upon psychoeducational basic skills testing, a child may do quite well on the math subtests, but do poorly on reading and other language-based subtests. Likewise, in the classroom, children with CAPD are likely to perform more poorly in classes that are highly dependent on verbal language skills or are presented primarily via lecture format. On speech-language testing, children with CAPD may or may not exhibit a language disorder; however, they are very likely to do poorly on measures that tap auditory perceptual skills. In addition, depending on the underlying processing deficit, they may show decreased performance in areas such as vocabulary, sequencing, auditory discrimination, and phonological decoding or awareness skills. Conversely, syntax, semantics, and phonological abilities may appear fine; however, children may exhibit difficulty with nonverbal auditory abilities (such as musical aptitude, clapping or marching in rhythm, and singing) along with pragmatic difficulties and expressive or receptive prosodic deficits.

Cognitively, children with CAPD may exhibit normal or high IQ scores; however, verbal scores will most frequently be lower than performance scores. It should be noted, however, that **not all children with CAPD exhibit normal IQ scores. Therefore, we recommend that greater attention be given to any relative disparities between verbal and performance scores.** Often, children with CAPD will be classified as "learning disabled," because academic achievement does not meet intellectual capacity. Furthermore, it is possible that performance scores may be lower than verbal scores in cases of right-hemisphere dysfunction, which may affect auditory perception of nonlinguistic auditory input, such as prosody and communicative intent.

Information obtained from classroom teachers will frequently indicate that children with CAPD are distractible in the classroom and require a high degree of externally imposed organization in order to perform well. In addition, difficulty following multistep directions will often be noted. Children may be withdrawn or sullen and refuse to participate in classroom discussions, or may participate, but respond with comments that are inappropriate or demonstrate a lack of understanding of the discussion content. They may say "Huh?" or "What?" a lot, and discrimination errors may be noted in which the children appear to understand what is said, but fail to respond in the correct manner. When taking spelling tests, children with CAPD may either exhibit difficulty spelling in general, or may correctly spell words that sound like the target word, but are not. In particular, the current use of "invented spelling" (i.e., spelling words the way they sound) in lower grades may provide an indicator of children's phonological representation and sound-symbol association abilities. Finally, **if a child exhibits equal difficulty with routine tasks that rely on procedural memory, such as putting away his or her coat or going to the circle for the Pledge of Allegiance at the beginning of each day, as he or she does with novel instructions, the question of a possible higher-order executive or organizational disorder, rather than an auditory processing deficit, should be raised.**

Although some children with CAPD exhibit no significant neurologic or otologic sequelae, family history of learning disorders, or history of neurological trauma, it has been my observation that many children with CAPD do have a positive history of early chronic otitis media. In addition, if pressed, the parents often will acknowledge that either the father or the mother also had difficulties in school, were "slow readers," or struggled in some way academically. The child may have poor music and singing skills, although drawing and art skills will often be good.

Overall, the screening team should look for a general pattern in which skills and behaviors that rely upon listening and verbal language are relatively depressed when compared to those academic and personal pursuits that do not rely upon the auditory system. McFarland and Cacace (1995) discussed the need for modality specificity when defining and assessing central auditory processing abilities. Although auditory processing deficits are often accompanied by some difficulties in other modalities (discussed in subsequent chapters) when reviewing information gathered during the screening process, the screening team nevertheless should look for difficulties in those areas that particularly relate to audition, both linguistic and nonlinguistic.

Finally, it should be recognized that few children with CAPD will exhibit all of the above characteristics. It is not the task of the screening team to diagnose CAPD, but rather to calculate the likelihood, based on all of the data collected, that a CAPD is present. Methods of diagnosing and defining disorders of central auditory processing will be discussed in Chapters 5 and 6.

The key red flags to be on the alert for during the screening process, as discussed in this section, are summarized in Table 4-4. The following case studies are provided to illustrate the use of the multidisciplinary assessment results in the determination of the likelihood of CAPD being present. All of the children discussed below had a history of chronic otitis media, which was one of the key factors that led to their being referred for central auditory screening.

Case Study #1

J.P. was a 7-year-old boy with a history of possible pervasive developmental delay (PDD). At an early age, J.P. was diagnosed with autism; however, this diagnosis had recently been questioned by his medical and educational team. At the time of central auditory screening, J.P. was receiving a variety of special education services, including speech-language intervention, learning resource services, and occupational and physical therapy.

Table 4-4
Common Indicators of CAPD

- Behaves as if peripheral hearing loss is present, despite normal hearing
- Demonstrates significant scatter across subtests within domains assessed by speech-language and psychoeducational tests, with weaknesses in auditory-dependent areas
- Verbal IQ scores often lower than performance scores
- Requires high degree of external organization in the classroom
- Exhibits difficulty following multistep directions
- Exhibits poor reading and spelling skills
- May refuse to participate in class discussions or respond inappropriately
- May be withdrawn or sullen
- Exhibits a positive history of chronic otitis or other otologic or neurologic sequelae
- May exhibit poor singing and music skills
- Motor skills (gross and fine) may be deficient

Behaviorally, J.P. exhibited the following traits in the classroom and at home:

- Extreme distractibility, especially under conditions of excess visual or auditory activity in the environment
- Sensitivity to loud sounds, including the vacuum cleaner and the fire alarm
- Difficulty following even simple directions
- Preference for watching television rather than reading or playing outside
- Difficulty initiating and completing tasks in all classes and at home
- Need for frequent repetition (however, he did not ask others to repeat, he merely stared at them uncomprehendingly until they rephrased the information presented)
- Social isolation, preferring to engage in tasks alone or in a parallel play, rather than interactive, manner
- Inconsistent attention to verbal input, especially when engaged in another task (such as watching television)

J.P.'s cognitive evaluation (WISC-III) revealed:

- Verbal and performance cognitive capacity relatively evenly developed, with significant scatter among subtests
- Significant weaknesses in the areas of visual-motor integration, visual tracking, spatial perception, following directions, abstract verbal reasoning, and solving verbal math problems
- Significant strengths in the areas of auditory comprehension of simple sentences and stories and memory for digits
- Poor verbal and nonverbal reasoning abilities

Psychoeducational testing (W-J III) indicated that J.P. exhibited:

- Poor basic math calculation abilities
- Poor reading and spelling abilities for both sight word and word attack skills
- Difficulty with letter, number, and color identification
- Relatively evenly developed academic abilities across all domains

Speech and language testing revealed:

- Below-average receptive and expressive vocabulary skills
- Difficulty understanding complex language forms
- Excellent comprehension of verbally presented information using simple linguistic units

- Weak oral expression, including immature sentence forms and difficulty formulating sentences based on abstract concepts
- Good ability to answer questions relating to concrete details of a story or passage, but difficulty drawing inferences or determining what will happen next
- Articulation errors, including tongue thrust and difficulty with [s], [th], and [z]
- Poor sound blending and auditory figure/ground abilities

Additional findings from other members of the multidisciplinary team indicated that J.P. exhibited:

- General fine and gross motor difficulties, including difficulty cutting with scissors, copying simple patterns, kicking a ball, heel- and toe-walking, clapping in rhythm, and all other tasks assessed
- Lack of a clear hand preference
- Some delay in adaptive living skills, such as dressing himself when fastening buttons was required, simple meal preparation, and bathing independently

On auditory questionnaires (CHAPS), J.P.'s teachers reported that J.P. had difficulty in all acoustic environments if information presented was particularly complex or if visual or auditory distractors were present. In contrast, J.P.'s parents reported that J.P. performed auditory tasks much better in quiet listening environments. Because of J.P.'s distractibility, a trial with Ritalin was suggested by his physician. During this trial, J.P. exhibited:

- Significant improvement in auditory discrimination, sound blending, following simple directions, and other auditory-related tasks
- No improvement in visual-spatial or motor abilities, with the exception of visual figure/ground abilities

Impressions:

Results of the multidisciplinary evaluation suggested that J.P. did not exhibit a CAPD as a primary contributing factor to his difficulties. Specific evidence to suggest that CAPD was not a primary concern included articulation errors that were developmental (rather than acoustic) in nature, relative weaknesses in nonauditory areas (visual-spatial, motor), strengths in auditory comprehension, and improvement in phonological awareness and related auditory abilities when medicated with Ritalin. Of particular interest was J.P.'s difficulty identifying numbers and colors in addition to letters. Although problems with sound-letter identification are often seen in cases of CAPD, number and color identification typically is intact by age 7 and these skills are not dependent on auditory function. Finally, J.P.'s delay in adaptive living skills and other, nonauditory areas provided clear evidence that a CAPD was not a primary contributing factor in this case. Indeed, it appeared that auditory processing might be an area of relative strength for this young boy. As such, it was recommended that further exploration of J.P.'s visual-spatial, motor, and sensory integration issues be undertaken. In addition, because of the improvement noted in auditory-related skills with Ritalin, J.P.'s physician recommended that he continue with the medication, even though he did not meet all of the diagnostic criteria for AD/HD.

Case Study #2

C.M., a 10-year-old boy, presented with a history of language processing and academic difficulties. At the time of screening, he was receiving special education services under the dual classification of learning disability and speech-language disorder, as well as occupational therapy for fine motor concerns. The following behavioral traits were noted:

- Difficulty initiating work independently and remaining on task in academic classes
- Difficulty remembering day-to-day routines, including sequence of classes in the academic day, combined with consistent, daily difficulty finding materials (e.g., books, writing utensils, paper) in his desk or backpack
- Occasional use of immature language forms or clowning behaviors, especially when frustrated or during social communication situations
- Difficulty following directions
- Off-topic contributions to classroom discussions
- Difficulty comprehending verbally presented information, with frequent requests for repetition, especially in noisy or distracting environments
- Use of verbal rehearsal (repetition of information) as a memory strategy
- Difficulty sitting still for even a relatively short period of time, with a tendency to play with objects in his reach or crawl onto (or under) the table; frequent verbal redirection was required

Cognitive assessment (WISC-III) conducted with C.M. indicated:

- Overall cognitive abilities in the low average range
- Verbal ability slightly (but not significantly) better than performance ability
- Scatter in nonverbal tasks, with strengths in areas requiring memory for visual detail and sequencing steps in a story (i.e., WISC-III: Picture Completion, Picture Arrangement, Symbol Search) and weaknesses in copying designs (graphomotor skills)
- More evenly developed verbal skills, with weaknesses only in the areas of solving verbal math problems and social judgment

Psychoeducational testing (W-J R) revealed:

- Difficulty with any task (visual or auditory) when fluid reasoning, generalization, or making inferences was required
- Auditory and visual memory difficulties (both short- and long-term)
- Difficulty with any task requiring a motor output response
- Weaknesses in oral reading and written language, with a relative strength in simple math calculation

Speech and language assessment indicated:

- Age-appropriate receptive and expressive vocabulary
- Significant difficulty with a variety of receptive and expressive language tasks, including categorization, reasoning (e.g., same versus different, drawing inferences), word retrieval, sentence formulation, semantic relationships, and critical thinking skills
- Excellent phonological awareness and spelling (both word attack and sight word) abilities when each was assessed separately, accompanied by poor reading comprehension
- Poor performance on all SCAN subtests (Competing Words, Auditory Figure/Ground, and Filtered Words)

It was noted by both the psychologist and speech-language pathologist that C.M.'s performance on all tests was inconsistent in that he would sometimes miss easy items while, at the same time, completing far more difficult tasks accurately. This inconsistency suggested that the results were a minimal estimate of C.M.'s true functioning abilities. Behavioral questionnaires (CHAPS) filled out by C.M.'s teachers indicated that C.M. exhibited difficulty with auditorily presented information when not paying attention, when extremely complex language forms were used, or when involved in other tasks, regardless of acoustic environment. No other specific auditory difficulties were noted.

Impressions:
Although it was clear that C.M. had difficulty with a variety of auditory-related tasks, he also had difficulty with tasks that could not be considered auditory in nature. Indeed, C.M. appeared to exhibit overall language processing difficulties, both receptively and expressively. Evidence to support this contention included the wide variety of language areas impacted, including sentence formulation, word retrieval, critical thinking and reasoning skills, and so forth. Moreover, C.M. exhibited some possible signs of an attention-related confound, including being easily distracted both auditorily and visually and exhibiting difficulty remaining in his seat. The fact that C.M. exhibited his weakest cognitive performance on tasks requiring motor output and nonverbal cognitive areas, combined with the fact that he had difficulty remembering day-to-day procedures and demonstrated significant inconsistency within measures, suggested the possibility of a higher-order executive function or language confound. Although he performed poorly on the SCAN, there was some question raised by the speech-language pathologist as to whether he really understood the directions. The presence of poor reading comprehension abilities in the face of excellent decoding and sight word abilities provided additional evidence of a higher-level language-based deficit. It was concluded that although processing verbal information (or language processing) was clearly an area of difficulty for C.M., it was unlikely that a primary CAPD was the key factor in his deficit. Therefore, comprehensive central auditory testing was not recommended at the time. Rather, it was recommended that attention be given to higher-order linguistic, metalinguistic, and metacognitive skills to improve C.M.'s overall language, reasoning, and problem-solving skills. (*Note*: Subsequent central auditory testing conducted for follow-up research purposes to assess accuracy of screening conclusions indicated no evidence of a CAPD in this case.)

Case Study #3

K.R. was a 15-year-old girl with a history of language delay and academic difficulties. Of particular concern was her social and emotional well-being, as she exhibited a history of bedwetting and related behaviors indicative of anxiety. K.R.'s parents had not requested an educational evaluation prior to the time of this screening because of their fear that she would be "labeled" and suffer additional social/emotional harm. However, she was receiving private speech therapy for an articulation deficit, which will be discussed subsequently, as well as private tutoring for reading and related difficulties. Independent speech-language, cognitive, and psychoeducational testing was conducted prior to central auditory screening.

According to parent report, K.R. exhibited:

- Extremely slow response time to verbally presented questions or requests for information
- Chronic bedwetting dating from infancy
- Withdrawal from communicative situations and preference for motor or visual activities, such as solitary sports (bowling, track, gymnastics) and art
- Anxiety and depression, including frequent crying, acting-out behaviors, possible recreational drug use (suspected by her parents but never confirmed), and possible sexual promiscuity (again, never confirmed)
- Poor ability to express herself verbally or in writing accompanied by an expressed dislike for recreational reading
- Lack of follow-through on verbally presented directions or instructions
- Quiet, difficult-to-understand speech
- History of articulation deficit related to infantile suckle and tongue thrust

Cognitive evaluation (WISC-III) undertaken at age 15 indicated:

- Average verbal cognitive abilities and above average to superior performance abilities
- Relative weaknesses in general fund of knowledge and verbal comprehension abilities, with a strength in visual-spatial perception
- Reticence to guess when she wasn't sure of the answer, particularly during verbal activities

Psychoeducational testing (W-J III) revealed that K.R. exhibited:

- Average academic achievement abilities in all broad areas, with excellent performance in mathematics
- Superior abilities in fundamental skills subserving reading (i.e., word attack, phonological awareness, word identification and discrimination, sight word abilities, reading speed, reading accuracy) accompanied by poor reading comprehension abilities
- Inconsistent classroom performance, with grades ranging from As to Ds and no clear pattern of performance (e.g., Ds in Spanish [reliant on auditory skills] and art [despite very

good art ability]; As in social studies [a lecture-based class] and physical education)

The psychologist who performed cognitive and psychoeducational testing noted that K.R.'s responses were often quite delayed and that she seemed to have some difficulty sustaining attention to tasks, especially those that she deemed "boring." Furthermore, because K.R.'s older brother had been diagnosed with attention-deficit disorder, the possibility of ADD was raised in this case. However, K.R.'s parents did not follow through on recommendations for a medical consultation. Because of K.R.'s slow response time to verbally presented information, a speech-language evaluation was undertaken. This assessment revealed:

- Overall expressive and receptive vocabulary abilities in the high average range
- Slow rate of speech, possibly suggesting slow language processing or formulation speed
- Very low speaking volume (which she was able to control upon demand) accompanied by insufficient breath control during speaking
- Relative weaknesses in reasoning, concepts and directions, semantics, word association, and social judgment (pragmatics); however, overall language abilities were in the average range
- Good auditory discrimination abilities combined with poor auditory memory for words, nonwords, digits, and sentences
- Average dichotic listening and filtered words performance, but poor auditory figure/ground (speech-in-noise) abilities as assessed by the SCAN-C

Based on these findings, it was concluded that K.R. exhibited an "auditory processing deficit" impacting auditory memory, speech-in-noise skills, and receptive language abilities. However, it should be noted that the terms *language processing* and *auditory processing* were used interchangeably by the private speech-language pathologist, psychologist, and parents in this case. On the CHAPS, neither K.R.'s parents, teachers, therapists, nor K.R. herself reported any difficulty in auditory skills, regardless of acoustic environment, except when extremely complex language forms or multistep directions were used. Nevertheless, the speech-language pathologist suggested the use of an assistive listening device in the classroom, a suggestion the school district was reluctant to follow until further exploration of K.R.'s central auditory abilities was undertaken.

Impressions:

It was concluded that a fair amount of data existed to suggest that K.R. did not exhibit a primary CAPD. Indeed, those areas most closely related to auditory processing appeared to be areas of relative strength for K.R., including phonological awareness, discrimination, dichotic listening, and related skills. In contrast, K.R.'s comprehension of verbal (and written) information did appear to be impacted, suggesting the presence of a higher-order language-based disorder. Further complicating K.R.'s case was the presence of behaviors that were not consistent with either language or auditory processing deficit, including chronic bedwetting, depression, anxiety, anti-social tendencies, and issues related to vocal volume and breath control. The lack of a clear pattern in academic performance also was an area of concern that seemed to suggest an underlying factor not related to language or cognitive abilities. For these reasons, it was concluded that comprehensive central auditory assessment was not warranted in this case; however, further exploration of language processing issues was recommended. Most important, psychological follow-up for the social/emotional concerns was felt to be critical.

Despite these conclusions, K.R.'s parents continued to be convinced that CAPD was at the root of all of her difficulties. Therefore, comprehensive central auditory assessment was undertaken at their expense. Results of the assessment indicated no evidence of central auditory dysfunction. The recommendations listed above were made again; however, at the time of this writing, it is unknown whether K.R.'s parents have taken steps to follow through on the suggestions made by the multidisciplinary team.

These case studies all have concerned children for whom a CAPD does not appear to be present, or does not appear to be a primary contributing factor to learning or communication difficulties. The following case studies illustrate situations in which central auditory evaluation did, indeed, appear warranted.

Case Study #4

A.L. was an 11-year-old girl who was receiving special education services under the classification of speech and language impairment. She had previously been classified as learning disabled in the areas of reading and written language as well, but her most recent evaluation had suggested that she no longer met state criteria for that classification. A.L. had been diagnosed with AD/HD at a young age and was taking Adderall daily. The use of medication was extremely successful in controlling A.L.'s attention-related difficulties; however, concerns regarding specific areas remained even when medicated. Behaviorally, A.L.'s teachers and parents reported that she exhibited:

- Good ability to sustain attention (when medicated) and to complete tasks once they were initiated in the classroom and at home
- Some difficulty understanding during lecture-based classes despite good effort, especially in noisy environments
- Reticence to join in group discussions and difficulty answering questions posed in the classroom
- Frequent requests for repetition or clarification of verbally presented instructions or information, but good follow-through once they were understood
- Dislike for reading, both recreationally and for classroom assignments
- Frustration during conversational situations in backgrounds of noise

A.R.'s cognitive evaluation (WISC-III) indicated:

- Overall cognitive capacity in the average range, with performance abilities somewhat (but not significantly) better than verbal abilities
- Significant scatter in subtests, with strengths in visual-abstract perceptual skills and weaknesses in following directions, solving verbal math problems, and auditory comprehension

Psychoeducational testing (W-J III) revealed:

- Very slow oral and silent reading rate, particularly as related to sound-symbol association and word attack (phonological decoding) abilities, leading to poor reading comprehension
- Good math calculation and abstract reasoning skills
- Poor spelling skills accompanied by relatively good written language abilities
- Good academic performance in "nonauditory" classes such as art, physical education, and mathematics (however, solving math word problems was an area of difficulty for A.R.) along with below-average performance in lecture-based classes such as social studies
- Good performance during science experiments and labs, with poor performance on tests covering information presented in lecture

Speech and language evaluation indicated:

- Average to low-average receptive vocabulary and language abilities accompanied by good expressive language skills
- Difficulty comprehending sequenced directions
- Poor phonological awareness, speech-sound and word discrimination, and short-term auditory recall abilities

On the CHAPS, A.R.'s teachers reported that A.R. exhibited signs of frustration and difficulty in noisy environments, and did much better in quiet or when multimodality cues were added. She also exhibited the most difficulty with linguistically complex material, particularly in backgrounds of noise.

Impressions:

Based on these findings, it was determined that a CAPD affecting speech-sound discrimination and related abilities may well be impacting A.R.'s comprehension and learning in the classroom. Analysis of patterns across cognitive, psychoeducational, and speech/language evaluations indicated difficulties in those areas that are thought to be subserved, at least in part, by auditory processing skills. These include phonological awareness and decoding, comprehension of lecture-based academic information, reading rate and accuracy, and related abilities. For this reason, it was suggested that a comprehensive central auditory evaluation be conducted. When this evaluation was undertaken, it was found that A.R. did, indeed, exhibit diagnostic findings consistent with CAPD affecting phonological representation and speech-sound processing. Methods of assessing and interpreting central auditory tests will be addressed in subsequent chapters.

As we will see later in this book, not all types of CAPD affect speech-sound processing per se. Rather, some forms of CAPD impact those auditory skills thought to be subserved by areas of the brain not traditionally considered to be phonologic- or language-related in nature, including the right hemisphere.

The following case illustrates a situation in which comprehensive central auditory assessment was indicated by the screening process, despite the presence of a pattern of findings that was very different from that seen in A.R.'s case.

Case Study #5

At 9 years of age, L.F. had few friends and preferred to engage in solitary pursuits. At the time of screening, he was not receiving special education services largely because of good basic academic achievement in most areas; however, a multidisciplinary evaluation was indicated because of concerns noted in mathematics class and social/emotional concerns.

Behaviorally, L.F. exhibited:

- Some distractibility and impulsivity, especially when engaged in social communication situations
- Poor sense of humor, with difficulty in both understanding and delivering the punch lines of jokes
- Frequent complaints of mistreatment by others, especially related to being teased or yelled at on the playground
- Difficulty sequencing multistep directions, despite an ability to perform each step of the process accurately
- High anxiety level in social situations
- Restricted facial and vocal affect, leading to a wooden or "flat" expression and voice quality
- Dislike of creative writing, art, imaginative play, and music activities and preference for reading science fiction stories and playing video games or rule-governed board games
- Tendency to take things too literally and to be overwhelmed easily when creative problem solving was required

L.F.'s cognitive evaluation (WISC-III) indicated:

- Overall cognitive capacity in the superior range, with verbal abilities slightly (but not significantly) better developed than performance abilities and some scatter in subtests
- Relative weaknesses in auditory comprehension involving social judgment, part-to-whole synthesis (e.g., object assembly), abstract verbal reasoning abilities, and abstract visual abilities (e.g., block design)
- Relative strengths in fund of general knowledge, short-term auditory memory, vocabulary, and processing speed

Psychoeducational testing (W-J R) revealed:

- Excellent reading speed, accuracy, and comprehension, despite poor sight word reading abilities
- Relatively evenly developed academic achievement across all other areas, except for a significant weakness in math computation

Speech and language testing indicated:

- Superior receptive and expressive vocabulary abilities

- Above-average receptive and expressive language abilities, with the exception of sequencing multistep directions
- Difficulty with abstract reasoning and storytelling skills, generation of creative ideas, and expression of ideas and emotions
- Good story comprehension and ability to answer questions related to the details of a passage accompanied by difficulty identifying the main theme or concept of the same story or passage
- Poor pragmatics and social communication skills
- Poor use of vocal prosody accompanied by relatively flat facial affect

On the CHAPS, L.F.'s parents reported quite different findings from those of his teachers. Although his parents reported that he had difficulty in virtually every auditory-related arena, regardless of acoustic environment or complexity of information, his teachers reported virtually no auditory difficulties except when sequencing of particularly complex information was required.

Impressions:

Results of the multidisciplinary team evaluation indicated that L.F. may exhibit a CAPD specifically relating to the processing of nonlinguistic, intonation-related auditory information that allows one to determine what is *meant* versus what is *said*. The overall pattern of difficulties exhibited by L.F. suggested a strong possibility of right-hemisphere dysfunction or nonverbal learning disability affecting his abstract reasoning, part-to-whole synthesis, math calculation, and related skills. The auditory difficulties he appeared to be experiencing likely were merely one part of a larger entity affecting various aspects of his social communication and learning. A comprehensive central auditory evaluation was recommended to explore further these auditory manifestations. Results of the evaluation confirmed the suspicion of right-hemisphere-based CAPD. Information regarding diagnostic indicators of this type of auditory deficit, as well as directions for management, will be provided in subsequent chapters.

Once it is decided that a central auditory evaluation is indicated, it still remains to be determined whether the child is capable of participating in such testing and whether the information obtained from central auditory assessment will add significantly to the management program for the child.

Is the child capable of participating in comprehensive central auditory assessment?

Even if the likelihood of the presence of CAPD has been determined and it is felt that further evaluation is necessary, it may be determined that, for one reason or another, the child in question cannot be tested using present assessment tools.

As discussed in Part One, a mental age of 7 or 8 is required for most tests of central auditory processing. Therefore, comprehensive behavioral evaluation of very young children is not possible at the present time, although electrophysiologic measures of central auditory function may be quite useful in this population, as will be discussed in later chapters. Likewise, although children with hearing loss may also exhibit concomitant central auditory processing disorders, many of the assessment tools in current use require normal or near-normal peripheral hearing sensitivity.

Finally, the presence of significant cognitive, attention, or behavioral disorders may interfere with a child's ability to participate in comprehensive central auditory testing. Normal cognitive capacity is not necessary for participation in central auditory evaluation; however, the child must be able to follow the instructions and deliver the appropriate response required of each test used. In cases of children with very low cognitive ability, extreme hyperactivity that is uncontrolled by medication, or emotional or behavioral disorders that may result in refusal to cooperate, it may be impossible to administer a behavioral battery of central auditory processing tests.

It should be noted that, **by deciding not to refer for comprehensive assessment based on these reasons, the screening team is not implying that a CAPD is not present. Rather, it should be acknowledged that although the child may exhibit CAPD, the presence of such a disorder cannot be confirmed at the present time.** More important, intervention should not be withheld simply on the basis of an inability to test reliably. Although a deficit-specific management program cannot be developed without the identification of the underlying dysfunctional process, many management strategies may be employed that address the child's most significant presenting complaints. A later chapter on management will delineate various intervention strategies that may be implemented in these situations. Results of the multidisciplinary team assessment, as outlined in this chapter, are invaluable in determining relative areas of functional weakness and guiding directions for intervention and management in these cases.

Would results of comprehensive central auditory assessment add information that is likely to affect the overall assessment and management of the child's learning and communication difficulties?

On occasion, children will be referred for CAPD screening who, after having been determined to be eligible for special education services in the area of learning disabilities or language delay, are already receiving comprehensive special education services that target their disability areas. For example, the child with reading difficulties, as well as difficulty hearing in noisy environments, may undergo daily therapy with a reading specialist who focuses on auditory discrimination and speech-to-print skills. In addition, environmental modifications may already be in place for the purpose of improving the child's access to auditory information in the classroom. **It is possible that comprehensive central auditory evaluation, even if results of such an evaluation confirm the presence of a CAPD, may result in little or no contribution to the overall management of the child. In this situation, the screening team may prudently decide not to refer for comprehensive central auditory assessment at the present time because the cost of such testing, in terms of time and money, may outweigh the potential benefit.**

This having been said, readers should be cautioned that not all central auditory processing disorders are alike and, depending on the underlying dysfunctional process, recommendations for management will differ greatly. Therefore, clinicians should avoid at all costs blanket statements regarding what is an appropriate management strategy for all children with CAPD. Chapter 6 will discuss interpretation of central auditory assessment results, and management will be covered in subsequent chapters. Clinicians should be familiar with the range of possible profiles within the larger category of CAPD, as well as differential, deficit-specific management recommendations, before determining that intervention strategies currently in place for a given child are adequate.

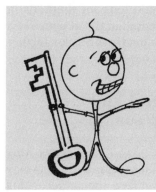

KEY CONCEPT

The clinician should avoid at all costs blanket statements regarding management approaches appropriate for all children with CAPD.

Table 4-5

Key Factors in Determining the Need for Comprehensive Central
Auditory Assessment

- Completeness of current evaluations

  Have the child's overall cognitive, learning, and language abilities been assessed? Are there any medical or other factors that should be considered prior to central auditory assessment?

- Likelihood of the presence of CAPD

  Does the child exhibit patterns across multidisciplinary evaluation results and behavioral observations that are consistent with probable CAPD?

- Ability to evaluate the child

  Does the child have the necessary cognitive, attention, or related ability to participate in a behavioral comprehensive central auditory evaluation?

- Need for additional management recommendations

  Will the results of a comprehensive central auditory assessment contribute significantly to the child's overall educational plan?

In conclusion, data collected from the screening process should be reviewed for trends across findings that suggest the presence of CAPD. Prior to referral for a comprehensive central auditory assessment, it should also be ascertained that sufficient assessments of cognitive, speech/language, and related abilities have been performed, that the child has the capacity to participate in the assessment procedure, and that the comprehensive evaluation will add sufficient additional information to the child's educational picture to justify the time and effort spent in such a pursuit. Finally, in those cases in which complete assessment procedures cannot be performed but a CAPD is likely to be present, the screening team should look for methods in which intervention strategies may be implemented in the absence of a confirmation of CAPD. Key factors in determining the need for further central auditory assessment are outlined in Table 4-5.

Final Considerations in Central Auditory Processing Disorders Screening

The importance of screening for CAPD has been discussed in this chapter, as have the methods through which screening for CAPD may be accomplished. However, it must be recognized that a screening program, no matter how efficient and well-organized, is of no use unless a clear, workable plan for follow-through is implemented as well. In particular, a comprehensive diagnostic assessment program must be in place and the outcomes of the screening process must be monitored.

In many geographical areas, resources for diagnosis and treatment may not be available, due either to lack of funding or lack of trained professionals to carry out the necessary steps involved in performing comprehensive central auditory evaluation and making recommendations for management. If the implementation of a CAPD screening program is under consideration, the availability of follow-up services for children identified by screening should be carefully investigated. As stated by Musiek, Gollegly, Lamb, and Lamb (1990), **even though procedures exist to diagnose most central auditory processing disorders, it should not be assumed that they will be available in a given locale.** Comprehensive central auditory evaluation is necessary to confirm and define the disorder, as well as for developing a deficit-specific management program. Therefore, **implementation of a screening program without the means of diagnostic and therapeutic follow-through is nothing short of a futile expenditure of time and effort.**

Unfortunately, considerable education on the part of special education professionals and audiologists is needed regarding the nature of CAPD and central auditory assessment for an appropriate service delivery program to be implemented. I have encountered many regions throughout the country in which a screening program, such as the one described in this chapter, has been put into place without appropriate means of follow-through, and is used for diagnostic purposes. **It cannot be overemphasized that the procedures discussed in this chapter are for screening purposes only, and complete diagnostic procedures are a vital, integral portion of the overall CAPD service delivery system.**

A second consideration is that of monitoring the outcome of any screening program. Data should be collected regarding the number of children referred for screening, the number referred for comprehensive evaluation, and the number ultimately identified as exhibiting CAPD. These numbers can serve as benchmarks for outcome measures and can be used to monitor quality assurance, effectiveness, and efficiency of the given program and its individual team members. These numbers can also be compared more globally to national normative values for similar programs, once such values are available. In this manner, overall effectiveness of the screening program may be established and directions for further modifications in the process may be suggested.

Finally, the success of any screening program depends on cooperation from all persons involved. Therefore, efforts should be made to ensure coordination among all facets of the screening program, from administrative support to funding, data collection, decision making, and follow-through. Only in this way can a CAPD screening program achieve its ultimate goal: the identification of children with CAPD.

Summary

This chapter has reviewed several basic considerations in screening for CAPD. The need for a CAPD screening program is evidenced by the estimated prevalence of auditory processing disorders in the educational setting and the potential impact of such a disorder on children's learning. The primary purpose of CAPD screening is to determine the need for referral for additional diagnostic testing.

Screening for CAPD should be approached from a multidisciplinary team perspective so that information can be collected that will reflect the whole child. In determining the need for further evaluation, the team should be on the alert for general trends across data that suggest relative difficulty in academic, cognitive, and behavioral areas that are most dependent on audition. In addition, the team should ascertain that further evaluation will add sufficient additional information to justify the time and effort involved in such a pursuit, and that the child in question is capable of participating in comprehensive central auditory evaluation procedures.

Finally, the implementation of a screening program will be of no use unless adequate resources are available for appropriate follow-through. Therefore, CAPD screening is just one component, albeit a vital one, of the entire CAPD service delivery system.

Review Questions

1. What is the primary purpose of screening for CAPD?

2. What four questions should be answered by the CAPD screening?

3. Discuss the justification factors that help to document the need for a CAPD screening program.

4. Why should a multidisciplinary team approach be utilized in CAPD screening?

5. List the core members of the CAP screening team and discuss the relative contribution of each.

6. Discuss the reason(s) why the screening tools discussed in this chapter should never be used for diagnostic purposes.

7. Identify several speech-language, psychoeducational, and cognitive test tools that may provide valuable information to the CAP screening team.

8. Discuss the behavioral, academic, language, and cognitive characteristics typically associated with CAPD.

9. What should be done if a child is suspected of having a CAPD, but a comprehensive central auditory assessment cannot be performed due to age, cognitive ability, or other reasons?

10. Discuss the factors necessary to ensure the success of a CAP screening program.

CHAPTER

FIVE

Overview of Central Tests

Once the likelihood of the presence of a central auditory processing disorder has been determined, it falls to the audiologist to perform assessments that will determine whether a CAPD is present and, if so, attempt to quantify and qualify the disorder. This chapter provides a basic overview of central tests. The rationale for use of a test battery approach to assess auditory processing skills in children and the issues of validity and reliability of central tests will also be considered. Administration protocols for specific test tools as well as suggestions for choosing the components of the test battery based on individual need will be provided in Chapter 6.

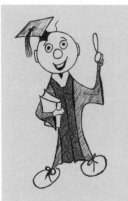

Learning Objectives

After studying this chapter, the reader should be able to:

1. Discuss the rationale for a test battery approach to CAP assessment.
2. Distinguish between validity and reliability of central tests and discuss the importance of test validity in central assessment.
3. Describe the major categories of central tests and discuss the purpose of each.

Rationale for Test Battery Approach

A question I often hear is, "What is the best test of central auditory processing?" This is a difficult, if not impossible, question to answer as there is no one test that is sufficient in scope to address the complexities of the CANS. As seen in Part One, the CANS is a highly redundant, complex system. Therefore, it is logical that the assessment of the CANS would, likewise, be redundant and complex.

The question to be answered by the central assessment is of paramount importance. If the question is simply, "Is a central auditory processing deficit present?" then the use of one or two valid test tools may be all that is needed to obtain an adequate answer. However, **if central assessment is undertaken with an eye toward identification of the underlying deficient processes and development of a deficit-specific management plan, then the assessment procedure must tap a variety of mechanisms.**

It is my opinion that the simple identification of the presence or absence of CAPD is insufficient. As will be seen in the next chapter, the outcome of a central assessment should be the development of an auditory profile that delineates the child's auditory strengths and weaknesses. Using this profile, a management program that will build upon the individual child's strengths and assist in overcoming the weaknesses may be designed. Therefore, the use of different tests that assess different processes is necessary. Again, it should be emphasized that knowledge of the underlying neuroanatomy and neurophysiology is essential in order to choose those test tools that will best provide clinicians with the information necessary to interpret the assessment results and make recommendations for management.

An additional purpose of CAP testing is the differentiation of site of lesion or dysfunction. It is my contention that this issue cannot be separated from that of describing auditory processing abilities in the clinical population. The identification of site of lesion, or level of dysfunction within the brain, will have a significant impact on recommendations for management, including the need for medical referral. Clinicians should be aware that, although rare, neurological disorders requiring medical intervention can and do occur in the school-age population. Therefore, clinicians engaging in central assessment must continually be on the lookout for symptoms that may indicate the need for neurological or other medical referral. Again, in order to investigate fully the system in question, it will be necessary to utilize tests that assess different processes and different levels and to examine the test results for trends and comparisons across assessment tools.

Finally, as stated by Musiek and Lamb (1994), the audiologist's job is the evaluation of hearing. Hearing does not end with the peripheral auditory system. Rather, peripheral acuity is merely the first step in the overall process of hearing. Therefore, from a philosophical perspective, **it is the audiologist's responsibility to assess all factors that affect hearing in the child or adult, and this includes evaluation of the central auditory system. The utilization of several test tools which assess a variety of processes represents the state of the art in current CAP assessment and should become the standard of care.**

It should be noted that I have been discussing specifically those tests designed for the evaluation of the CANS. However, when one considers comprehensive CAP assessment, the results of cognitive, speech/language, educational, and other measures should not be forgotten. Indeed, these findings will play a large role in interpreting CAP assessment findings as well as making recommendations for management. Therefore, in a very practical sense, the assessment of central auditory processing abilities in the school-age child should be a multidisciplinary one, and the screening tools discussed in the previous chapter will become an essential part of the overall CAP test battery.

In conclusion, one single test is not sufficient to explore dysfunction fully in any sensory system. When evaluating the peripheral auditory system, a test battery approach is utilized, including pure-tone air- and bone-conduction testing, word recognition measures, immittance testing, and other measures deemed necessary. Comprehensive assessment of central auditory processing abilities is certainly no exception. **Only through the use of a well-chosen test battery, in conjunction with information supplied by associated professionals and other individuals in a multidisciplinary manner, will audiologists engaged in central auditory assessment be able to delineate those processes that are dysfunctional; evaluate the impact of the dysfunction on children's educational, medical, and social status; and make appropriate recommendations for deficit-specific management that will address an individual child's needs.**

Test Validity and Reliability

The clinical validity and reliability of tests of central auditory function are often called into question, and rightly so. However, it is my experience that these issues are often poorly understood and frequently confused. An understanding of the meanings of these terms as well as the methods through which validity and reliability of a given test tool are determined will assist clinicians in critically evaluating literature pertaining to specific test tools on the market, wisely choosing tools for clinical use, and increasing confidence in the interpretation of results of a comprehensive assessment.

The terms *validity* and *reliability* are not interchangeable, although both are important when evaluating the clinical utility of a given test tool. Very simply, validity refers to a test's ability to assess that condition(s) it purports to assess. **In other words, in order to determine the clinical validity of a test procedure, it must be demonstrated that the test typically will be abnormal in those subjects who present with the specific disorder in question and that the test typically will be normal in those subjects who do not present with the disorder. Reliability is the degree to which the test will yield the same results within the test session or upon repeat testing.**

Figure 5-1 provides an example of a decision matrix to use in determining the validity of diagnostic test tools. A *true positive* is a positive finding in subjects who do, in fact, have the disorder or disease, or an indication of the test's ability to identify correctly the presence of the disorder (hit). Conversely, a *false positive* is a positive finding on the test in subjects who do not have the disorder (false alarm). Likewise, a true negative is a negative finding in subjects who do not

TEST RESULT

	ABNORMAL	NORMAL
DISORDER PRESENT	True Positive (hit)	False Negative (miss)
DISORDER ABSENT	False Positive (false alarm)	True Negative (correct rejection)

Figure 5-1. Sample decision matrix for determining the validity of diagnostic test tools.

have the disorder, or an indication of the test's ability to identify correctly the absence of the disorder (correct rejection). Finally, a false negative is a negative finding in subjects who do, in fact, have the disorder (miss) (Turner & Nielsen, 1984).

The sensitivity of a diagnostic test is the number of true positives (hits) over the total number of true positives and false negatives (hits and misses). Therefore, *sensitivity* refers to the degree to which the test is able to identify correctly the presence of a disorder. The number of true negatives (correct rejections) over the total number of false positives and true negatives (false alarms and correct rejections) is referred to as *specificity,* or the test's ability to identify correctly those subjects who do not have the disorder. *Efficiency* refers to the test's overall degree of both sensitivity and specificity, or the test's ability to identify correctly both the presence and the absence of a disorder.

As sensitivity of a test increases, specificity decreases, and vice versa. The reason for this is quite simple. **The more sensitive a test is,**

the more likely it is to result in false alarms. The reverse is also true: the more specific a test is, the more likely it will be that some subjects who have the disorder will be missed.

In making clinical decisions regarding the choice of test tools, clinicians will need to choose those tools that will best meet the needs of the individual situation. Therefore, depending on the question to be answered, the necessary degree of sensitivity and specificity of the test tool may change. For example, if the clinician is concerned that the presence of a life-threatening disorder is quite possible, it may be more prudent to err on the side of the conservative. In this situation, the clinician may decide that it would be better to have a false alarm than to miss the disease altogether. Therefore, the clinician is likely to choose a highly sensitive test tool even though the chance of a false positive finding may be greater.

On the other hand, if the disorder in question is unlikely to occur in the given population, specificity may be more important than sensitivity. Let us consider the current audiological issue of universal newborn hearing screening. As the likelihood of finding a significant hearing loss in a well newborn is quite low, choosing a test that yields a smaller degree of false positives may be more desirable, as this would reduce the incidence of unnecessary referrals for further audiological evaluation.

The question to be answered by the diagnostic test is the critical factor. If the issue is to identify the disorder correctly *at all costs*, regardless of the number of false alarms, then the sensitivity of the test tool will be of paramount importance. If, however, one is charged with the task of identifying only those patients who do, in fact, have the disorder, even if it means missing some, then specificity will be the issue to consider. **In the majority of clinical situations concerning central auditory assessment, clinicians will want to choose those test tools that have the greatest sensitivity and specificity, or those that are most efficient, even though this will mean that some false alarms will occur and some subjects who do exhibit CAPD will be missed.**

A final, crucial issue in determining test validity is the standard against which test findings are compared. For example, if measures of validity are conducted for a test of central auditory processing using a population of children with *language impairment* and the test is shown to be highly efficient, the findings would suggest that the test is valid for language impairment. The question of validity for disorders of central auditory processing cannot be adequately answered because the number of children in the validation sample who actually present with disorders of the CANS is unknown. The act of establishing validity for one type of disorder does not necessarily imply validity for other, related disorders. For this reason, I suggest that, **when considering validity of any tool that purports to assess central auditory process- ing, clinicians should examine critically the population upon which validation studies were conducted.** For a test to be considered a valid test of central auditory processing, data should be available that demonstrate validity utilizing a population with known CANS disor- ders or lesions. Only in that way can clinicians be sure that the test tool in question is a measure of central auditory processing and not some related disorder.

Over the years, there have been many who have questioned the appropriateness of using individuals with CANS lesions as the "gold standard" for determining the validity of central auditory test tools. Certainly, this practice does have its drawbacks. For example, there is no direct one-to-one relationship between structure and function in the human brain. Rather, complex skills are mediated by complex neu- roanatomical substrates. This, combined with the inherent variability of brain function among individuals, makes it difficult to draw firm conclusions from localized lesions. Historically, difficulties related to localizing and defining precisely the extent of lesions in the neurologi- cal population (difficulties that, with the advent of more advanced neuroimaging techniques, may be largely solved) have merely added to this problem. In addition, there is the very basic, but very real, fact that lesioned brains are not normal, and drawing conclusions regard- ing normal function from abnormal brains should be approached with caution. Finally, the majority of lesion studies have been completed using adults, yet the results of these studies have been applied to the pediatric population for purposes of localizing site of dysfunction and interpreting central auditory test outcomes. This has led some to question the validity of using these central auditory tests with the pediatric population, especially because evidence of documented brain lesions is largely absent in the majority of children with CAPD.

Nevertheless, the study of brain lesions and the dissociations of function associated with them has been the primary means of deter- mining the underlying neurophysiology of brain function for virtually all neuroscience fields, including neuropsychology, cognitive neuro- science, language, and auditory neuroscience. Put quite simply, the best way to understand the function of a particular brain region is to look at what a person *can't* do when that particular region is lesioned. The fact that some children with auditory difficulties exhibit patterns of performance on tests of central auditory function that precisely mirror those of known CANS lesions cannot be put down to coinci- dence, but must be taken as evidence of dysfunction in the central auditory system. Furthermore, it is inappropriate to use other popula-tions—such as children with learning or language disabilities—for the validation of central auditory test tools in the pediatric population for the simple reason that not all children with learning or language disor-ders do, indeed, exhibit central auditory dysfunction. Therefore, stud-ies of individuals with known lesions of the CANS continue to be the gold standard against which tests of central auditory processing are validated, and remain invaluable to the process of developing and evaluating central auditory test tools.

As mentioned previously, reliability refers to the repeatability of test results. Reliability of a given test tool is best estimated by using a sample population similar to the test population for which the test was designed (Franzen, 1989). A variety of factors may affect test relia-bility. For our purposes, we will separate these factors into two gener-al categories: procedural variables, or those that relate to the test itself, and patient variables, or those that relate to the patient or disor-der (Table 5-1).

Procedural variables, otherwise known as errors of measurement (Heise, 1969), may include issues such as calibration of equipment, practice effects, ceiling effects found when a test is too easy, and other variables directly related to the measurement being studied. One example of a procedural variable that should be familiar to most audiologists is that of the use of too few items, such as during stan-dard word recognition testing. It is generally known within our field that, for years, debate raged regarding the use of full versus half lists of phonetically balanced, monosyllabic word lists for clinical word recognition testing. Although few of us would argue that the use of a ten-word list would provide sufficient test-retest reliability, the deci-sion to use twenty-five or fifty words differs from clinic to clinic. Also,

Table 5-1

Some Factors That May Affect Test Reliability

Procedural Variables	Patient Variables
Equipment calibration	Age
Practice effects	Degree and stability of hearing loss
Ceiling effects	Overall health
Floor effects	Attention
Use of too few items	Intelligence and linguistic ability
Other test-related factors	Presence of related disorder(s)

although the use of half lists for word recognition testing may be adequate for testing many populations, it may not be adequate for other, more involved, populations. Therefore, the use of fewer items on a test may affect test-retest reliability of word recognition measures in certain populations.

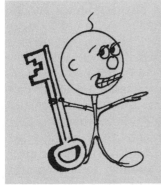

KEY CONCEPT

Just because a test has demonstrated validity for one type of disorder (e.g., learning disabilities), it cannot be inferred that the test is valid for a related disorder (e.g., CAPD).

Many procedural variables that affect test reliability, once identified, may be modified in order to improve reliability. For example, if the use of too few items is a critical factor, then the addition of more items will provide a solution. Practice effects may be controlled for by allowing the patient or subject to practice those items prior to testing or by choosing stimuli for which large practice effects are not found. Increasing the difficulty of the test may control for ceiling effects, whereas making the test easier may control for floor effects in those tests in which difficulty of the test is a critical factor. Regular calibration of test equipment will control for procedural variables related to equipment standardization. Variables related to test administration and scoring can be avoided by establishing specific test protocols. In any case, **it is important that clinicians identify possible sources of test-related variability and make all efforts to correct or control for these variables when possible.**

A second source of variability that may affect test reliability is the patient or disorder itself (Heise, 1969). As discussed in Chapter 3, the age of the patient being tested will have a significant impact on central test-retest reliability. The younger the population, the more variability noted, so that reliability of many central tests is quite poor when administered to children younger than approximately age 7. Age-appropriate normative data are required through age 11 or 12. Variability also increases with aging in adults, so that age- (and gender-) appropriate normative data may be required for certain central auditory test tools in the adult population as well (Bellis & Wilber, 2001).

Degree, symmetry, and stability of peripheral hearing loss, if present, may have significant impacts on the reliability of many central tests. Issues such as overall health, attention, linguistic abilities of the patient, intelligence, and the presence of additional, related disorders may all affect central test reliability (Jerger & Jerger, 1975; Musiek & Lamb, 1994).

It has been suggested that the reliability of central tests may be difficult to determine using a population of subjects with CAPD due to the dynamic nature of central disorders as well as to the high degree of variability among these subjects (Musiek & Chermak, 1994). The argument was that, due to neuroplasticity and the fact that CNS pathology results in constant change within the brain, reliability continues to be an important issue in CAPD assessment. Although this may well be the case, a review of the literature shows that very little research has been reported in which the reliability of specific CAP assessment tools in populations with known CAPD was studied. Therefore, **the issue of reliability of central auditory tests is an area of further, much-needed research. Furthermore, clinicians involved in central assessment must be familiar with possible sources of variability within the clinical population. Finally, central auditory assessment, interpretation of test results, and measures of treatment efficacy must take these factors into account.**

To summarize, validity is a test's ability to measure what it purports to measure, whereas reliability refers to the repeatability of test results. An understanding of issues surrounding validity and reliability of central tests is critical in order to determine the clinical utility of specific test tools as well as for the administration and interpretation of tests of central auditory function.

Overview of Central Tests

Historically, tests of central auditory function have been categorized in a variety of ways. For example, the ASHA Committee on Disorders of Central Auditory Processing (ASHA, 1990) divided central tests into monotic, dichotic, and binaural tests. Katz (1994) discussed non-speech-based, monosyllabic, spondaic, and sentence procedures, and Bellis and Ferre (1996) separated tests of central auditory function into two broad categories: those that add information to the signal and those that take away information from the signal. More recently, there has been a trend toward categorizing central auditory tests on the basis of the process(es) they assess or the manner in which the auditory signals are delivered to the ears. For example, ASHA (1996),

Bellis (1996), Bellis and Ferre (1999), and Chermak and Musiek (1997) categorized behavioral tests of central auditory processing as follows: dichotic speech tests, monaural low-redundancy tests, temporal ordering tests, and binaural interaction tests. The Bruton conference consensus statement on central auditory assessment listed the following categories of behavioral central auditory assessment tools necessary for a minimal test battery: a dichotic task, a frequency or duration pattern sequence test, and a temporal gap detection test (Jerger & Musiek, 2000).

Schow and colleagues (Schow & Chermak, 1999; Schow, Seikel, Chermak, & Berent, 2000; Domitz & Schow, 2000) undertook exploratory and confirmatory factor analyses of several central auditory test tools in common clinical use in an attempt to determine a minimal auditory processing assessment (MAPA) battery that would tap into those processes identified in the ASHA (1996) consensus definition of central auditory processing and the 2000 Bruton conference consensus statement (Jerger & Musiek, 2000). They also addressed the issue of sensitivity and specificity of various combinations of test tools. Their results clearly demonstrated that no one test alone was sufficient to screen for, let alone diagnose, CAPD. Further, they found that the most commonly used CAPD test tools could be represented by four primary factors or processes: auditory pattern temporal ordering (APTO), monaural separation/closure (MSC), binaural separation (BS), and binaural integration (BI). They also demonstrated that this factorial construct remained most stable when subtests from the SCAN (Keith, 1986) were not included in the battery, as many of these subtests loaded on several different factors. For a discussion of the use of the SCAN and its upper extensions in diagnosis of CAPD, readers are referred to Chapter 4. It is important to note that the authors did not include a measure of temporal gap detection in their analyses.

For purposes of this chapter, I categorize behavioral tests of central auditory processing according to the general auditory task required of each (i.e., dichotic speech tests, temporal processing tests, tests of monaural low-redundancy speech, and binaural interaction tests). In later chapters regarding choosing and administering components of the test battery (Chapter 6) and interpreting test results (Chapter 7), the tests will be discussed in terms of the underlying process(es) and factors represented by each.

Tests of phonological awareness, phonemic synthesis, auditory comprehension of language, and similar measures will not be included in this chapter, as they cannot be considered diagnostic tests of central auditory function. For a discussion of these test tools, readers are referred to Chapter 4.

Finally, two caveats must be emphasized. First, we must realize that, when using any behavioral or psychophysical measure, we can never truly assess individuals' *perceptions*. Rather, we are always assessing individuals' *behavioral responses* to what they perceive. As such, we must always keep in mind that any behavioral test of central auditory function is, at its core, really a test of organized and planned *output*, from which we make inferences about what individuals perceive. Second, although this discussion concerns itself exclusively with auditory tests, we must acknowledge the possible importance of developing and administering analogous measures in other modalities (e.g., visual) for purposes of differentially identifying auditory versus pan-sensory processing deficits (Cacace & McFarland, 1998; Jerger & Musiek, 2000; McFarland, Cacace, & Setzen, 1998).

Dichotic Speech Tests

As discussed in Chapter 2, dichotic listening involves the presentation of stimuli to both ears simultaneously, with the information presented to one ear being different from that presented to the other. Dichotic speech tasks differ from each other in terms of the stimuli utilized as well as the task required of the listener. Stimuli used in dichotic tests range from digits and nonsense syllables to complete sentences. **Depending on the test itself, listeners may be required to repeat everything that is heard (binaural integration) or to direct their attention to one ear and repeat what is heard in that ear only (binaural separation).** In addition, some tests of dichotic listening require listeners to perform a directed attention task in which they repeat what is heard in one ear first, followed by the stimuli presented to the other ear.

Dichotic stimuli may be viewed on a continuum from least to most difficult. In general, the more similar and closely aligned the stimuli presented to the ears are, the more difficult the dichotic task will be. In addition, the issue of degree of linguistic loading of dichotic stimuli must be taken into account. As seen in Chapter 3, a greater right-ear advantage (REA) will be observed in children when more complex, linguistically loaded dichotic stimuli are used than with the use of less complex stimuli. As the child matures, the REA will decrease, reaching adult values by approximately age 11 to 12.

One of the most common dichotic tests in use today is the Dichotic Digits Test (DDT). Kimura (1961a) first utilized triads of digits presented dichotically for the assessment of central auditory function. More recently, a revised version of Kimura's procedure was introduced in which two digits from 1 through 10 (excluding 7) are presented to each ear simultaneously (Musiek, 1983a). The listener is required to repeat all four digits heard. On the continuum of least to most difficult, the DDT may be considered to be somewhat in the middle, as the stimuli are very closely aligned but lightly linguistically loaded. **The DDT has been shown to be sensitive to brainstem and cortical lesions (Musiek, 1983a), as well as to lesions of the corpus callosum** (Musiek, Kibbe, & Baran, 1984). In addition, the test is quick and easy to administer and score and appears to be relatively resistant to peripheral hearing loss (Musiek, 1983a; Musiek, Gollegly, Kibbe, & Verkest-Lenz, 1991).

A more difficult task than the DDT is the Dichotic Consonant-Vowel (CV) test developed by Berlin and colleagues (Berlin et al., 1972). In this test, stimuli consist of six CV segments (pa, ta, ka, ba, da, ga). Single CV segments are presented to each ear using a dichotic paradigm and the listener is asked to choose both segments heard from a printed list. Although the test is very lightly linguistically loaded, its difficulty lies in the high degree of similarity among the CV segments as well as the close acoustical alignment of the stimuli (Niccum, Rubens, & Speaks, 1981). In addition, the test may be administered so that the presentation of a CV segment to one ear may lag behind the presentation of a different CV segment to the other ear by 15, 30, 60, or 90 msec in order to investigate the effect of lag time on listener performance (Berlin et al., 1975). **The Dichotic CV test has been shown to be sensitive to cortical lesions; however, as in many central tests, laterality of dysfunction cannot be determined by the test results** (Berlin et al., 1975; Olsen, 1983). It should be noted that the difficulty of this test may preclude its use in some populations (Mueller & Bright, 1994). My own experience indicates that this test is often too difficult for young children, and variability is high in the school-age population. Furthermore, because of the auditory distortions introduced by peripheral hearing loss that affect phoneme discrimination, the Dichotic CV test should only be used with listeners exhibiting normal peripheral hearing sensitivity.

One of the most widely used dichotic speech tests is the Staggered Spondaic Word Test (SSW), first described by Katz in 1962. This test involves the dichotic presentation of spondees in such a manner that the second syllable of the spondee presented to one ear overlaps the first syllable of the spondee presented to the other ear. The ear-specific spondees and the overlapping spondee form separate words. For example, when the word *upstairs* is presented to the right ear and *downtown* is presented to the left ear, the overlapping syllables will result in the dichotic presentation of the word *downstairs*.

Specific details regarding administration and scoring of the SSW will be provided in Chapter 6. **The SSW has been shown to be sensitive to brainstem and cortical lesions** (Katz, 1962). In addition, the test is relatively resistant to peripheral hearing loss (Arnst, 1982; Katz, 1968), and is simple enough for use with a variety of ages (Katz, 1977).

Two commonly used dichotic procedures use sentences as stimuli. The first is the Competing Sentences Test (CST), developed by Willeford in 1968 (Willeford & Burleigh, 1994). The test consists of simple sentences presented dichotically. The target sentence is presented to one ear at a quieter level than the competing sentence, which is presented to the other ear. The listener is instructed to repeat the sentence heard in the target ear only and ignore the competing sentence, which assesses the process of binaural separation of auditory information. **The sensitivity of the CST as compared to other dichotic measures in the identification of cortical lesions has been questioned by a number of researchers (Lynn & Gilroy, 1972, 1975; Musiek, 1983b). However, it has been suggested that dichotic sentence tasks such as the CST may be valuable in investigating neuromaturation and language processing abilities** (Porter & Berlin, 1975; Willeford & Burleigh, 1994). As will be discussed in the following chapter, the utility of the CST in central auditory assessment appears to depend, at least in part, on the way in which the test is scored. Although Willeford and Burleigh (1994) suggested a relatively lax scoring criterion in which responses are judged to be incorrect only if they are grossly wrong or the listener fails to respond at all, the use of a more strict quadrant scoring method results in significantly less variability in children. Finally, the degree of variability of performance on competing sentences tests appears to be affected by the linguistic content of the sentences. For example, a version of the CST that has recently been made commercially available from Auditec of St. Louis yields very different normative values (lower scores and greater variability in adults) than does the original Willeford CST (Hexamer & Bellis, 2000). Because the two tests are identical in terms of test administration, this finding appears to be due to differences in the linguistic content between the two tests and, indeed, listeners report that the Auditec sentences are far more difficult than are the Willeford sentences. This topic will be addressed further in Chapter 6.

A second dichotic sentence procedure is the Synthetic Sentence Identification test with Contralateral Competing Message (SSI-CCM), described by Jerger and Jerger (1974, 1975). Stimuli for the SSI-CCM are ten third-order approximations of English sentences. The stimuli resemble nonsense sentences, thus lightening the linguistic load of the test. The sentences are presented to the target ear while a competing message consisting of continuous discourse is presented to the contralateral ear. The listener is required to choose from a printed list which of the ten sentences was heard. Like the CST, the SSI-CCM assesses the process of binaural separation of auditory information. **The SSI-CCM has been found to be useful in differentiating brainstem from cortical pathology** (Jerger & Jerger, 1975; Keith, 1977). The SSI with Ipsilateral Competing Message (SSI-ICM), in which both the sentence and the competing message are presented to the same ear, will be discussed in the section dealing with monaural low-redundancy speech tests.

A modification of the SSI-CCM entitled the Dichotic Sentence Identification test (DSI) was introduced in 1983 by Fifer and colleagues (Fifer, Jerger, Berlin, Tobey, & Campbell, 1983). The test uses the SSI sentences presented dichotically and requires the listener to identify both sentences heard from a printed list of all ten sentences, thus tapping the process of binaural integration. The DSI was initially devised in hopes of providing a dichotic speech test that would be resistant to the effects of peripheral hearing loss. Although more research is needed into its clinical utility, **the DSI appears to show sensitivity to disorders of the CANS** (Mueller, Beck, & Sedge, 1987), **while being minimally affected by peripheral hearing loss** (Fifer et al., 1983). Therefore, the DSI may be a promising tool for the evaluation of central auditory function in the hearing-impaired population.

Monosyllabic words may also be used as stimuli in dichotic listening tasks. In the SCAN: A Screening Test for Auditory Processing Disorders (Keith, 1986), as well as in the revision of the original test (SCAN-C Test for Auditory Processing Disorders in Children—Revised; Keith, 2000a) and the adolescent/adult version (SCAN-A; Keith; 1994b), the Competing Words subtest is a directed attention dichotic task using monosyllabic words. During presentation of the first list, the listener is instructed to repeat the stimulus heard in the right ear first, followed by the left ear. During presentation of the second list, the instruction to the listener is reversed. **The SCAN test paradigm is reported to assist in determining ear differences related to neuromaturation** (Keith, 1986). The SCAN is a popular screening tool for CAPD due to its ease of administration; however, its validity as a diagnostic tool for CAPD has been called into question in recent years (e.g., Musiek et al., 1990). Schow et al. (2000) demonstrated that the Competing Words subtest of the SCAN—unlike other dichotic listening tests discussed in this section—appeared to assess multiple factors, rendering its utility for central auditory assessment questionable.

A second dichotic procedure using monosyllabic words has been presented in recent years. The Dichotic Rhyme Test (DRT) was introduced by Wexler and Hawles (1983) and modified by Musiek, Kurdziel-Schwan, Kibbe, Gollegly, Baran, and Rintelmann (1989). The DRT is composed of rhyming, consonant-vowel-consonant words, each beginning with one of the stop consonants (p, t, k, b, d, g). Each pair of words differs only in the initial consonant, (e.g., ten, pen). As such, the stimuli are almost perfectly aligned so that fusion takes place and the listener most often hears and repeats just one of the two words presented. **The DRT has been shown to be particularly sensitive to detection of dysfunction in the interhemispheric transfer of information via the corpus callosum** (Musiek, Kurdziel-Schwan, Kibbe, Gollegly, Baran, & Rintelmann 1989). Unfortunately, the DRT is not commercially available at the present time, despite its demonstrated utility in identifying disorders of interhemispheric integration.

In conclusion, dichotic listening tasks involve the presentation of a different stimulus to each ear simultaneously. They may be viewed in a variety of different ways, including type of stimuli used, level of difficulty, degree of linguistic loading, and the task required of the listener. Types of dichotic speech stimuli include CV segments, digits, monosyllabic words, spondaic words, and sentences, with the use of CV segments being the most difficult task due to the limited amount of linguistic information combined with the close temporal alignment of stimuli presentation. Sentence stimuli are considered to be heavily linguistically loaded whereas digits or CV segments carry a much lighter linguistic load. Finally, depending on the instructions given to the listener, dichotic tasks may assess the processes of binaural integration, binaural separation, or a combination of both (directed attention). Dichotic speech tasks have been shown to be sensitive to cortical and corpus callosal dysfunction, as well as, to a lesser degree, brainstem lesions, and are in wide clinical use today. Other dichotic measures currently in development or used primarily for research purposes also hold great promise for use as central auditory assessment tools. For example, it has been suggested that comparing performance on nonverbal (tonal) dichotic measures to that on dichotic speech measures may provide a means of assessing both right-to-left and left-to-right interhemispheric transfer of auditory information (e.g., Bellis, 1999; Bellis & Wilber, 2001). In addition, methods of evaluating language (including semantic) processing using a dichotic paradigm in combination with auditory electrophysiologic recording have recently been described (e.g., Jerger, Greenwald, Wambacq, Seipel, & Moncrieff, 2000). However, the ultimate clinical utility of these new dichotic paradigms in the evaluation of CAPD remains to be investigated. A summary of the dichotic speech tasks discussed in this section is presented in Table 5-2.

Table 5-2

Summary of Selected Dichotic Speech Tests

Test	Process(es) Assessed	Sensitive to
Dichotic Digits	Binaural integration	Brainstem, cortical, and corpus callosal lesions
Dichotic Consonant-Vowels	Binaural integration	Cortical lesions
Staggered Spondaic Word Test	Binaural integration	Brainstem and cortical lesions
Competing Sentences Test	Binaural separation	Neuromaturation and language processing
Synthetic Sentence Identification Test With Contralateral Competing Message	Binaural separation	Cortical versus brainstem lesions
Dichotic Sentence Identification Test	Binaural integration	Brainstem and cortical lesions
Dichotic Rhyme Test	Binaural integration	Interhemispheric transfer

Temporal Processing Tasks

In Chapter 3, we discussed the effects of various pathologies, particularly lesions of the cerebral hemispheres or the corpus callosum, on temporal processing abilities. For the most part, nonspeech stimuli such as tones or clicks are utilized in the evaluation of temporal ordering abilities. As mentioned in Chapter 3, temporal processing is critical to perception of speech and music. Temporal processing tasks, particularly temporal integration, two-tone ordering, gap detection, and brief tone tasks, have been used for many years in order to investigate lesion effects on temporal aspects of audition (Carmon & Nachshon, 1971; Cranford et al. 1982; Efron, 1985; Efron & Crandall, 1983; Jerger et al., 1972; Lackner & Teuber, 1973; Swisher & Hirsh, 1972; Thompson & Abel, 1992a, b). A test of auditory temporal gap detection that has recently become commercially available is the

Random Gap Detection Test (RGDT; Keith, 2000c). In this test, stimuli (clicks and brief tones of octave frequencies from 250 through 4000 Hz) are presented in pairs and the silent interval between each pair randomly increases and decreases in duration from 0 to 40 ms. Listeners are required to indicate whether they hear one stimulus or two. The gap detection threshold is defined as the smallest interval at which the listener consistently identifies two stimuli. The test is quick and easy to administer, and does not require any special equipment other than an audiometer and compact disk player. Although validity of the RGDT for CAPD has not yet been assessed, similar gap detection paradigms have been shown to be sensitive to cortical, particularly left temporal lobe, dysfunction (Lackner & Teuber, 1973).

Despite the fact that other measures of temporal processing such as temporal integration, brief tone tasks, and two-tone ordering have been shown to be sensitive to central auditory dysfunction, they are not in common clinical use today. This likely arises from the lack of readily available commercial versions of these tasks. Similarly, although between-channel gap detection may provide a more ecologically valid measure of temporal processing important for speech perception than within-channel gap detection tests such as the RGDT, as discussed in Chapter 2, there is currently no such test designed for general clinical use. As such, the development of commercially available tests of a variety of temporal processes is an area of research in the field of central auditory assessment that deserves increased attention.

A second type of temporal processing task involves the perception of temporal order of more than two consecutive acoustic stimuli, or temporal pattern perception.

The Frequency Patterns (or Pitch Pattern Sequence) Test (FPT), was initially designed to investigate both pattern perception and temporal sequencing abilities (Pinheiro & Ptacek, 1971; Ptacek & Pinheiro, 1971). The test consists of 120 pattern sequences. Each sequence is made up of three tone bursts: two of one frequency and one of another. The frequencies utilized are 1122 Hz and 880 Hz. Thirty items are presented to each ear, and listeners are instructed to report verbally each pattern heard. Six patterns are possible: high-high-low, high-low-high, high-low-low, low-high-low, low-low-high, and low-high-high. The test taps the processes of frequency discrimination, temporal ordering, and linguistic labeling. **The FPT is useful in the detection of disorders of the cerebral hemispheres, although laterality information cannot be obtained from this test** (Musiek & Pinheiro, 1987; Pinheiro, 1976; Pinheiro & Musiek, 1985). **In addition, the test has been shown to be sensitive to corpus callosal dysfunc-**

tion in that patients with disruptions in the interhemispheric transfer of auditory information exhibit improvement in performance when the linguistic labeling component of the test is removed by requesting the listener to hum the pattern rather than verbally describe it (Musiek et al., 1980). **Finally, results of the FPT may provide information regarding neuromaturation in the child with learning disability by indicating the degree of myelination of the corpus callosum** (Musiek, Gollegly, & Baran, 1984).

A related test of temporal ordering is the Duration Pattern Test (DPT). Described by Pinheiro and Musiek (1985), the DPT is similar to the FPT except that the frequency of the tones is held constant at 1000 Hz and duration is the factor to be discriminated. Short (250 msec) and long (500 msec) tone bursts are presented in sequences of three-tone patterns and, like the FPT, the listener is asked to describe verbally the pattern heard (e.g., short-short-long, long-short-long, etc.). **The DPT appears to be sensitive to cerebral lesions while remaining unaffected by peripheral hearing loss** as long as the stimuli are presented at a frequency and intensity that can be perceived by the listener (Musiek, Baran, & Pinheiro, 1990). The DPT assesses the processes of duration discrimination, temporal ordering, and linguistic labeling. Additional research is needed to delineate the functional implications of poor performance on the DPT versus the FPT. In my clinical experience, some listeners do poorly on both tasks whereas others may have difficulty with only one of the two tests. Normative data, presented in Chapter 6, suggest that the DPT is a more difficult task than is the FPT. Further, preliminary data collected in my clinic suggest that listeners who perform poorly on both tests may exhibit difficulty in both receptive and expressive prosody, while listeners who perform poorly on just the DPT may exhibit only receptive prosodic deficits. This topic will be discussed further in Chapter 7; however, it is important to emphasize that these two tests of auditory temporal pattern perception are not interchangeable.

Finally, an additional test of auditory pattern perception that is also a dichotic nonspeech task was developed by Blaettner et al. (1989). The Psychoacoustic Pattern Discrimination Test (PPDT) assesses discrimination of temporal changes through the use of dichotically presented sequences of noise bursts or click trains. The listener is required to indicate discrimination of a monaural change in the pattern by pressing a button. Preliminary information indicates that, like other temporal patterning tasks, **the PPDT is sensitive to lesions of the cerebral hemispheres, including the auditory association areas.** In addition, abnormal findings on the PPDT have been found to correlate with abnormal findings on middle or late evoked potential measures. Although the PPDT holds great promise as a test for temporal processing, a drawback to the procedure is that it is not readily available in standardized format for clinical use at the present time.

To summarize, despite the use of temporal processing tasks in research and the importance of temporal processing in speech and music perception, very few tests of temporal processing are currently available for widespread clinical use. Those that are available include the Random Gap Detection Test, Frequency Patterns Test, and the Duration Pattern Test. The RGDT is a measure of auditory temporal gap detection. The FPT and the DPT assess the processes of discrimination (frequency or duration, respectively), temporal ordering, and linguistic labeling. Both of these tests are currently available on compact disc (Musiek, 1994). Another test of temporal processing is the Psychoacoustic Pattern Discrimination Test, which assesses temporal patterning abilities without the need for linguistic labeling or verbal report. All of these tests appear to be relatively resistant to the effects of peripheral hearing loss as well as being sensitive to cerebral pathology. The temporal processing tests discussed in this section are summarized in Table 5-3.

Table 5-3

Summary of Selected Tests of Temporal Processing

Test	Process(es) Assessed	Sensitive to
Random Gap Detection Test (RGDT)	Temporal resolution	Cortical, particularly left temporal lobe, lesions
Frequency Patterns Test (FPT)	Frequency discrimination, temporal ordering, linguistic labeling	Cortical lesions, interhemispheric transfer
Duration Patterns Test (DPT)	Duration discrimination, temporal ordering, linguistic labeling	Cortical lesions, interhemispheric transfer
Psychoacoustic Pattern Discrimination Test (PPDT)	Temporal discrimination	Cortical lesions, including auditory association areas

Monaural Low-Redundancy Speech Tests

Due to redundancy within the auditory system (*intrinsic redundancy*) as well as in spoken language (*extrinsic redundancy*), normal listeners are typically able to achieve closure and make auditory discriminations even when a portion of the auditory signal is missing or distorted. This ability is often compromised in listeners with central auditory dysfunction. Electroacoustically modifying the temporal, frequency, or intensity characteristics of the acoustic signal reduces the amount of extrinsic redundancy and, because central pathology results in a reduction of intrinsic redundancy, auditory closure cannot be achieved. Therefore, **although listeners with CAPD will typically perform quite well when auditory stimuli are presented in ideal listening environments, such as during standard phonetically balanced word recognition testing, they will often demonstrate significant problems when the task is made more difficult by distorting the signal in some way.** This section will discuss three methods of reducing the redundancy of the speech signal in order to assess central auditory function: low-pass filtering, time compression, and addition of reverberation. In addition, because the primary effect of the addition of noise is a reduction in the redundancy of the speech signal, speech-in-noise tasks also will be discussed in this section.

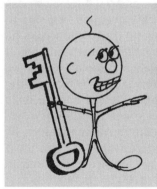

KEY CONCEPT

Tests that reduce the redundancy of the speech signal primarily tap the process of auditory closure.

Low-pass filtering of the speech signal has been employed to assess the integrity of the CANS since 1954 (Bocca, Calearo, & Cassinari, 1954). A number of studies have investigated the utility of low-pass filtered speech in the detection of CANS dysfunction, and readers are referred to Rintelmann (1985) for a review. This section will describe two readily available, standardized filtered speech tests in clinical use today: the Ivey filtered speech test included in the Willeford central test battery (Willeford, 1977) and filtered NU-6 lists.

The Ivey filtered speech test of the Willeford central test battery is probably the most widely used low-pass filtered speech test in clinics today. The test consists of two fifty-item lists of the Michigan consonant-nucleus-consonant (CNC) words with a 500 Hz cut-off and 18 dB/octave filter. The filtered words tend to be intelligible to normal listeners; however, listeners with central pathology perform poorly on this test.

In addition to the Ivey test, low-pass filtered versions of the Northwestern University No. 6 (NU-6) word lists are available *(Tonal and speech materials for auditory perceptual assessment*, 1992; Wilson & Mueller, 1984). Low-pass versions of the test utilizing cut-off frequencies of 500, 700, 1000, and 1500 Hz may be used. Normative values for the 500, 700, and 1000 Hz cut-offs may be found in Wilson and Mueller (1984). The use of the 1500 Hz cut-off frequency is described in Bornstein, Wilson, and Cambron (1994). It should be noted that, **when the 500 Hz cut-off is used, normal listeners have a great deal of difficulty with this test, indicating that this cut-off frequency probably would not be clinically feasible for use in a CAP test battery** (Wilson & Mueller, 1984). Bornstein et al. (1994) also described the use of a high-pass filtered (2100 Hz cut-off) version of the NU-6. Further research into the use of the 1500 Hz low-pass and 2100 Hz high-pass NU-6 lists with listeners having neurological involvement remains to be completed. It is important to note that several tests of low-pass filtered speech are currently commercially available through Auditec of St. Louis, using several cut-off frequencies, male and female speakers, and different word lists. Each of these stimulus factors will affect the difficulty of a particular test. Although low-pass filtered speech tests have, in general, been shown to be sensitive to central auditory dysfunction, it is critical that separate age-specific normative values be developed for each test individually. Normative values for the most commonly used tests of low-pass filtered speech are presented in Chapter 6, and indicate that the male-speaker, 1000 Hz, NU-6 version is easier for both children and adults than the female-speaker version of the same word list at the same frequency cut-off. The recent addition of low-pass filtered phonetically balanced kindergarten (PBK) lists provides a possible means of evaluating monaural low-redundancy speech in young children or listeners with limited vocabulary; however, this test, too, remains to be normed and validated.

Findings for low-pass filtered speech in general indicate that this procedure is sensitive to a variety of central disorders, including

brainstem and cortical dysfunction. These tests, like the other monaural low-redundancy speech tasks to be discussed in this section, primarily tap the process of auditory closure (ability to fill in the missing components) of degraded auditory information.

A second method of reducing the redundancy of the speech signal is time compression. In this technique, the temporal characteristics of the signal are altered by electronically reducing the duration of the speech signal without affecting the frequency characteristics (Fairbanks, Everitt, & Jaeger, 1954). Normative studies using time-compressed versions of the NU-6 word lists (30–70% compression) indicate that normal listeners demonstrate a reduction in word recognition scores as the degree of compression increases, culminating in a marked deterioration in performance with 70% compression (Beasley, Forman, & Rintelmann, 1972; Beasley, Schwimmer, & Rintelmann, 1972). Findings in subjects with neurological dysfunction indicate that **time-compressed speech tasks are most sensitive to diffuse pathology involving the primary auditory cortex**, particularly at the higher degrees of compression (Baran et al. 1985; Kurdziel, Noffsinger, & Olson, 1976; Mueller et al., 1987).

Reverberation is the persistance of an acoustic signal, or echo, that occurs in an enclosed space. This term may be familiar to many clinicians, as it is reverberation that is most bothersome in rooms with poorly controlled acoustic characteristics and a preponderance of hard surfaces that enable sound to "bounce" for a period of time following the cessation of the signal. The degree of reverberation is defined by the time required for a signal to decay 60 dB following offset of the signal (Wilson, Preece, Salamon, Sperry, & Bornstein, 1994). As reverberation time increases, recognition of subsequent words decreases (Helfer & Wilber, 1990). Thus, reverberation provides an additional method of reducing the redundancy of a speech signal for the purposes of central assessment.

Studies of the effects of signal distortion on word recognition abilities indicate that **a combination of disortion techniques results in greater effects than does the use of one disortion technique alone** (Harris, 1960). This is known as the *multiplicative effect.* Wilson, Preece, Salamon, Sperry, and Bornstein (1994) reported on the use of time compression combined with electronically induced, 0.3-second reverberation for central auditory assessment. The addition of reverberation to time-compressed speech resulted in the expected decrease in word recognition performance in a group of normal listeners; however, further research is needed using neurologically disabled populations. It should be noted that the data provided by Wilson, Preece, Salamon, Sperry, and Bornstein (1994), as well as my own clinical experience, suggest that a **65% time compression condition appears to be difficult even for normal listeners. This suggests that a time compression rate of 45% may be more appropriate for clinical use.**

A final method of reducing the redundancy of the speech signal is to embed the signal in a background of noise. Although speech-in-noise tests have been shown to be at least marginally sensitive to a wide variety of disorders of the CANS and related disorders (Chermak, Vonhof, & Bendel, 1989; Dayal, Tarantino, & Swisher, 1966; Heilman, Hammer, & Wilder, 1973; Morales-Garcia & Poole, 1972; Olsen, Noffsinger, & Kurdziel, 1975; Sinha, 1959), lack of standardized test tools and material-specific normative data have resulted in conflicting findings and questionable test reliability. Therefore, Mueller and Bright (1994) suggested that **speech-in-noise tests may well be the most misused tests of central auditory function.**

Of primary importance is the collection of normative data regarding whatever materials and signal-to-noise ratios are used in testing. Typically, monosyllabic words combined with the ipsilateral presentation of white or speech spectrum noise at signal-to-noise ratios of 0 to +10 dB are utilized. Some clinics also use "cafeteria" noise or multi-talker babble as the competing signal. The Synthetic Sentence Identification test with Ipsilateral Competing Message (SSI-ICM) (Jerger & Jerger, 1974), which presents the third-order SSI sentences described previously along with ipsilateral continuous discourse, is an example of a commercially available speech-in-noise test. **The SSI-ICM has been shown to be useful in the identification of lesions of the low brainstem** (Jerger & Jerger, 1974, 1975). An additional test of speech in noise designed specifically for small children is the Pediatric Speech Intelligibility (PSI) Test (Jerger, Jerger, & Abrams, 1983). In this test, stimuli are presented at various S/N ratios, and the child is required to point to the picture representing the target message. The PSI is one of the few speech-in-noise tests with well-established normative values for various S/N ratios. A similar test, the Selective Auditory Attention Test (SAAT; Cherry, 1980), also requires listeners to identify a target that is embedded in competing signals. Although the SAAT was designed to be administered in a diotic mode, it may also be presented monaurally by routing both the target and the competition to the same earphone.

Recently, Jerger et al. (2000) reported on what they termed a "more ecologically valid" measure of speech in noise. The authors employed a quasi-dichotic sound-field procedure in which listeners heard different portions of the same fairy tale from each of two speakers placed to their right and left. The listeners' task was to identify the presence of an inappropriate word—or a semantic incongruity—

embedded in the message delivered by one of the two speakers. This was a directed attention task in which listeners were instructed to attend to one speaker at a time. Topographic electrophysiologic maps of brain activity were obtained which indicated processing negativities at approximately 400 and 900 ms following presentation of target words. The negativity occurring at 900 ms (termed the N900) was relatively symmetrical between hemispheres in the authors' group of young, normal listeners. The authors suggested that this paradigm may provide a means of evaluating speech-in-noise abilities in a manner that more closely resembles real-world listening and that, further, can be verified via physiologic means. Additional research into the clinical utility of this paradigm for central auditory assessment remains to be completed.

There are several additional tests of speech-in-noise that are commercially available; however, most of them were designed to evaluate listeners with hearing impairment, particularly as relates to benefit from amplification. As such, their employment in central auditory assessment has yet to be investigated.

Clinicians engaged in speech-in-noise testing should be warned that, **due to the great variability in scores seen in normal and lesioned listeners, speech-in-noise test results should be interpreted with caution.** In a study using NU-6 words presented in white noise at 0 dB signal-to-noise ratio, Olsen et al. (1975) found that a reduction in word recognition performance of at least 40% was required before the findings were considered to be significant. Even using this criterion, site of lesion could not be determined from the test results, and a number of listeners with temporal lobe lesions continued to perform within normal limits on the task. Therefore, I would recommend that speech-in-noise tests only be used in conjunction with other, standardized tests of central auditory function.

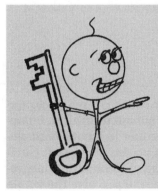

KEY CONCEPT

Clinic-specific normative data should be collected for all speech-in-noise tests employed. Data obtained for one test should not be assumed to be appropriate for another.

Table 5-4

Summary of Selected Monaural Low-Redundancy Speech Tests

Test	Process(es) Assessed	Sensitive to
Low-Pass Filtered Speech	Auditory closure	Brainstem and cortical lesions, especially primary auditory cortex
Time-Compressed Speech with and without reverberation added	Auditory closure	Brainstem and cortical lesions, especially primary auditory cortex
Synthetic Sentence Identification with Ipsilateral Competing Message (SSI-ICM)	Auditory figure/ground, auditory closure	Low brainstem lesions
Speech-in-Noise Tests (including PSI and SAAT)	Auditory figure/ground, auditory closure	Low brainstem and cortical lesions

In summary, the inclusion of a monaural low-redundancy speech test in the central auditory test battery may be useful for the identification of central dysfunction. Methods of reducing redundancy of a speech signal include band-pass filtering, time compression, addition of reverberation, and addition of competing noise. All of these tasks assess a listener's ability to achieve auditory closure of degraded auditory information. Finally, the clinician should use caution when engaging in speech-in-noise testing due to the lack of standardization and high degree of variability inherent in this type of task. Types of monaural low-redundancy speech tests are summarized in Table 5-4.

Binaural Interaction Tests

Tests of binaural interaction generally assess the ability of the CANS to process disparate, but complementary, information presented to the two ears. **Unlike dichotic listening tasks, the stimuli utilized in binaural interaction tasks typically are presented either in a nonsimultaneous, sequential condition, or the information presented to each ear is composed of a portion of the entire message, necessitating integration of the information in order for the listener to perceive the whole**

message. This is considered to be a function primarily of the low brainstem, as discussed in Chapter 2. Several binaural interaction tasks have been used clinically, including rapidly alternating speech perception, band-pass and CVC binaural fusion tasks, interaural difference limen tasks, and the masking level difference (MLD).

Rapidly alternating speech perception (RASP) is a procedure in which sentence material is switched rapidly between ears at periodic intervals, resulting in the alternating presentation of unintelligible, sequential bursts of information. In normal listeners, this rapidly alternating presentation of a speech message is easily understood. However, some listeners with brainstem lesions demonstrate difficulty with the task (Lynn & Gilroy, 1977). The most commonly used version of the RASP was developed by Willeford (Willeford & Bilger, 1978). In their study, the authors found the test to be simple, even for very young children. **Subsequent studies suggested that the RASP may not be sensitive to anything other than grossly abnormal brainstem pathology** (Lynn & Gilroy, 1977; Musiek, 1983c; Willeford & Burleigh, 1994). **Because of the availability of other tests that demonstrate greater efficiency with regard to brainstem pathology, such as the ABR and MLD, there is some question as to the clinical utility of the RASP in central assessment.**

Binaural fusion tasks involve the presentation of different portions of a speech stimulus to each ear, necessitating fusion of the information in order for the listener to perceive the entire word. Information may be band-passed so that only the high-frequency portion of the stimulus is presented to one ear and the low-frequency components are presented to the other, or CVC words may be utilized in which the consonants are presented to one ear and the vowel to the other in a sequential fashion.

Matzker (1959) used bisyllabic, phonetically balanced word lists for assessing binaural resynthesis. In his test, the low-pass band (500–800 Hz) was presented to one ear while the high-pass band (1815–2500 Hz) was presented to the other. The forty-one-word list was presented three times: twice using the filtered bands and once, during the second presentation, diotically so that fusion was not required. His results indicated that **listeners with cortical lesions performed normally on the binaural fusion task whereas listeners with brainstem pathology had difficulty with the resynthesis of the auditory information.**

Smith and Resnick (1972) maintained that the use of monosyllabic words would reduce the redundancy of the signal and thereby improve the sensitivity of binaural fusion tasks. In their study, monosyllabic, CVC words were band-passed and presented using a variation of Matzker's resynthesis paradigm. Test results were interpreted by comparing the results of the diotic presentation of the stimuli with the two presentations requiring fusion. Diotic scores were significantly higher than resynthesis scores in four out of four cases of brainstem pathology.

Presently, several band-pass filtered, binaural fusion tests are available commercially through Auditec of St. Louis and other sources. For some of them, such as the band-pass filtered NU-6 list, normative data have been collected (Wilson & Mueller, 1984). Age-appropriate norms for selected binaural fusion tasks will be presented in Chapter 6. Overall, **studies examining these tasks suggest that they are somewhat sensitive to brainstem lesions** (Lynn & Gilroy, 1977; Musiek, 1983c; Noffsinger et al., 1972). **In addition, abnormal binaural fusion or resynthesis performance has been seen in children with dyslexia or learning disability** (Welsh, Welsh, & Healy, 1980; Welsh, Welsh, Healy, & Cooper, 1982; Willeford, 1977).

An additional binaural fusion task is the Segmented-Alternated CVC fusion task developed by Wilson, Arcos, and Jones (1984) as a tool to assess central auditory function while remaining relatively unaffected by peripheral hearing loss. In this test, CVC words are segmented so that the consonant segments are delivered to one ear and the vowel is delivered to the other ear in an alternating manner.

The concept of evaluating interaural time or intensity just noticeable differences (jnds) has existed for several years; however, it has not gained wide popularity as a clinical tool. Pinheiro and Tobin (1969, 1971) utilized an interaural intensity difference (IID) paradigm in which the degree of intensity difference between ears needed for lateralization of a signal was evaluated. Their results indicated that **subjects with central involvement demonstrated greater IIDs in the ear ipsilateral to the lesion.**

More recently, Levine et al. (1993a, b) described an interaural jnd task in which tonal stimuli were either high- or low-pass filtered and presented in pairs to both ears simultaneously. Either the onset time (time jnd) or the intensity (level jnd) of one half of the stimulus pair was altered in one ear. The listener was required to indicate when the signal lateralized to one side or the other. **The results of high-pass time jnd evaluation were found to be closely correlated with ABR results and, thus, appeared to be a good behavioral measure of brainstem integrity.** However, their test paradigm and that of Pinheiro and Tobin (1969) require greater acoustic control of the stimulus than is possible utilizing standard audiometric equipment. Therefore, clinical utility of these test paradigms is questionable at this time.

A final test of binaural interaction is the masking level difference

Table 5-5

Summary of Selected Binaural Interaction Tests

Test	Process(es) Assessed	Sensitive to
Rapidly Alternating Speech Perception (RASP)	Binaural interaction	Questionable sensitivity to gross brainstem lesions
Binaural Fusion	Binaural interaction	Gross sensitivity to brainstem lesions
Interaural Just-Noticeable Differences	Binaural interaction, lateralization	More information needed re: neurological populations
Masking Level Differences (MLD)	Binaural interaction	Brainstem lesions

(MLD), described in Chapter 2. **MLDs may be obtained to speech or tonal stimuli, and have been shown to be highly sensitive to brainstem dysfunction.** Many commercial audiometers have the built-in capability to conduct MLD testing. MLD paradigms using spondaic word stimuli are also available on compact disk. However, tonal MLDs have been shown to be a better diagnostic indicator of central auditory dysfunction in children than speech MLDs (Sweetow & Reddell, 1978).

Overall, and with the exception of the MLD, the clinical utility of the majority of binaural interaction tests has been questioned on the bases of sensitivity and ease of administration. Noffsinger et al. (1984) have suggested that the three primary responsibilities of the auditory brainstem are sound transmission, binaural integration of sound, and the control of reflexive behavior. These three areas may be tested reliably using the ABR, MLD, and acoustic reflex paradigms, respectively. Therefore, the need for additional behavioral tests of brainstem integrity is questionable at this time and, indeed, the tests discussed in this section are not considered to be in widespread clinical use. A summary of binaural interaction tests discussed in this section is provided in Table 5-5.

Other Behavioral Measures

The previous discussion centered on those categories of central auditory test tools that are typically identified as components of the behavioral central auditory assessment test battery. There are, however, additional measures that appear to shed light on auditory function in some children with presumed auditory-based learning or language deficits. In addition, some behavioral measures exist that can help us assess higher-order functions such as auditory attention and vigilance—an assessment that aids in the differential diagnosis of auditory versus attention-related disorders. Finally, the use of measures in other modalities that are analogous to the auditory tasks discussed in this chapter may be useful in exploring the degree of auditory modality specificity in CAPD, an area that needs a great deal of additional investigation. This section will provide a brief discussion of some of these measures which, although not in common clinical use today, may find a solid spot in the central auditory armamentarium in coming years.

Research completed in the auditory neuroscience laboratory at Northwestern University has suggested that some children with learning difficulties may exhibit fundamental deficits in the ability to make fine-grained acoustic discriminations necessary for normal speech perception. Recently, Kraus and colleagues reported on a novel auditory discrimination paradigm that can be used with even relatively young children and that illuminates the listener's ability to make these fine-grained auditory discriminations (Kraus, Koch, McGee, Nicol, & Cunningham, 1999). In their paradigm, a computer-based parameter estimation by sequential tracking (PEST) procedure is used in which the minimal difference required to tell whether two consonant-vowel (CV) minimal contrast pairs are different is measured.

Two primary CV combinations are of interest: /da/ versus /ga/, which requires discrimination of a very rapid spectro-temporal change in the formant transition, as discussed in Chapter 1; and /ba/ versus /wa/, which involves a more slowly moving durational difference. In the PEST procedure, which used a two-alternative, forced-choice paradigm, listeners are instructed that they will hear two pairs (or sets) of syllables and are to indicate by pushing a button the interval in which the syllabi were different. One interval always has a matching pair (e.g., /da/-/da/), and the other always has a different pair (eg., /da/-/ga/), with the interval in which the difference occurs changing randomly. A software program controls the algorithm that systematically alters the special characteristics of the stimuli so that they are rendered more difficult to discriminate following correct responses and easier to discriminate following incorrect responses, eventually converging at a threshold level. The just noticeable difference (jnd), or discrimination threshold, is defined as the smallest acoustic difference needed for a listener to make correct responses 67% of the time.

The authors have shown that some children with learning or language deficits exhibit larger jnds for the /da/ versus /ga/ contrast, but not for the /ba/ versus /wa/ contrast, as compared to children with no history of disorder. Further, this difficulty in behavioral discrimination is also reflected in the electrophysiologic mismatch negativity response (MMN) of the same children (Kraus et al., 1996). As discussed in Chapter 1, the /da/ versus /ga/ contrast appears to rely on precise temporal coding at the level of the auditory cortex whereas the /ba/ versus /wa/ contrast appears to rely more on signal encoding at the thalamic level (King et al., 1995). Because the /ba/ versus /wa/ contrast is far less vulnerable to disruption by cortical dysfunction, it serves as a good control to ensure that the child (or adult) being tested did, indeed, understand the task. Further in investigation into the use of this paradigm with individuals exhibiting known lesions of the CANS, along with comparisons of this paradigm with other behavioral tasks of central auditory function, are needed. However, this measure may prove to be a valuable addition to the central auditory test battery.

A limited supply of the PEST software has been made available by the research team, and normative values for discrimination thresholds in children have been published (Kraus et al., 1999). It should be noted, however, that the paradigm requires a great deal of additional psychophysical stimulus delivery and response equipment that is not generally available in audiology clinics. Therefore, this procedure is not in general clinical use at the present time.

A second procedure that may ultimately show promise in evaluation of very fine-grained auditory function presumed to be important for speech perception is the backward masking paradigm described by Wright et. al (1997). In this paradigm, the child's ability to detect brief auditory stimuli in the presence of an auditory masker that occurs following the stimuli is measured. The authors demonstrated that some children with language learning impairments have severe difficulty with this task under stimulus conditions that resemble those in running speech. That is, continuous speech involves rapid sequential presentation of sounds with different acoustic spectra. Some children with language learning impairments demonstrate deficits in the ability to detect sounds that are followed rapidly by other sounds, providing a possible auditory basis for some language or auditory comprehension disorders. This paradigm has not been investigated in individuals with known CANS lesions, nor is it commercially available at the present time.

The differential diagnosis of attention-deficit hyperactivity disorder (AD/HD) and CAPD is a topic of considerable importance, and will be addressed in Chapter 7. However, it is important to note that several measures are available to assist in determining how well a child or adult can sustain attention to auditory stimuli. One of these, the Auditory Continuous Performance Test (ACPT; Keith, 1994a), was discussed in Chapter 4. Briefly, this test, like most vigilance tests, evaluates the listener's ability to respond consistently to a target when it occurs randomly in a long series of nontarget stimuli. Similar measures also exist using visual stimuli, and their employment as part of a behavioral central auditory assessment can be very useful in determining whether a generalized attention-related deficit exists when the presence of an attention confound is suspected.

Finally, in deference to the modality specificity issues raised by Cacace and McFarland (1998) and others, the Bruton consensus conference document (Jerger & Musiek, 2000) suggested that a comparison of performance on analogous auditory and visual tasks should be considered when assessing central auditory function. However, to date, there are few, if any, commercially available visual-based versions of the tests discussed in this chapter. I have reported on visual-motor interhemispheric transfer task that can, along with auditory measures of interhemispheric function, be used to assess corpus callosum function (Bellis & Wilber, 2001). In addition, several clinics, including my own, are in the process of developing visual analogs to many of the auditory tasks discussed in this chapter. For example, temporal ordering tasks, such as Frequency and Duration Patterns, can easily be converted to the visual modality using color, size, brightness, or placement on a computer screen and having the subject linguistically label the pattern seen (e.g. red-red-black, big-small-big). This would assist in determining whether pattern perception difficulties seen in some children with CAPD are restricted to the auditory modality or whether they also exist in the visual modality as well.

Along these same lines, McFarland, Cacace, and Setzen (1998) described several auditory and visual temporal-order discrimination tasks and demonstrated that temporal order perception in normal subjects does appear to be reliant on sensory modality-specific mechanisms. As such, dissociation of function in auditory versus visual modalities may be exhibited by at least some children with CAPD; however, this remains to be confirmed. Virtually any of the auditory tasks described in this chapter can be converted into the visual modality, but this area requires a great deal of development, standardization, validation, and additional investigation before its clinical utility in differential diagnosis of CAPD can be determined.

Sensitivity and Specificity of Behavioral Central Auditory Measures

I began this chapter with a discussion of issues relating to validity of behavioral central auditory test tools. I also discussed some of the difficulties inherent in determining sensitivity and specificity of these measures. In general, Chermak and Musiek (1997) report that the efficiency (sensitivity and specificity combined) of these behavioral measures range from poor (approximately 68%) to good (near 90%) for some test tools, depending on the measure, site of lesion, extent of lesion, and a variety of other factors. In general, low-pass filtered speech tests seemed to fare relatively poorly, whereas Duration Patterns and Dichotic Digits appeared to be more efficient at detecting CANS lesions. However, a great deal of research is still needed, and that which is available often suffers from poor subject control, lack of standardized pass/fail criteria, and similar issues.

In addition, most central auditory tests demonstrate sensitivity to dysfunction in certain regions of the CANS, but not to dysfunction in other regions. For this reason, it follows that children with CAPD will show deficits in some, but not all, central tests administered, depending on the type of auditory disorder that is present. Therefore, the determination of absolute sensitivity/specificity of these test tools may prove to extremely difficult at best (Domitz & Schow, 2000). To my knowledge, no study has been completed that systematically evaluated the efficiency of various *combinations* of these test tools in identifying known CANS lesions, although some studies have verified the existence of patterns of test findings in cases of region-specific CANS dysfunction. This issue will be discussed further in relation to central auditory assessment interpretation in Chapter 7.

Because of these difficulties, Chermak and Musiek, (1997) advised that, presently, sensitivity/specificity information should be viewed with caution and used primarily as a general guide to central auditory test selection. Clinicians should avoid placing too much emphasis on this issue until more information is obtained.

Electrophysiological Procedures

No discussion of central auditory tests would be complete without mention of electrophysiological procedures. These procedures were discussed in some detail in Chapter 3. More and more attention in recent years has been given to the use of electrophysiology for pediatric central auditory assessment. Advantages of electrophysiologic measures over behavioral central tests include their utility in very young children or hard-to-test populations, the ability to obtain responses that are not reliant on subject cooperation or behavioral response, and the fact that they provide a noninvasive means of assessing CANS function objectively. Despite these advantages, however, clinicians should be aware of what information these types of measures do and no not provide.

Fundamentally, auditory electrophysiology assesses the ability of CANS neurons to fire synchronously in response to acoustic stimuli. Chapter 1 discussed the importance of precise temporal firing of populations of neurons in speech encoding. Therefore, any disorder that disrupts neural synchrony would, likewise, be expected to affect the ability to process speech. As such, auditory electrophysiology may be thought of as a means of capturing a glimpse of neurophysiologic encoding at its most basic level.

On the other hand, not all cases of CAPD will be reflected by abnormalities in neural synchrony. Chermak and Musiek (1997) estimated that 65% to 70% of central auditory processing disorders are due to neuromorphological disorder, 25% to 30% might be due to delayed neuromaturation, and under 5% are due to neurologic disease or insult. For the vast majority of these, we are unable to confirm precisely the presence of an abnormality, although recent advances in neuroimaging techniques may aid us in this endeavor in the near future. Clinical experience shows, however, that many individuals with CAPD exhibit normal auditory electrophysiologic responses, at least for those measures that are in common clinical use. Further, we must always keep in mind that, although auditory evoked potentials provide an index of neural synchrony in the CANS, they do not share a one-to-one correspondence with auditory behavior; that is, they do not tell us how well the individual is able to process and use the synchronous neural information. Therefore, the finding of an electrophysiologic abnormality may confirm the presence of CANS dysfunction, but it sheds little or no light on the nature of the auditory disorder that an individual exhibits, nor does it provide directions for management that can be designed to address the individual's functional difficulties.

That having been said, there are many situations in which auditory electrophysiologic recording adds greatly to the central auditory assessment process. The ABR evaluates integrity of the brainstem auditory pathways and, as such, will typically be normal in children with higher-order learning, language, or auditory deficits. However, in those cases in which possible brainstem involvement or auditory neuropathy is suspected, the ABR is an invaluable diagnostic tool. Sensitivity of the ABR is best for tumors of the VIIIth nerve (up to 90%); however, its sensitivity for other brainstem lesions is somewhat lower (Musiek & Lee, 1995).

The middle latency response (MLR) has recently been given a great deal of attention in assessment of CAPD. Because of intersubject variability in MLR peak latencies and amplitudes, it appears that the best indicators of CAPD using the MLR are either presence or absence of response or through a comparison of response amplitudes obtained over right versus left scalp electrode sites (Kraus, Ozdamar, Krier, & Stein, 1982; Marvel, Jerger, & Lew, 1992). When the response is significantly smaller (> 50%) over one site than the other, this is termed an electrode effect (Musiek, Baran, & Pinheiro, 1994), and is an indicator of CANS dysfunction. Ear effects—or smaller responses to stimulation of one ear than the other, regardless of electrode recording site—may also be somewhat useful in CAPD diagnosis (Shehata-Dieler, Shimizu, Solimon, & Tusa, 1991).

The LEP, including the P300, can also be a valuable indicator of CANS dysfunction at the cortical level. Again, interpreting the obligatory LEP responses (i.e., the P1, N1, and P2) in terms of presence versus absence, electrode effects, or ear effects appears to provide the most sensitive indicator of CAPD, as absolute latency and amplitude of these responses demonstrate significant intersubject variability (Musiek et al., 1994). Finally, absence of the P300 occurs in some cases of CAPD, but it also occurs in cognitive, attention, and other higher-order disorders as well. It is possible that the use of speech stimuli in obtaining the LEP may provide greater insight into neurophysiologic asymmetries than the use of tonal stimuli (Bellis et al., 2000).

As discussed in Chapter 3, the mismatch negativity (MMN) may provide an indication of basic sensory encoding of acoustic change at the thalamocortical level; however, its utility in central auditory assessment remains debatable at the present time. In addition, there are many other auditory event-related potential paradigms that appear to show promise in evaluating CANS integrity, some of which may provide more valuable indices of functional implications of CANS dysfunction. However, these are primarily experimental at the present time, and do not enjoy widespread clinical use.

A topic of some controversy is whether electrophysiological measures are a necessary part of central auditory assessment. The Bruton conference consensus statement included the ABR and MLR in its recommendations for what constitutes a minimal test battery for the diagnoses of CAPD (Jerger & Musiek, 2000). Similarly, Parthasarathy

(2000) stated unequivocally that auditory electrophysiologic measures should be included in every central auditory test battery, as they provide objective evidence of CANS dysfunction. One primary argument in favor of the use of these measures is that behavioral tests can be confounded by motivation, attention, and other non-auditory-related factors. Although this argument has some merit, these factors can be identified and controlled for during testing by careful ongoing analysis and interpretation of patterns of test results during behavioral assessment, a topic that will be discussed further in Chapter 7.

In my own experience, I have found auditory electrophysiology to be an extremely valuable tool in some cases, but of very little value in others. When a child is too young to be tested using behavioral tests of central auditory function, auditory evoked potentials may uncover objective evidence of CANS dysfunction. These data can then be used along with information from other professionals working with the child (e.g., speech and language, psychology, education) to develop auditory-based intervention goals for the child in question. However, we must acknowledge that the results of electrophysiologic evaluation do not give us a precise understanding of the types of auditory processes that are affected in the child, and we must proceed on a best-guess hypothetical basis when devising management plans.

In older children and adults who can be tested using behavioral means, I have found that results of the behavioral central auditory assessment provide far greater insight into the types of auditory processing deficit the individual exhibits and the functional impact of the deficit than do results of electrophysiologic testing. Thus, my ability to devise a management plan that is specific to the individual's disorder is not enhanced by the use of auditory evoked potentials. In these cases, the use of auditory electrophysiology is of little practical value beyond physiologic confirmation of CANS dysfunction. Moreover, because many cases of CAPD do not result in electrophysiologic abnormalities, normal auditory evoked responses do not rule out or refute the presence of an auditory processing deficit.

Finally, we must consider the issue of cost versus benefit. If a measure, such as evoked potentials, is not likely to shed much light on the nature and functional impact of the disorder, and we have other tools at our fingertips that will provide greater direction for intervention and management, we must ask whether gratuitous inclusion of auditory electrophysiologic measures is worth the cost in terms of time and money. If, however, objective documentation of CANS dysfunction is a primary goal of the assessment, if we suspect some type of neurologic disorder that may require medical follow-up, or if behavioral tests cannot be completed for some reason, then the benefits of evoked potential testing likely outweigh the costs.

Nevertheless, the documentation of neurophysiologic abnormalities continues to be important in many situations. In addition, in some cases, auditory electrophysiology may provide the only means by which we can assess CANS function. Therefore, clinicians should be familiar with electrophysiological measures of auditory function and make every attempt either to provide such services or to locate a source to which patients can be referred for such testing.

In conclusion, while I do not advocate the addition of electrophysiological measures to all central auditory evaluations, it should be recognized that they may provide useful information in certain situations. Therefore, electrophysiology should be considered an integral part of the central auditory test battery.

Summary

This chapter has discussed the topics of test validity and reliability, as well as provided an overview of behavioral and physiologic central auditory assessment tools. The clinical validity of a given test tool may be calculated by evaluating the sensitivity and specificity of the test related to a specific standard. When tests of central auditory function are considered, it is suggested that the tests' ability to identify documented CANS lesions be the standard for determination of test validity. Reliability is determined by assessing the repeatability of test results in specific populations.

A variety of assessment tools is available within each of the categories discussed in this chapter, and each category is designed to assess different processes. Therefore, a comprehensive central auditory processing evaluation should include tests from more than one category as well as associated measures of speech/language, cognitive, and educational abilities, in a test battery approach. Only in this manner can an auditory profile delineating auditory strengths and weaknesses be developed and appropriate, deficit-specific recommendations for management made.

Review Questions

1. List and discuss three reasons why a test battery approach to central auditory assessment should be utilized.

2. Define the following terms related to test validity:

false positive	true positive
false negative	true negative
sensitivity	specificity
efficiency	

3. Define test reliability and provide examples of procedural and patient variables that may affect test reliability.

4. List and give a brief description of five dichotic speech tests.

5. What auditory processes do the dichotic speech tasks described above evaluate?

6. List and give a brief description of three tests of temporal ordering.

7. What auditory processes do the temporal ordering tests described above evaluate?

8. List and give a brief description of four methods of reducing the redundancy of a speech signal for purposes of central auditory assessment.

9. Discuss the limitations of speech-in-noise testing.

10. What auditory process does monaural low-redundancy speech testing evaluate?

11. List and give a brief description of four methods of assessing binaural interaction abilities.

12. Discuss the limitations of binaural interaction tests in general.

13. Identify additional behavioral measures that may, with time, prove to be useful additions to central auditory assessment.

14. Discuss the value of including electrophysiological procedures in central auditory assessment.

CHAPTER

SIX

Comprehensive Central Auditory Assessment

his chapter provides readers with information necessary to plan and carry out comprehensive evaluations of central auditory function. Because of the practical nature of the information contained herein, readers may be tempted to skip the earlier chapters in this book and approach central auditory assessment from a "cookbook" perspective, using this chapter as a guide. However, I cannot overemphasize the importance of understanding the scientific bases of central auditory assessment. Therefore, **I strongly recommend that the information provided in the previous chapters be studied carefully and internalized prior to entering the assessment arena.** With an understanding of the scientific underpinnings, as well as the nature of the various types of central auditory assessment tools, this chapter can serve as a resource for information regarding specific assessment protocols. Test interpretation will be covered in Chapter 7.

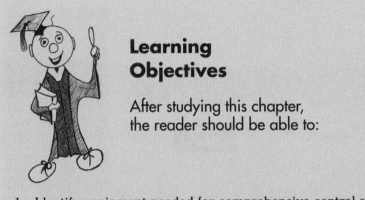

Learning Objectives

After studying this chapter, the reader should be able to:

1. Identify equipment needed for comprehensive central auditory assessment.
2. Identify components of the assessment procedure.
3. Discuss methods of choosing components of the central auditory test battery.
4. Delineate assessment protocols for several commonly utilized tests of central auditory function.

Required Equipment

Although screening procedures for CAPD can be and often are administered utilizing little more than a portable cassette tape deck, a table, and two chairs, **behavioral diagnostic tests of central auditory function should always be conducted in a sound booth so that adequate acoustic control of stimuli can be maintained.** A two-channel audiometer is required for many of the test procedures that will be discussed in this chapter. In addition, clinicians will need to procure a good quality tape player or a compact disc player. I recommend that both types of equipment be available, as several commonly used tests are available only on magnetic tape, while others can be found on compact disc, which provides higher quality and fidelity of auditory stimuli than can be obtained through the use of magnetic tape (Noffsinger, Wilson, & Musiek, 1994). As in all audiological assessment, equipment should be calibrated regularly and maintained in good working order.

The Assessment Procedure

Prior to central auditory assessment, full evaluation of the peripheral auditory system should be conducted. The Bruton conference consensus statement recommendations (Jerger & Musiek, 2000) emphasized that pure-tone audiometry, word recognition performance-intensity (PI) functions, immittance audiometry, and otoacoustic emissions (OAEs) be included as part of any central auditory assessment. Although some question the need for OAEs and word recognition PI functions in cases of clearly normal peripheral hearing sensitivity, it is clear that the integrity of the peripheral auditory system must be established before any evaluation of central auditory function is undertaken. In my own clinic, these assessments are always completed as part of the screening process before consideration for central auditory assessment, along with multidisciplinary measures of speech and language, cognition, and learning, as discussed in Chapter 4.

Comprehensive central auditory assessment should be undertaken in such a manner as to maximize the child's abilities while controlling for confounding factors such as environmental distractions, attention, and fatigue. If at all possible, children should not undergo central auditory assessment when overly tired or ill. I have found it useful to schedule younger children in the morning so that they enter the clinic fully rested and alert.

The first portion of any central auditory assessment should be an interview with the child and accompanying parent(s) or caregiver. Often, children and parents arrive at the clinic with varying degrees of apprehension. Before beginning formalized assessment, it is advisable to explain the evaluation process fully so that they know what to expect and their apprehension can be minimized.

A complete history should be taken at the time of the interview, to include information related to the child's medical and educational history, auditory symptoms, and general behavior. Parents and children should be asked about those skills that require multimodality coordination or interhemispheric integration, such as art, music, and motor coordination. In addition, the presence of a family history of learning or hearing problems should be identified. In many cases, clinicians will hear, "Well, Johnny's father doesn't really think that this testing is all that important. After all, *he* had the same kinds of problems in school when he was Johnny's age." This comment may suggest a possible familial transmission of auditory processing or learning disorders.

Like the assessment itself, the interview should be individualized. At times, clinicians may need to ask several, detailed questions in order to draw information from a reluctant parent or child. Conversely, one or two questions may prompt a descriptive monologue including a wealth of applicable information. **Regardless of the amount of information obtained from screening procedures and questionnaires, the face-to-face interview is necessary, as previously unknown details often will emerge.** In addition, clinicians will be able to get a feel for the parent's (and child's) attitudes toward the possible disorder as well as its impact on social, emotional, and other aspects of the child's life.

Before beginning the assessment, clinicians should make sure that factors that may affect a child's ability to attend, including hunger, thirst, or needing to go to the bathroom, have been eliminated. Any extraneous environmental distractions should be kept to a minimum. For this reason, I typically suggest that parents not accompany the children into the sound suite for testing, except in select circumstances. Instead, I advise parents to wait, and I assure them that they will be called when testing is completed and that the results of the evaluation will be explained to them at that time.

The time required to complete the assessment will depend on the individual situation. Children undergoing evaluation should be monitored carefully for signs of fading attention or fatigue, and frequent breaks should be offered. In some cases, a complete evaluation may be completed within forty-five minutes. When additional test procedures are deemed necessary or frequent breaks are required, testing may require as long as two to three hours.

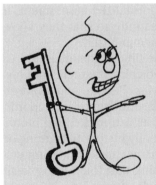

KEY CONCEPT

Every effort should be made to minimize or eliminate any extraneous factors that may adversely affect the child's ability to attend during central auditory testing.

When the test session has been completed, clinicians should sit down with the parents and child once again and explain the components and results of the evaluation as well as make preliminary recommendations for management. Questions and concerns should be addressed at this time. This practice helps to foster the parents' and child's understanding of the disorder and assists in ensuring that follow-through will occur, but does not take the place of a written report. Suggestions for report writing and imparting information to parents and educational professionals will be provided in Chapter 10.

In summary, the assessment procedure should include an interview with the parents and child, the assessment itself, and a discussion of evaluation results and preliminary recommendations for management. Therefore, clinicians will need to schedule comprehensive central auditory assessments so as to ensure that sufficient time is available for all portions of the assessment procedure. This practice may be time-consuming, perhaps discouraging some clinicians for whom caseloads are already overwhelming. However, fostering an atmosphere of relaxation and thoroughness will help to increase the productivity of the test session itself, as well as assist in ensuring understanding of the disorder and follow-through on management recommendations.

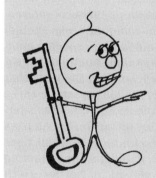

KEY CONCEPT

Clinicians should set aside ample time for a complete interview, assessment procedure (including breaks as needed), and post-test counseling.

Choosing the Test Battery

In the previous chapter, the rationale for a test battery approach to central auditory assessment was presented. However, the question of which tests would be appropriate for inclusion in a central auditory test battery remains. The ASHA (1996) consensus statement lists several auditory behaviors that comprise central auditory processing. It stands to reason that, when assessing central auditory function, one would choose a battery that taps as many of these identified processes as possible. However, the ASHA (1996) document did not define precisely how the available test measures correspond to the identified underlying auditory phenomena.

Schow et al. (2000) undertook a confirmatory factor analysis to elucidate this issue more clearly. As mentioned in Chapter 5, they identified four general factors represented by the central tests that were included in their analysis. They then related these factors directly to at least four of the auditory behavioral phenomena identified by the ASHA (1996) consensus statement. These factors included (1) Auditory Pattern Temporal Ordering (APTO), which can be assessed by tests such as Frequency and Duration Patterns; (2) Monaural Separation/Closure (MSC), which tests of monaural low-redundancy speech, such as low-pass filtered speech and similar measures, appear to tap; (3) Binaural Separation (BS), which is measured by dichotic tests involving directed attention; and (4) Binaural Integration (BI), for which dichotic tests involving nondirected attention and report of both ears is required.

Three additional, more complex, yet measurable auditory behaviors were also identified by Schow et al. (2000). These behaviors are presumed to be a component of many of the test procedures listed above and include (1) localization/lateralization or binaural interaction, (2) auditory discrimination, and (3) other temporal tasks, including gap detection. Although the authors did not include specific auditory tests that directly tap these three areas in their analysis, largely because of the lack of clinically available tools, some of the tests that were discussed in the previous chapter appear to fall into these three categories. For example, localization/lateralization and binaural interaction can be assessed using Binaural Interaction tasks such as Binaural Fusion or the MLD; however, the need for more efficient tests in this category is apparent. The new PEST paradigm for obtaining jnds to fine-grained acoustic differences developed by Northwestern University's auditory neuroscience laboratory may prove to be an excellent measure of auditory discrimination at its most basic level. Finally, the advent of the RGDT allows for a clinically available means of assessing temporal gap detection.

Although much more research still needs to be done regarding which combination(s) of clinical test measures tap those auditory behaviors identified by ASHA (1996) most efficiently, we now have an empirically derived framework in place for choosing components of the central auditory test battery. This framework is much the same as that suggested by Bellis (1996), Bellis and Ferre (1999), and Chermak and Musiek (1997). Before I discuss the components of the framework, however, it should be noted that the report of the Bruton consensus conference (Jerger & Musiek, 2000) suggested that, at minimum, a test battery for central auditory assessment could include only three behavioral measures of central auditory function: a dichotic task, a temporal patterning task, and a gap detection task, along with physiologic measures such as immittance audiometry, OAEs, and ABR/MLR. In light of the ASHA (1996) recommendations and the Schow et al. (2000) confirmatory factorial analysis, I feel that this minimal battery is *too* minimal. That is, it does not provide sufficient means of assessing each of the auditory behavioral phenomena set forth in the ASHA (1996) definition of central auditory processes.

That having been said, and using the categorization of central auditory tests that was provided in Chapter 5, I recommend that the components of the comprehensive central auditory test battery be chosen from the following general areas:

- A dichotic listening task that involves directed attention (BS)
- A dichotic listening task that involves report of both ears (BI)
- A temporal patterning test such as Frequency or Duration Patterns (APTO)
- A test of monaural low-redundancy speech, such as LPFS, Compressed Speech with or without reverberation, or one of the other measures discussed in the previous chapter (MSC)
- A temporal gap detection test, such as the RGDT (other temporal processes)
- A binaural interaction test, such as binaural fusion or the more sensitive MLD (binaural interaction)
- An auditory discrimination task such as the Northwestern PEST paradigm (however, readers should note that this task requires additional equipment not typically available in audiology clinics)
- Physiologic measures of auditory function, such as ABR, MLR, and late event-related potentials (*Note:* I do not include immittance audiometry and OAEs in this category because, as discussed in the previous chapter, these are measures of peripheral auditory integrity and, as such, should be completed prior to considering central auditory assessment).

Before moving on to a discussion of how to choose the tests to include in an assessment from the above list, some mention should be made of what I have come to term *assessment in a box procedures*. By this I mean auditory tests that are packaged together, require little acoustic control or even auditory equipment beyond a portable cassette or compact disc player and headphones, and include manuals for cookbook-style interpretation of results. The most commonly used example of this type of test battery is the SCAN and its revisions and upper extensions.

It is clear why these types of test tools are attractive to clinicians, especially those who are just beginning to explore the field of CAPD. They remove the uncertainty of having to choose components of the test battery; lessen the inconvenience involved in procuring various types of test materials from several sources, devising scoring sheets, and locating normative data; require less knowledge and experience with CAPD to administer; and render interpretation far easier and more straightforward. For these reasons, assessment tools such as the SCAN may be the most commonly used "diagnostic tests" of central auditory processing today.

However, there are significant concerns regarding the use of these types of assessment tools. Primary among these are issues related to reliability and validity. The SCAN has been criticized for rather weak test-retest reliability in young school-age children (Cacace & McFarland, 1998). Of even more concern is the high correlation found between the SCAN and nonauditory tests of vocabulary function. For example, the SCAN correlates with the Peabody Picture Vocabulary Test—Revised (PPVT-R) nearly as strongly as it does with itself (Keith, Rudy, Donahue, & Katbamna, 1989), which raises a question as to whether it measures anything different than the PPVT-R.

Moreover, each subtest of the SCAN has been shown to tap into multiple auditory behavioral factors, rendering its interpretation in terms of functional processes affected in a given child difficult at best (Schow et al., 2000). Domitz and Schow (2000) found that the SCAN exhibits very poor sensitivity for CAPD (approximately 45%), rendering it unacceptable even for screening use. The addition of a temporal processing measure did not improve its sensitivity. Finally, inclusion of the SCAN subtests in confirmatory factor analysis yielded a lesser degree of uniformity in the overall construct, suggesting that the general framework for categorizing central auditory tests delineated above is much more stable when the SCAN subtests are not included (Schow et al., 2000). Therefore, as was recommended in Chapter 4, the SCAN should be used for screening purposes only. Even then, results of the SCAN should be considered in light of additional information from the multidisciplinary team when attempting to determine whether a child *may* exhibit an auditory processing deficit. For comprehensive central auditory assessment, I recommend that tests be chosen from the framework proposed above, a process that involves knowledge of the various tests, the process(es) assessed by each, test administration, and test interpretation. These factors, in turn, ultimately rely on the clinician's knowledge of the underlying neurophysiology of auditory processing, a topic that was emphasized heavily in Part One of this book.

Although the decision regarding how many and precisely which central tests to utilize should be based upon each individual case, I suggest the following rule of thumb: **because it is desirable to ensure that the test battery assesses different processes as well as different levels of the CANS, it would be prudent to include at least one test from each category.** An exception to this rule may be electrophysiological procedures, which should be recommended when the individual situation warrants their inclusion. **In addition, it is often helpful to include two tests of dichotic listening: one that is considered to be linguistically loaded (such as Competing Sentences or Staggered Spondaic Words), and one that carries a lighter linguistic load (such as Dichotic Digits).** The reason for this is that, as discussed in Chapter 3, children may perform quite differently on dichotic speech tasks, depending on the degree of linguistic loading.

The decision regarding which test(s) within each category to utilize also will depend on the individual situation. Clinicians will want to choose tests that have demonstrated validity and reliability and for which normative data are available for the age of the child. For example, older children and adolescents may perform quite reliably on the Dichotic CV test, but this test is likely to be much too difficult for younger children. In this case, a test such as Dichotic Digits, which is simpler and can be administered to children as young as age 7, may be a more appropriate choice.

An additional factor in choosing test battery components is the question to be answered by the assessment. As discussed in the previous chapter, if the goal is to identify the presence of a CAPD *at all costs*, then clinicians will want to include a greater number of tests, even though the possibility of a false positive result will be greater. In the majority of central auditory evaluations, however, it is recommended that clinicians choose those tests that are the most efficient in terms of validity, time, and ease of administration.

Finally, it should be emphasized that **central auditory assessment is a dynamic process requiring ongoing interpretation *during* the evaluation process.** The assessment situation should be entered into with a basic "game plan" based on preassessment information in mind; however, that plan may, and often will, change, depending upon the situation.

For example, a child may be referred for comprehensive central auditory assessment with the primary complaint of severe difficulty understanding speech in noise and preliminary screening information that indicates a strong likelihood of CAPD. Based upon this history, the clinician cannot predict which process or processes may be dysfunctional in this child. Therefore, the assessment plan will include a test from each category of central tests, as recommended above. However, it may be noticed during testing that, on a test of auditory closure such as low-pass filtered speech, the child performs at a borderline-normal level. In this case, the clinician may decide to include a more difficult test of auditory closure, such as Time-Compressed Speech with reverberation, in order to tap the process of auditory closure more fully. In addition, a speech-in-noise test may be given for the purpose of obtaining descriptive data, although, as was seen in the previous chapter, speech-in-noise tests should be interpreted with caution and age-appropriate normative data must be available for the specific materials utilized.

In other words, individualization of the assessment procedure requires ongoing interpretation of the data, rather than simply collecting the data during assessment, and then scoring and interpreting the test results after the child has left the clinic. Decisions regarding additional assessment tools to include, as well as judgments of response reliability, must be made continually throughout the assessment procedure.

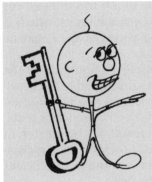

KEY CONCEPT

Data collected during the assessment procedure should undergo ongoing qualitative and quantitative interpretation during, rather than after, the assessment process.

Test Administration

This section describes recommended assessment protocols for several commonly used tests of central auditory function. I do not intend to suggest that the following protocols are the only manner in which these tests may be administered. In addition, some tests of central auditory function will not be discussed in this section. The measures I have chosen are, for the most part, those that are in relatively common clinical use, are easily available, and for which some sort of standardized normative data have been collected. Unless otherwise specified, the age-specific normative data presented for tests in this chapter are based on my own data collected from more than 250 listeners age 7 to adult from four clinic sites. When available, normative data presented in the respective test manuals or in the literature are also included. Normal cutoffs are based on two standard deviations below the mean unless otherwise noted, as recommended in Jerger and Musiek (2000) and Domitz and Schow (2000). Many commonly used test tools still require more in-depth normative data collection for various ages, including older adults. For information regarding statistical analysis and procedures related to the collection of normative data, readers are referred to Chapter 11.

Dichotic Speech Tests

When administering any dichotic speech test, several procedural factors should be considered. By definition, a two-channel audiometer is required for dichotic listening. Because dichotic speech tests are interpreted in terms of ear effects, it is recommended that clinicians monitor only one channel at a time and keep careful track of which ear the monitored channel is being routed to so that scoring errors may be avoided. Finally, the administration of most dichotic speech tests require that the stimuli be delivered to both ears at equivalent intensities. Therefore, it is recommended that these tests only be administered in cases of bilaterally symmetrical hearing sensitivity. A summary of the dichotic speech tests described in this section is presented in Table 6-1.

Dichotic Digits (DD)

There are three commercially available versions of the Dichotic Digits (DD) test: single, double, and triple digits. In the majority of situations, double digits will be the task of choice as it is sufficiently challenging while remaining simple enough even for young children. However, for cases in which double digits prove to be too difficult, single digits may be administered.

It is recommended that the DD test be administered at 50 dB SL (re: spondee threshold), or, in cases of peripheral hearing loss, at the most comfortable loudness level (MCL). Listeners are instructed that they will be hearing different numbers in each ear at the same time and should repeat all of the numbers heard, regardless of order. The

Table 6-1

Summary of Selected Dichotic Speech Tests: Test Administration

Test	Stimuli	Presentation Level	Scoring
Dichotic Digits	20 presentations of 4 digits each (2 to each ear)	50 dB	% correct
Dichotic Consonant-Vowels	30 pairs of CV segments per ear	55 dB	% correct per ear
Staggered Spondaic Words	spondaic words presented in staggered format in 4 conditions: RNC, RC, LC, and LNC	50 dB	% of errors per ear; in each condition; and total
Competing Sentences	25 sentence pairs	target: 35 dB; competing: 50 dB	% correct per ear
Synthetic Sentence Identification Test With Contralateral Competing Message	10 third-order approximations of English sentences	primary: 30dB; competing: varies from 30–70 dB	% CORRECT per ear
Dichotic Sentence Identification	same as SSI	50 dB (re: PTA)	% correct per ear, and interaural difference
Dichotic Rhyme Test	30 pairs of rhyming CVC words	50 dB	% correct per ear

first three stimulus presentations are for practice. The test consists of 20 stimulus presentations or, for double digits, 80 digits in all (40 per ear). The test is scored in terms of percent correct per ear (for double digits, each digit is worth 2.5%).

The following normative values for children are provided in the accompanying test maual; however, as with all tests of central auditory function, clinicians are strongly urged to collect their own age-appropriate normative data. Age-specific normal cutoffs for the double digits version of the Dichotic Digits test (Frank E. Musiek, Dartmouth-Hitchcock Medical Center) are as follows:

7 years to 7 years, 11 months: 55% left, 70% right
8 years to 8 years, 11 months: 65% left, 75% right
9 years to 9 years, 11 months: 75% left, 80% right
10 years to 10 years, 11 months: 78% left, 85% right
11 years to 11 years, 11 months: 88% left, 90% right
12 years to adult: 90% left and right

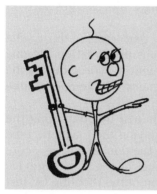

KEY CONCEPT

When administering dichotic speech tests, clinicians need to monitor the channels carefully to avoid errors in scoring and interpretation.

It should be noted that the adult normative cutoff of 90% for this test may need to be adjusted as more information is collected regarding Dichotic Digits performance in aging adults. Recent research by Bellis and Wilber (2001) suggested that separate normative values may be required for men over age of approximately 35 and women older than age 55. In addition, the DD test has been shown to be relatively resistant to cochlear hearing loss in adults when a criterion level of 80% for both ears is used (Musiek, 1983a).

Dichotic Consonant-Vowels (CV)

The recommended intensity for administration of the Dichotic CV test is 55 dB HL (75 dB peak equivalent SPL). All listeners should have hearing sensitivity within normal limits. The test consists of thirty pairs of CV segments. A response form is given to the listeners, and they are instructed to indicate the segments heard.

Testing begins with monotic presentation of the stimuli so that the listener may practice. When the listener is able to identify fourteen out of sixteen CVs presented monaurally, test administration may begin. The test is given in three manners: (1) no lag (simultaneous) condition, (2) 90 msec lag condition to one ear, and (3) 90 msec lag to the other ear. Like the DD test, Dichotic CVs are scored in terms of percent correct per ear, as well as double correct (occurrences in which stimuli presented to both ears are reported correctly).

Three measures may be obtained: (1) right-ear advantage (REA), (2) lag effect, and (3) auditory capacity effect. The REA is computed by comparing right-ear scores to left-ear scores during the simultaneous presentation condition. Unlike more linguistically loaded tests of dichotic listening, the REA for Dichotic CVs does not show a significant maturational effect in normally hearing children ages 7 to 15 (Roeser, Millay, & Morrow, 1983).

The lag effect is computed by comparing performance during the 90 msec lag conditions to that for simultaneous presentation. Normal listeners tend to show a significant improvement in scores during the left-ear 90 msec lag condition, whereas listeners with temporal lobe lesions do not.

Finally, auditory capacity may be determined by computing the double correct scores. The manual accompanying the magnetic tape version of the Dichotic CV test indicates that the double correct score improves from approximately 22% at age 7 to 43% at age 15. Normative values for the compact disc version of the Dichotic CV test indicate that the 90th percentile for single-ear performance (right or left) during the simultaneous presentation condition is at 56.7%. Therefore, **performance below 50% in an adult would be indicative of possible disorder** (Noffsinger, Martinez, & Wilson, 1994). Again, it should be stressed that each clinic needs to develop age-appropriate, normative data for the Dichotic CV test.

Staggered Spondaic Words (SSW)

The SSW is administered at 50 dB SL (re: pure tone average [PTA] or spondaic threshold); however, in cases of intolerance, the presentation level may be reduced to as low as 25 dB SL without significantly affecting test results. If a conductive hearing loss of 20 dB or greater is present, the presentation level to the affected ear should be lowered to 30 dB SL.

As described in Chapter 5, SSW stimuli are arranged in a manner such that spondaic words are presented in four conditions: (1) right noncompeting (RNC), (2) right competing (RC), (3) left competing (LC), and (4) left noncompeting (LNC). These four conditions are shown in Table 6-2 using the first item of the SSW test. Stimuli presentation is alternated between left leading and right leading; therefore, it is critical that clinicians carefully monitor which channel is routed to which ear and note this information on the score sheet. Listeners are required simply to report the words heard.

Table 6-2

Sample Item from the Staggered Spondaic Test

RNC	RC	
up	stairs	
	down	town
	LC	LNC

Note: RNC = Right Noncompeting; RC = Right Competing; LC = Left Competing; LNC = Left Noncompeting.

The scoring procedure for the SSW is somewhat involved. Scores obtained include the Raw SSW Score (R-SSW), which indicates the percentage of errors obtained in each of the four conditions (RNC, RC, LC, and LNC); percentage of errors by ear; and total percentage of errors. These numbers are converted to the C-SSW score, using a correction chart provided with the test forms, for interpretation. In addition, scores may be interpreted quantitatively in terms of total-ear-condition (used only for site of lesion testing with adults), and qualitatively in terms of response bias (such as reversals, order effects, and ear effects), as well as listener behavior during testing (including response time). Because scoring and interpretation for the SSW are complex, readers are referred to the manual that accompanies the test for detailed information (Katz, 1986).

This scoring procedure was developed primarily to relate SSW test results to the subtypes of CAPD proposed by Katz and his colleagues (Katz, Smith, & Kurpita, 1992; Masters, Stecker, & Katz, 1993), commonly referred to as the Buffalo Model. However, the Buffalo Model, like all theoretical models of CAPD subtyping, including my own, is not universally accepted. Therefore, the SSW can alternatively be scored just like any other dichotic test. Indeed, factor analysis of SSW "subtests," along with those of other tests, has shown that the RC and LC scores of the SSW primarily assess binaural competition or integration (BI), similar to other dichotic tests of binaural integration (Schow & Chermak, 1999). The noncompeting scores of the SSW do not appear to load onto any auditory processing factor at all, and seem to assess general word recognition in quiet.

As such, the SSW can be employed and interpreted in the same manner as the other tests of binaural integration discussed in this section. What is needed, however, is the development of age-appropriate normative values based on this interpretation paradigm and including normal cutoffs for right-ear and left-ear values separately under competing conditions as well as values for magnitude of the REA for children of various ages.

Competing Sentence Test (CST)

The CST consists of twenty-five sentence pairs. The target signal is presented to one ear at 35 dB SL (re: PTA) and the competing signal is presented to the opposite ear at 50 dB SL. Ten target sentences are presented to one ear, followed by ten to the other. The remaining five stimulus items may be used for practice or in order to assess the listener's ability to repeat both sentences when they are presented dichotically at equal intensity levels (50 dB SL). During administration of the CST, clinicians need to monitor carefully the channel through which the target sentence is being presented and to make sure that the intensity levels are correct for each ear. Listeners are required to repeat the target sentence only and ignore the competing message in the other ear.

Willeford and Burleigh (1994) suggested that the CST be scored liberally when used with children. Paraphrasing of the target sentence is allowed. Responses are scored as incorrect when the child's response includes significant intrusions of words from the competing message or the child fails to respond at all. Using this scoring method, normative values in children ages 5 to 10 indicate scores of 100% in the "strong" (usually right) ear, whereas scores in the "weak" (usually left) ear may range from 0 to 100%, improving with increasing age of the child. **These findings suggest a significant effect of maturation on the CST, with the ear advantage decreasing as a function of an increase in the age of the child.** However, in my own experience, this liberal approach to scoring has resulted in confusion on the part of clinicians, as well as a significant lack of standardization among clinics using the CST.

For this reason, I use the following, more stringent, scoring method with the CST, adapted from F. E. Musiek (personal communication, June 1994). Each of the 10 target sentences is assigned a value of 10 points and is divided into quadrants, each worth 2.5 points, or 25% of the total sentence score. The child's response is scored in terms of quadrants correct. Therefore, scores of 10, 7.5, 5, 2.5, or 0 are possible for each sentence, with a possible score of 100 for all 10 sentences. Table 6-3 provides an example of how sample responses to the first item of the CST may be scored.

The total ear score is achieved simply by adding the 10 sentence scores, resulting in a percent correct score for that ear. For example, the following sentence scores may be obtained: (1) 10, (2) 7.5, (3) 10, (4) 10, (5) 2.5, (6) 5, (7) 10, (8) 7.5, (9), 10, (10) 2.5. The total ear score

Table 6-3

Scoring of Sample Responses to the First Item of the Competing Sentences Test

Item 1		
TARGET:	I think we'll have rain today.	
COMPETING:	There was frost on the ground.	
Responses:	I think we'll have rain today.	Score: 10
	We'll have rain today.	Score: 7.5
	I think we'll have frost today.	Score: 7.5
	There was rain today.	Score: 5
	I think we have frost on the ground.	Score: 5
	There was frost today.	Score: 2.5
	I think there was frost on the ground.	Score: 2.5
	There was frost on the ground.	Score: 0
	I don't know.	Score: 0

is computed simply by adding the scores. Therefore, in this example, the ear score would be: 10 + 7.5 + 10 + 10 + 2.5 + 5 + 10 + 7.5 + 10 + 2.5 = 85, or 85%.

Using this scoring method I have developed the following normative values (2 standard deviations below the mean):

7 years to 7 years, 11 months: 35% left, 80% right
8 years to 8 years, 11 months: 39% left, 82% right
9 years to 9 years, 11 months: 74% left, 90% right
10 years to 10 years, 11 months: 88% left, 90% right
11 years to 11 years, 11 months: 90% both ears
12 years to adult: 90% both ears

As can be seen from these values, right-ear scores on the CST reach adult values by age 9 years, whereas left-ear scores demonstrate a maturation effect until age 11. I have found that scoring the test in this manner reduces the variability of scores within the age groups being tested, as well as provides a less ambiguous method of scoring the CST.

Synthetic Sentence Identification with Contralateral Message (SSI-CCM)

Both the ipsilateral and contralateral versions of the SSI test use the same sentence stimuli: ten third-order approximations of English sentences. The competing message consists of continuous discourse (a male speaker reading a story about the life of Davy Crockett). During administration of the SSI-CCM, it is recommended that the primary message be presented at 30 dB HL to one ear. The competing message presented to the other ear may be varied from 30 dB HL (0 dB signal-to-noise ratio [S/N]) to 70 dB HL (-40 dB S/N). Listeners are given a list of all ten sentences, and they are required to identify the sentence heard by number.

The score is reported in terms of percent correct per ear. The CCM score is considered to be either the score obtained in the most difficult condition (-40 dB S/N), or the average of the S/N conditions tested. If a score of 100% is achieved in the -40 dB S/N condition for a given ear, no further test conditions are necessary. The degree of asymmetry between ears on the SSI-CCM is generally a better indicator of central auditory dysfunction than is absolute test performance. Adults with normal hearing tend to perform at or near 100% in all conditions as do most listeners with brainstem lesions. Listeners with temporal lobe disorders tend to do poorly in the ear contralateral to the lesion (Jerger & Jerger, 1975).

It is recommended that the SSI only be administered in cases of normal hearing sensitivity at 500, 1000, and 2000 Hz.

Dichotic Sentence Identification (DSI)

The DSI test consists of the presentation of thirty pairs of the SSI sentences. It was designed for use with hearing-impaired listeners; however, **the listener's PTA should be no poorer than 50 dB for administration of the DSI.** The test stimuli are presented at a level of 50 dB SL (re: PTA of 500, 1000, and 2000 Hz). Listeners are given printed lists of the sentences, and instructed that they will hear two sentences presented simultaneously and are to indicate (by number) which sentences were heard. Results are scored in terms of percent correct per ear, which may be computed by multiplying the number correct by 3.33.

The test may be interpreted in terms of individual ear performance as well as interaural difference. Normative values for the DSI are based on the degree of hearing loss, with **individual ear scores of 75% or better considered to be within normal limits, regardless of PTA.** As the PTA increases, the normative values decrease, so that listeners with a PTA of 49 dB may achieve an individual ear score of only 23% and still be considered to have performed within normal limits.

Normative values for interaural difference scores are, likewise, based on the PTA of the poorer ear, and are as follows:

< 39 dB poorer ear PTA— < 16% difference between ears

< 40 dB to > 59 dB poorer ear PTA— < 39% difference between ears

Detailed information regarding normative values for the DSI may be found in its accompanying test manual, as well as in Fifer et al. (1983).

Dichotic Rhyme Test (DRT)

It is recommended that the DRT be administered at 50 dB SL (re: spondee threshold). The test consists of the presentation of thirty pairs of rhyming CVC words. Because of the close temporal alignment of the stimuli, listeners typically hear and report just one word for each stimulus presentation, resulting in an individual ear score near 50%. **As in all dichotic speech tests, it is critical that clinicians monitor one channel at a time and carefully note to which ear each channel is routed.**

Scores are expressed in terms of percent correct per ear. My normative data indicated no significant effect of age or ear on the DRT. Normative values (2 standard deviations *above and below* the mean) were 32–60% per ear. Scores below or above these values for a given ear are considered abnormal. It should be noted that my findings indicated a slightly smaller range of scores than those of Musiek, Kurdziel-Schwan, Kibbe, Gollegly, Baran, and Rintelmann (1989), who reported normative values of 30–73% for the right ear and 27–60% for the left ear in a group of 115 normal-hearing adults.

Once again, I should mention that the Dichotic Rhyme test is not commercially available at the present time. However, it is a useful tool to evaluate interhemispheric function, and is a good means of beginning the central auditory assessment because of the simplicity of the task for the listener. Therefore, the previous information was presented in the hopes that this test will soon be made clinically available.

Temporal Processing Tests

As discussed in the previous chapter, temporal processing skills may be assessed in a variety of ways; however, many of these methods require a degree of acoustic control that is not typically available from a standard audiometer. Therefore, this section will describe three tests of temporal processing that are currently commercially available: the Random Gap Detection Test, Pitch Patterns, and Duration Patterns. Readers are referred to the References at the end of this

Table 6-4
Summary of Selected Tests of Temporal Processing

Test	Stimuli	Presentation Level	Scoring
Random Gap Detection Test (RGDT)	Tone and click pairs with randomly varying ISIs from 0 to 40 ms	55dB HL	Average of gap detection thresholds for all stimuli; > 20 ms is considered abnormal
Frequency Patterns Test (FPT)	Sixty patterns of triads of tones differing in frequency	50 dB HL	% correct
Duration Patterns Test	Sixty patterns of triads of tones differing in duration	50 dB HL	% correct

book for sources of additional methods of evaluating temporal processing abilities. Table 6-4 provides a summary of the three tests discussed in this section.

Random Gap Detection Test (RGDT)

In the RGDT (Keith, 2000), several pairs of tonal or click stimuli are presented to the listener, who is required to indicate whether one or two sounds are heard. Subtest 1 is a practice and preliminary screening procedure consisting of 500 Hz tone pairs with interstimulus intervals (ISIs) presented in ascending order from 0 to 40 ms. The purposes of this preliminary procedure are to determine whether the listener is able to complete the task and to provide an opportunity for practice.

During Subtest 2, the standard test, ISIs from 0 to 40 ms are randomly presented to eliminate anticipatory responses. Stimuli consist of tonal pairs of octave frequencies from 500 to 4000 Hz. Subtests 3 and 4 consist of a practice session and a standard test, respectively, using click stimuli.

The test manual accompanying the RGDT recommends that the signals be presented binaurally at a comfortable listening level (i.e., 55 dB HL). Stimuli are routed from a compact disc player through a two-channel audiometer, and testing is conducted in a sound-shielded booth. Children can either respond verbally (i.e., "one" versus "two") or, alternatively, they can be instructed to hold up the number of fingers corresponding to the number of stimuli heard. RGDT thresholds are, first, calculated for each frequency by identifying the ISI at which the listener was able to identify two tones consistently. The average gap detection threshold is then calculated by averaging the threshold ISIs obtained for the various frequencies presented. The test takes approximately ten minutes to administer. Normative values collected from several clinics throughout the country indicate that gap detection thresholds greater than 20 ms should be taken as evidence of a temporal processing disorder.

Frequency (Pitch) Patterns

The Frequency Patterns test should be administered at an intensity of 50 dB SL (re: 1000 Hz threshold). The test consists of sixty test patterns, and stimuli can be presented monaurally or binaurally. Generally, it is appropriate to use half lists (thirty items) per ear; however, if scores are near the criterion for normal performance, making a clinical decision difficult, the full sixty-item list should be administered (Musiek, 1994). It is critical that detailed instructions be given to listeners and ample practice be provided to ensure comprehension of the task.

Listeners should be instructed that they will hear sets of three tones each that will vary in terms of pitch. Listeners are to report the tonal patterns heard (e.g., high-high-low, low-high-low). The clinician should then hum various patterns while visually cueing the listener. When the listener is able to perform the task with visual cues, the clinician should then hum various patterns without cueing the listener visually. If listeners are unable to perform the task without visual cues they should be reinstructed and given hummed patterns, both with and without visual cues, once again in order to determine whether the inability to perform the task is due to a lack of understanding of the test protocol or to a possible processing deficit. Once listeners have been instructed and are able to perform the task without visual cues, six practice items chosen randomly from the test itself may be given.

Test scores are expressed in terms of percent correct per ear. Only those patterns that are reported accurately are judged to be correct.

In situations where listeners are unable to perform the task without visual cues, or perform poorly on the task, they may be retested while humming or singing the pattern, thus removing the linguistic labeling component. In this manner, clinicians can compare listeners' performance on the two types of tasks, providing information regarding interhemispheric integration of auditory information. Some listeners will sing the responses from the outset. In this situation, they should be reinstructed simply to say, not sing, the required responses.

Normative values for the Frequency Patterns test suggest a cutoff score of 78% for young, normal-hearing adults (Musiek, 1994). My own clinic normative data, using thirty-item half lists, are in general agreement with this suggestion, with no significant effect of ear tested. My normative values (2 standard deviations below the mean) are as follows:

7 years to 7 years, 11 months: 35%
8 years to 8 years, 11 months: 42%
9 years to 9 years, 11 months: 63%
10 years to 10 years, 11 months: 78%
11 years to 11 years, 11 months: 78%
12 years to adult: 80%

It should be noted that **the high degree of variability found in very young children suggests that the Frequency Patterns test probably would not be an appropriate measure for children below age 7.**

A final issue regarding administration of the Frequency Patterns test, as well as the Duration Patterns test discussed in the following section, is whether reversals (e.g., saying "high-low-high" when the stimuli were "low-high-low") should be scored as incorrect responses. Although there are some who advocate not including reversals in the final error count, the test was designed to consider reversals as errors, and the age-appropriate normative values are based on this premise. The rationale for this recommendation is unclear at this time, particularly as labeling the tonal patterns in reverse order is just as likely in cases of cortical or interhemispheric dysfunction as are completely inaccurate responses. Moreover, although factor analysis has shown that both manners of scoring result in assessment of the same general processes, the practice of not including reversals in the final error count may certainly affect whether a given child passes or fails the task (Domitz & Schow, 2000). Because there is no satisfactory underlying rationale for counting reversals as correct, it is recommended that calculation of the final score include reversals as errors (F. E. Musiek, personal communication).

Duration Patterns

The Duration Patterns test is administered and scored in the same manner as the Frequency Patterns test, except that listeners are to respond in terms of the length of the stimuli (e.g., short-short-long,

long-short-long). Normative values suggest a cutoff of 73% for young, normal-hearing adults (Musiek, 1994). My own normative data collected from listeners age 7 to adult indicate that the Durations Pattern test is more difficult than the Frequency Patterns test. At all ages, normal cutoffs for Duration Patterns are approximately 7% to 10% lower than those of Frequency Patterns. Normal cutoffs are as follows:

7 years to 7 years, 11 months: 25%
8 years to 8 years, 11 months: 35%
9 years to 9 years, 11 months: 54%
10 years to 10 years, 11 months: 70%
11 years to 11 years, 11months: 71%
12 years to adult: 73%

These values suggest that the Duration Patterns task may be too difficult for young children, particularly those under approximately 9 or 10. For this reason, I typically administer only the Frequency Patterns test to young children. On the other hand, readers should remember that the two tests of auditory temporal patterning are not interchangeable and may well assess different processes. However, the functional implications of differential performance on these two tests have yet to be confirmed. I recommend, therefore, that both tests be administered whenever possible.

Finally, recent research indicates that aging in the adult may have a significant effect on temporal patterning performance (e.g., Bellis & Wilber, 2001). Therefore, it may be necessary to develop separate age- and gender-specific norms for the use of these tests in older adults.

It should be noted that, as long as the stimuli are detectable by the listener, both Frequency and Duration Patterns appear to be relatively resistant to mild to moderate degrees of cochlear hearing loss (Musiek, Baran, & Pinheiro, 1990).

Monaural Low-Redundancy Speech Tests

Monaural low-redundancy speech tests continue to be one of the most popular methods of assessing central auditory function, probably due to their ease of administration and scoring. All of the tests in this section are designed to be administered monaurally at a comfortable intensity level, listeners are instructed to repeat the words (and to guess if unsure), and the tests are scored simply by calculating the percent correct per ear. However, clinicians are reminded that normative values for these tests will differ, depending on the specific stimuli used. At the present time, a vast array of monaural low-redundancy speech tests are available. These tests vary in terms of speaker (male versus female), filter cutoffs, vocabulary level (e.g., NU-6 versus PBK), and a variety of other factors. To my knowledge, collection of age-specific normative data for all of these stimulus conditions has yet to be completed. Therefore, it is crucial that clinic norms be developed for each monaural low-redundancy speech test used.

With this caveat in mind, this section will provide information about the administration and scoring of the following general categories of monaural low-redundancy speech tests: low-pass filtered speech, compressed speech, compressed speech plus reverberation, and speech-in-noise tests. Because of the inherent distortion found in many peripheral hearing losses, **monaural low-redundancy speech tests should only be used for central auditory assessment in cases of normal peripheral hearing.** For a summary of the monaural low-redundancy speech tests discussed in this section, readers are referred to Table 6-5.

Low-Pass Filtered Speech (LPFS)

Two of the most commonly used LPFS tests today are the Ivey filtered words test, recommended by Willeford (1976, 1977), and the filtered NU-6 lists, available through Auditec of St. Louis and on the *Tonal and speech materials for auditory perceptual assessment* compact disc (1992). Although these are not the only filtered speech tests, my discussion will focus on these two tests.

As previously discussed, both low-pass filtered speech tests are to be administered monaurally at a comfortable intensity level. The listener is instructed to repeat the words heard, and the test is scored in terms of percent correct. For the Ivey test, normative data indicate a range of 74–98% for young, normal-hearing adults (Ivey, 1969). Normative values (2 standard deviations below the mean) for the low-pass filtered, NU-6 lists, using a cutoff frequency of 1000 Hz, indicate that normal performance for young adults is 75%, 80%, 83%, and 78% for NU-6 lists 1–4, respectively (Wilson & Mueller, 1984). My own clinic normative data using the Auditec male-speaker version of the 1000 Hz cutoff, low-pass filtered NU-6 words, at a presentation level of 50dB HL are as follows:

> 7 years to 7 years, 11 months: 62%
> 8 years to 8 years, 11 months: 70%
> 9 years to 9 years, 11 months: 68%
> 10 years to 10 years, 11 months: 72%
> 11 years to 11 years, 11 months: 75%
> 12 years to adult: 78%.

Table 6-5

Summary of Selected Monaural Low-Redundancy Speech Tasks:
Test Administration

Test	Stimuli	Presentation Level	Scoring
Low-Pass Filtered Speech			
Ivey	Michigan CNC words— male speaker; 500 Hz cut-off	50 dB	% correct per ear
NU-6	male speaker; 500, 700, 1000, and 1500 Hz cut-off	50 dB	% correct per ear
NU-6	NU-6 words— female speaker; 1500 Hz cut-off	50 dB	% correct per ear
Time Compressed Speech	NU-6 words—female speaker; 45% and 65% compression	50 dB	% correct per ear
Time Compression plus Reverberation	same as above with reverberation added	50 dB	% correct per ear
SSI-CM	10 third-order approximations of English sentences	primary: 30 dB; competing: varied between 20 dB and 50 dB	average of % correct at 0 dB S/N and –20 dB S/N

These scores are significantly better than those reported by Bornstein et al. (1994), who used the female-speaker version of the low-pass filtered NU-6 words. Their reported values for the 1500 Hz low-pass cutoff in a group of young, normal-hearing adults at a presentation level of 65 dB HL indicated a mean score of 66.5%, with a standard deviation of 8.5%. A primary difference between these two versions of the filtered NU-6 lists is that of gender: the female-speaker version of the low-pass filtered NU-6 word lists is more difficult than is the male-speaker version. Part of this difference likely arises from the fact that female speakers exhibit higher fundamental and formant frequencies. Thus, when low-pass filtering occurs, more of the information is eliminated from the words presented by female speakers. At the present time, I restrict myself to the use of the 1000 Hz, male-speaker version of the NU-6 word lists for children, primarily because they appear to be less affected by floor effects and because age-appropriate normative data are available. These findings underline the necessity of collecting test-specific normative data.

Time Compression and Time Compression plus Reverberation

Administration and scoring for Time Compressed Speech and Time Compressed Speech plus Reverberation are as previously discussed for low-pass filtered speech. The *Tonal and speech materials for auditory perceptual assessment* compact disc (1992) includes the NU-6 word lists (female speaker) at 45% and 65% time compression, both with and without 0.3 sec reverberation. As reported by Wilson et al. (1994), normative values for these conditions (2 standard deviations below the mean) for a group of young, normal-hearing adults are as follows:

45% compression (55 dB HL): 86.5%
45% compression plus reverberation (55 dB HL): 72.8%
65% compression (60 dB HL): 55.5%
65% compression plus reverberation (60 dB HL): 34.9%.

These findings indicate that **the 45% compression rate may be more useful as a clinical tool, because the 65% rate appears to be quite difficult even for adult normal listeners.**

Although the normative values presented above would seem to suggest that the Time-Compressed Speech tests are easier for listeners than low-pass filtered speech, this appears to be true only for adults. My own normative data using the 45% compression ratio, female-speaker NU-6 word lists, with and without reverberation suggest that significant floor effects and variability occur in children younger than approximately age 9. As such, I have been unable to establish clear normal cutoffs for this age group. For older children and adults, normative values are as follows:

45% compression (50dB HL):
　　9 years to 9 years, 11 months: 65%
　　10 years to 10 years, 11 months: 68%
　　11 years to 11 years, 11 months: 78%
　　12 years to adult: 85%

The addition of reverberation to the 45% compressed speech significantly impacts the normal cutoff values in children:

45% compression plus reverberation (50dB HL):
9 years to 9 years, 11 months: 52%
10 years to 10 years, 11 months: 59%
11 years to 11 years, 11 months: 62%
12 years to adult: 73%

The reason underlying the difficulty that children exhibit when compared to adults on this task is unclear at this time, and is an area for future research. Therefore, I typically use Time-Compressed Speech with and without reverberation with children as a confirmatory procedure. That is, if children perform at a borderline level on a test of low-pass filtered speech, I may administer the time-compressed measures to see how they fare when their auditory systems are taxed further. Often, children who perform at borderline on low-pass filtered speech tests find themselves completely unable to achieve auditory closure on the more difficult task, particularly when reverberation is added. This finding provides a guide for determining what types of acoustic environments are most problematic for the children in question.

Speech-in-Noise Tests

Of the many tests of speech-in-noise in use today, the most comprehensive normative and validity studies have been presented for the Synthetic Sentence Identification test with Ipsilateral Competing Message (SSI-ICM). Administration of the SSI-ICM is similar to that of the SSI-CCM, except that the primary signal and competing message are premixed at various S/N ratios for monaural presentation. Alternatively, clinicians may choose to mix the SSI-CCM into one earphone. The accompanying test manual suggests that the primary sentences be presented at 30 dB HL, and the S/N ratio be varied in 10 dB steps from 20 dB HL (+10 dB S/N) to 50 dB HL (–20 dB S/N). As in the SSI-CCM, the listener is given a printed list of the stimulus sentences and asked to indicate (by number) which sentence was heard. The individual ear score is calculated by taking the average of the percent correct at 0 dB S/N and –20 dB S/N.

The SSI-ICM score may be compared to the SSI-CCM score for interpretation purposes. Listeners with brainstem involvement tend to do poorly on the SSI-ICM as compared to the SSI-CCM. Again, it is important that listeners demonstrate normal hearing sensitivity in the frequency range of 250 through 2000 Hz for administration of the SSI-ICM.

Other speech-in-noise tests, including the PSI and SAAT, may be employed by clinicians involved in central auditory assessment. As discussed in the previous chapter, normative data should be collected for the specific stimuli, competing signal, and signal-to-noise ratios used, and interpretation of these tests should be undertaken with caution.

Binaural Interaction Tests

As previously discussed, many of the tests of binaural interaction have been criticized on the bases of ease of administration and sensitivity. For this reason, these tests do not enjoy widespread clinical use at the present time. This section discusses two types of binaural interaction tests that are currently available commercially and for which normative data have been established: binaural fusion tests and the masking level difference (MLD) (Table 6-6).

Binaural Fusion (BF) Tests

By definition, all tests of binaural interaction require a two-channel audiometer. To administer BF tests, the stimuli delivered to the two ears must be at equal intensity levels. This section discusses the administration of three BF tests: the Ivey adaptation of the Matzker BF test (Ivey, 1969), the compact disc band-pass version of the NU-6 BF test, and the CVC fusion task found on the *Tonal and speech materials for auditory perceptual assessment* compact disc (1992).

The Ivey BF test, recommended by Willeford (1977), consists of two lists of twenty spondees each. The stimuli are band-passed so that the low-pass segment of each word is presented to one ear and the high-pass segment is presented to the other. The listener is required to repeat the words heard, and the test is scored by calculating the percent correct.

Normative data were collected from adults using a presentation level of 25 dB SL (re: pure-tone thresholds at 500 and 2000 Hz), and from children using a presentation level of 30 dB SL (Ivey, 1969; Willeford & Burleigh, 1985). These normative studies, as well as that done by White (1977), indicated that the words included in List 2 were less familiar and, thus, resulted in lower scores in children than did the use of List 1. Therefore, Willeford and Burleigh (1985) suggested that 10% be added to the score obtained from the use of List 2 for compensation purposes.

Normative data (with 10% added to the List 2 scores for children) indicated cutoffs near or above 75% for children ages 6 through 8, near 80% for children age 9, and near 90% for 10-year-old children and adults (Willeford & Burleigh, 1985).

Table 6-6

Summary of Selected Binaural Interaction Tests: Test Administration

Test	Stimuli	Presentation Level	Scoring
Binaural Fusion			
Ivey	spondaic words; low-pass to one ear; high-pass to the other	25–30 dB SL	% correct per ear upon resynthesis
NU-6	NU-6 words; low-pass to one ear; high-pass to the other	30–35 dB SL	% correct per ear
CVC Fusion	segmented CVC words; consonants to one ear; vowels to the other	30 dB HL	% correct per ear
MLD	may be tonal or speech	levels and S/N ratios vary depending upon stimulus	SπNø threshold minus SøNø threshold

Administration of the monosyllabic BF task using the NU-6 word lists is similar to that of the Ivey BF test. As mentioned in the previous chapter, it has been suggested that the use of monosyllabic rather than spondaic words in BF testing may further reduce the redundancy of the signal and, thus, result in greater sensitivity (Smith & Resnick, 1972). The test should be administered at a comfortable listening level.

Results of normative studies demonstrated a performance-intensity function essentially identical to that of standard NU-6 word recognition performance, with a cutoff (2 standard deviations below the mean) of 86.6% at a presentation level of 36 dB HL for young, normal-hearing adults. When a presentation level of 30 dB HL was used, the normal cutoff was reduced to 66.4% (mean = 88.4%, standard deviation = 11.0%; Bornstein et al., 1994). Further research is needed in order to define normative values for children using the NU-6 word lists in a band-pass BF paradigm.

A final BF test that has recently been described by Wilson (1994) is the CVC fusion task included on the *Tonal and speech materials for auditory perceptual assessment* compact disc (1992). In this task, the carrier phrase and vowel segment of the word are presented to one ear and the consonant segments are presented to the other ear, thus preserving the spectral characteristics of the stimulus. Therefore, unlike the other BF tests discussed in this section, the CVC fusion task was designed to be relatively resistant to peripheral hearing loss. Normative data suggest a cutoff of 87.4% (2 standard deviations below the mean) at a presentation level of 30 dB HL for young, normal-hearing adults. My own normative values for this test suggest that 80% is an appropriate normal cutoff value for children who are 7 years to 11 years, 11 months, in age. Further research is needed using hearing-impaired and neurological populations. It should be noted that the utility of BF tests in central auditory assessment is questionable. As discussed in the previous chapter, these types of tests appear to be sensitive only to gross brainstem lesions. In my own practice, I use these tests only if time allows and if I am interested in a very gross test of brainstem function. Others use binaural fusion tests primarily as a means of demonstrating that the child is able to complete an auditory task successfully, especially if attention- or behavior-related confounds are suspected (Jeanane M. Ferre, personal communication).

Masking Level Difference (MLD)

A listener's performance on MLD testing will depend on the type of stimuli and masker and the specific administration protocols used. All MLD testing, however, is designed to compare the listener's signal threshold for a variety of masking conditions. A description of the masking conditions used in MLD investigations was provided in Chapter 2.

The MLD for pure tones may be as high as 10 to 15 dB, depending on the frequency of the signal and the characteristics of the masking stimulus. Many commercial audiometers are manufactured with the built-in capacity to perform pure-tone MLD testing, and readers are referred to the equipment manuals for specific administration protocols.

The MLD for speech is typically smaller than that for pure tones. This section describes administration of the premixed, spondaic MLD test included on the *Tonal and speech materials for auditory perceptual assessment* compact disc (1992). For this test, the listener is given a printed list of the ten spondees. First, testing in the SøNø condition is completed by routing one channel of the compact disc to one channel of the audiometer at a comfortable listening level (50 dB HL). The listener is asked to indicate which of the words was heard. Four words are presented for each of sixteen signal-to-noise ratios, increasing in 2 dB increments from 0 dB S/N to –30 dB S/N. It should be noted that, due to the competing noise, clinician monitoring of the stimulus words is impossible; therefore, the words have been embedded in noise bursts, which allow the clinician to keep track of when the stimulus is being presented.

Testing in the SπNø condition is done by routing each channel of the compact disc to the corresponding channel of the audiometer (left channel to left earphone, right channel to right earphone) at the same presentation level as the SøNø condition and, again, beginning with the 0 dB S/N condition. Testing continues until the listener fails to respond correctly to all words at two consecutive signal-to-noise ratios. Thresholds in both conditions are computed using the following equation:

Threshold = (dB HL) + 1 - (number of words reported correctly / 2)

The MLD is calculated simply by subtracting the threshold value obtained in the SπNø condition from that obtained in the SøNø condition.

Wilson, Zizz, and Sperry (1994) reported mean MLD values of 7.8 dB and 8.8 dB for presentation levels of 65 dB SPL (45 dB HL) and 85 dB SPL (65 dB HL), respectively, in a group of young, normal-hearing listeners. Standard deviations were on the order of 2.1 dB and 2.7 dB for the two intensity levels. Because 90% of the normal listeners studied exhibited MLDs larger than 5.5 dB, the authors suggested that MLDs smaller than 5.5 dB should be considered abnormal for normal-hearing listeners. Although this spondaic MLD paradigm is an easy-to-administer binaural interaction measure, readers should remember that tonal MLDs appear to be more sensitive to central auditory dysfunction in children (Sweetow & Reddell, 1978).

Electrophysiologic Tests

It is not within the scope of this book to present a complete discussion of administration and interpretation of auditory electrophysiologic measures. Therefore, what follows is a general guide to the use of these tools in the evaluation of central auditory function and reflects the most common test parameters used in my own clinic. I have included only those electrophysiologic measures that are in common clinical use at the present time. It should be noted that there is a lack of consensus regarding optimal stimuli, filter settings, and other testing and recording parameters, especially for the MLR and late event-related potentials. Therefore, the information provided in this section should be taken as a general set of guidelines only. Parameters discussed in this section are summarized in Table 6-7.

Table 6-7

Summary of Recording Parameters for Selected Electrophysiologic Tests

Test	Stimuli	Filters	Electrode Montage
Auditory Brainstem Response (ABR)	clicks or tone bursts; 11, 31, and/or 61 per second; 75 dB HL	100–3000 Hz	Cz/A1; Cz/A2
Middle Latency Response (MLR)	clicks or tone bursts; 11 per second; 70 dB HL	10–1500 Hz	C3/A1 or A2; C4/A1 or A2; Cz/A1 or A2
Late Event-Related Potentials (LEP)	tone bursts or speech syllables 60 dB HL	0.1–100 Hz	C3/Linked; C4/Linked; Cz/Linked; Lateral eye/ Supraorbital
P300	oddball paradigm using tone bursts or speech syllables; frequent:infrequent ratio 5:1	0.1–100 Hz	Cz/Linked or same as LEP

Auditory Brainstem Response (ABR)

When recording the ABR for neurologic purposes, it is recommended that a relatively high intensity level (i.e., 75 dB HL) be used to maximize the probability of obtaining waves I, III, and V. In my clinic, I record from a centrally located scalp electrode (i.e., Cz) referenced to both ipsilateral and contralateral earlobes (i.e., A1 [left] and A2 [right]). Stimuli consist of rarefaction click stimuli, although condensation or alternating polarity may be used if waveform morphology is poor using rarefaction clicks. Stimuli are presented at a rate of 11.1 or 31.1 per second (slow rate) and at 61.1 per second (fast rate), using a time window of 15 ms and filter settings of 100–3000 Hz.

Per convention, the ABR is interpreted in terms of presence versus absence of waves, absolute and interwave latencies, and waveform morphology and replicability. In addition, a comparison of fast- versus slow-rate responses yields an indication of auditory signal transmission through the brainstem auditory pathways when the system is stressed. Finally, a comparison of the amplitudes of wave V versus wave I may also provide clinically valuable information.

The ABR is sensitive to involvement of the auditory nerve and brainstem auditory pathways, and will also be abnormal in many cases of peripheral hearing loss. Further, the ABR can also be recorded using tonal stimuli. For further information regarding normative values for ABR parameters, readers are referred to Hood (1998).

Middle Latency Response (MLR)

The MLR is sensitive to dysfunction in the thalamocortical pathways. In my clinic, I use click or tone burst stimuli, presented at a rate of 11 per second or less, to elicit MLRs from scalp electrodes placed over left (C3) and right (C4) temporal lobes, as well as over midline (Cz). The earlobes serve as references to reduce the chance of post-auricular muscle (PAM) artifact that can occur with mastoid placement. Using this three-channel montage (Cz/A1 or A2, C3/A1 or A2, C4/A1 or A2), amplitude comparisons can be made for purposes of determining whether electrode or ear effects exist, as discussed in the previous chapter. Filter settings for the MLR are particularly important, as settings that are too narrow or that employ very sharp cutoffs can alter the MLR artificially. In my clinic, when employing the MLR for central auditory evaluation purposes, I use filter settings of 10 to 1500 Hz and a time window of 80 ms; however, other settings are acceptable. Responses are interpreted in terms of presence versus absence of response or significant electrode or ear effects. A 50% difference in amplitude between scalp electrode sites and ears is considered a sign of possible central involvement. Because sleep affects the MLR, especially in children, I perform all testing while the child is watching a video or engaged in another quiet activity. Alternatively, if a child must be asleep for testing to be completed, I monitor the ongoing EEG activity and only record during favorable sleep stages (Stage 1, 2, and REM), as discussed in Chapter 3.

Late Event-Related Potentials (LEP)

As discussed in Chapter 3, the appearance of the LEP will differ, depending on the age of the child. As such, it is important that clinicians be familiar with the effects of maturation on these responses. As with the MLR, LEP responses are recorded using a three-channel montage; however, I reference the C3, C4, and Cz active scalp electrode sites to linked earlobes. Further, I also use a fourth channel to monitor eye movements via electrodes placed above and beside the eye to reduce muscle artifact associated with eyeblinks. Although the topic of optimum filter settings for recording the LEPs is somewhat controversial, I have found the use of 0.1 to 100 Hz and a time window of 500 Hz to be adequate in most situations. Stimuli may consist of tone bursts or speech syllables presented at a rate of approximately 1 per second, and a finding of significant differences in the neurophysiologic response to tones versus speech may provide important clinical information regarding stimulus-specific signal encoding in the cortex. Because sleep will significantly affect the LEPs, all recordings are completed with the child fully awake and alert. Like the MLR, LEP responses are interpreted according to presence versus absence of response or electrode or ear effects.

Unlike the electrophysiologic responses discussed thus far, which can be passively elicited, recording of the P300 requires the child to pay active attention to the stimuli. Frequent and infrequent tone bursts or speech syllables are presented at a ratio of approximately 5 to 1 in an oddball paradigm, and the child is asked to count the infrequent stimuli. The P300 may be abnormally delayed, severely reduced in amplitude, or absent in some cases of auditory processing disorders. However, this response can also be affected by attention, cognition, and psychological factors that are not auditory-related.

For additional information on recording and interpreting middle and late auditory electrophysiologic responses, readers are referred to Katz (2002).

Summary

This chapter has described recommended procedures for comprehensive central auditory processing assessment, including equipment needed, components of the assessment process, choosing test battery components, and specific administration protocols and normative values for several tests of central auditory function in common clinical use today. It was not my intent to imply that the tests listed in this section are the only ones that may be utilized, or that the assessment protocols described herein are the only manner in which central auditory evaluation may be conducted. Rather, the purpose of this chapter was to provide clinicians entering into central auditory assessment practical information for immediate use in the clinical arena. Again, it should be emphasized that the information contained in the previous chapters should be studied carefully prior to attempting any evaluation of central auditory function.

Review Questions

1. List the equipment needed for comprehensive behavioral central auditory assessment.

2. List the steps that should be included in a comprehensive central auditory processing evaluation.

3. Discuss the factors that will affect the choice of which tests to include in a central auditory test battery.

4. Briefly outline the recommended stimulus presentation level, instructions to the listener, and method of scoring for the following behavioral tests of central auditory function:

Dichotic Digits	Dichotic CVs
Staggered Spondaic Words	Competing Sentence Test
SSI-CCM	Dichotic Sentence Identification
Dichotic Rhyme Test	Frequency Patterns
RGDT	Low-Pass Filtered Speech
Duration Patterns	SSI-ICM
Time-Compressed Speech	CVC Fusion
Band-pass Binaural Fusion	
Masking Level Difference	

5. Which of the above listed tests may be suitable for use in cases of peripheral hearing loss?

6. In review, identify the process or processes assessed by each of the above-listed tests.

CHAPTER

SEVEN

Interpretation of Central Auditory Assessment Results

Interpretation of central auditory assessment results may be undertaken with a variety of goals in mind and, depending on the desired outcome, the interpretation process may be involved and lengthy, or quick and simple. It is my contention that the simple identification of the presence of CAPD does not provide sufficient useful information upon which to base a rehabilitative program. Instead, interpretation should be entered into with the mind-set of a detective attempting to solve a complex mystery, and all aspects of the screening and assessment data should be analyzed so that the greatest amount of information may be obtained. To accomplish this task, clinicians must be able to relate the assessment findings to neuroscience, thus interpreting the given data in terms of how they deviate from the manner in which the typical CANS is supposed to function.

Because CAPD is a heterogeneous disorder, it is not possible to address all possible combinations of findings for interpretation purposes. Therefore, this chapter provides readers with a variety of ways in which the assessment data may be looked at, from simple identification of a disorder to the development of an auditory learning profile. In addition, types of management recommendations appropriate for specific assessment findings will be included; however, rehabilitative activities and management strategies will be provided in Chapters 8 and 9.

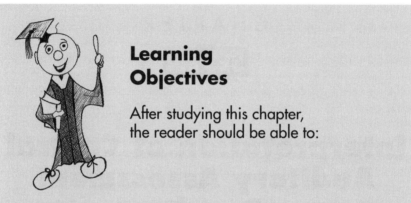

Learning Objectives

After studying this chapter, the reader should be able to:

1. Identify several questions that may be answered by the assessment results.
2. Discuss site-of-dysfunction interpretation of central auditory assessment results.
3. Discuss process-based interpretation of central auditory assessment results.
4. Identify and describe three primary and two secondary sub-profiles of central auditory processing disorders in children.
5. Discuss issues related to differential diagnosis of CAPD.

What Is the Question?

In Chapter 5, the rationale for a test battery approach to central auditory assessment was discussed. I emphasized that the question to be answered by the assessment process will have a major impact on the number and types of tests chosen. Logically, the question to be answered will also influence the manner in which test results are interpreted.

In its simplest form, the central auditory assessment should provide information regarding the presence or absence of some type of central auditory processing disorder, thus answering the common question of whether the child in question "has CAPD." As we will see in the following section, however, identifying of the presence of a central auditory disorder is not as simple as it as it appears on the surface. Nor does simple identification provide sufficient information to answer the question that will inevitably follow: Can we do anything about it and, if so, what?

To answer this question, several types of information must be obtained from the available assessment data. First, in order to develop a management plan that is as deficit-specific as possible, clinicians will need to determine what auditory process or processes are most likely dysfunctional in a given child. I call this procedure *process-based interpretation.* By identifying the dysfunctional process(es), we then can develop a management program that will build upon the child's auditory strengths while specifically targeting the weaknesses, thus resulting in greater efficiency and individualization.

Second, clinicians should be able to identify, as near as possible, the site of dysfunction within the CANS. This information is helpful in determining whether additional medical follow-up is indicated, as in the case of a possible neurological disorder or space-occupying lesion, as well as assisting in the development of management strategies. Interpreting test results in this manner also assists in increasing confidence in our conclusions by looking for logical patterns across measures of auditory processing, learning, language, and cognition that, when considered together, are consistent with dysfunction in one or more regions of the brain. In short, we look for patterns of dysfunction that "make sense" from a neurophysiologic and neuroanatomical standpoint, based on what we know about how the brain functions and which regions subserve various tasks. When our conclusions are consistent with the underlying neurophysiology of the system, we can be more confident that our diagnoses are accurate and our recommendations for management are appropriate and deficit-specific. When they are not consistent, however, we can use that information as an indication that we need to view our interpretations with caution, and should look further into the presenting difficulties of the child for other possible explanations. Therefore, once again it should be emphasized that it is imperative that clinicians be knowledgeable about the underlying science of brain function.

Finally, assessment results should be related to information from educational, cognitive, speech/language, social, and other disciplines. The use of subprofiles of auditory processing disorders is particularly helpful in determining the impact of a given CAPD on a child's quality of life, as well as providing direction for meaningful intervention.

In conclusion, **data from a central auditory assessment may be analyzed for the following four general purposes: identification of the presence or absence of a disorder, identification of underlying** processes that may be disordered, site-of-lesion (or site-of-dysfunction) information, and, in conjunction with academic and other measures, the development of a CAPD subprofile. By approaching interpretation of central auditory assessment results from a variety of perspectives, clinicians can help to ensure that the information obtained from the assessment is as applicable and meaningful as possible, so that a deficit-specific management program that addresses the individual child's difficulties may be developed.

Identification of Central Auditory Processing Disorders

The decision as to whether results of a comprehensive central assessment indicate that a CAPD is, in fact, present will depend on a variety of factors. Perhaps the most important is the criterion for abnormal performance chosen by the clinician. Depending upon whether the criterion chosen is strict or lax, the interpretation of results of a test battery, on the whole, may differ significantly.

Choosing a criterion level for abnormal performance involves deciding how many, and to what extent, individual test measures should be positive for the disorder before a determination that the disorder is present may be made. To illustrate, let us consider a situation in which five central tests are utilized together in a test battery approach. If we decide that performance outside the norm on any single test tool alone constitutes a positive finding on the entire battery, then this would be considered a *lax* criterion. If, on the other hand, results of all five tests must be abnormal for the battery to be positive, then the criterion is *strict*. Finally, if two, three, or four tests must be positive for CAPD before presence of disorder is determined, the criterion is said to be

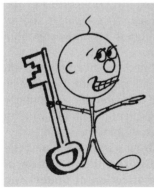

KEY CONCEPT

The decision whether to use a strict, lax, or intermediate criterion for test interpretation will have a significant effect on the ultimate outcome of the central auditory assessment.

intermediate. Obviously, the choice of a strict, lax, or intermediate criterion will have a significant impact on the interpretation of the entire test battery.

Just as it is important for clinicians to choose individual tests that exhibit the greatest sensitivity, it is critical that the criterion for abnormal performance yield as many hits as possible, while avoiding false positives and misses. What, then, would be the ideal criterion for identifying CAPD in the educational setting? Again, the answer to this question would depend on the ultimate goal of the assessment process.

One approach that has been advocated frequently is the use of an intermediate criterion in which failure (defined as performance < 2 standard deviations from the mean) on at least two tests of central auditory function (or, alternatively, performance < 3 standard deviations from the mean on one test) be required before a diagnosis of CAPD can be made. However, there is an inherent drawback to this type of approach. One of the purposes of using a test battery approach to central assessment is so that different tests that assess different processes may be included. **If each test within the battery assesses a different process under the central auditory processing umbrella, is it not possible that, in a given child, one underlying process may be disordered while the others remain quite functional, resulting in abnormal performance on only one test measure?**

Indeed, I find this frequently to be the case when assessing children for possible CAPD. Two children with similar presenting behavioral characteristics of CAPD may exhibit dysfunction in different underlying processes, singularly or in any combination. Therefore, the establishment of an intermediate criterion for interpretation in which two or more tests must be abnormal for the finding to be positive would be inadequate for identifying the presence of a single disordered process that, nonetheless, significantly impacts the child's ability to function and learn.

Furthermore, it is often difficult to equate performance on behavioral measures of central auditory processing to real-life difficulty in daily listening and learning situations. The effect of even a very mild deficit in one auditory area on one person's life may be very different than the effect of the same deficit on another's, depending on individual life circumstances. For example, persons who learn or work in very quiet environments and exhibit only mild difficulty on tests of auditory closure may find that their auditory deficits pose no more than an occasional, mild annoyance. However, others with the same mild deficit who learn or work in very noisy environments may find that their auditory disorders significantly interfere with their ability to perform daily tasks. Also important is the individual's linguistic competency and other top-down factors. A child with very good language, attention, and cognitive skills has significant strengths upon which to draw in compensating for an auditory deficit. But a child with weaker language or related skills will find that a similar auditory deficit results in a much greater degree of handicap. Therefore, we cannot always determine the functional impact of an auditory processing disorder from data such as how far below the norm a child performs on a given test or how many tests a child "fails." Instead, we must carefully consider our auditory test results in light of information from the rest of the multidisciplinary team in determining functional impact and directions for management.

For these reasons, I advocate a lax criterion for interpretation in which an abnormal finding on any given test tool, *combined with significant educational and behavioral findings*, may be considered as evidence of CAPD. **Therefore, in order for the presence of CAPD to be identified, it must be established that (1) one or more underlying auditory processes are disordered or delayed, and (2) the disorder or delay, in all likelihood, has a significant impact on the child's ability to function or learn.**

There are some inherent difficulties in this approach, particularly in the determination of significant impact. It is not always possible to establish a direct one-to-one relationship between a given presenting disorder and educational/behavioral findings. A child may exhibit concomitant physical or behavioral disorders, or disorders in other sensory processing systems, making it difficult or impossible to separate out the effects of the auditory complaint.

Nor is this separation of effects always necessary, or even desirable. When undertaking central auditory assessment from a whole-child approach, it is important to realize that the auditory disorder may be merely one piece in the overall puzzle. The clinician's task,

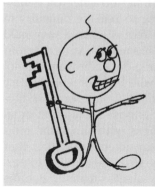

KEY CONCEPT

Simply identifying the presence of a disorder is not enough. Instead, the disorder must be qualified so that insightful intervention and educational planning can occur.

therefore, is not simply to identify the presence of an auditory disorder but to describe the disorder and help in determining which aspects of the child's overall presenting picture may be attributed, at least in part, to the given disorder. It is in these latter two tasks that process-based interpretation and the development of subprofiles of CAPD, to be discussed later in this chapter, come into play.

In conclusion, the identification of CAPD will depend on the criterion established for abnormal performance on a central auditory test battery. I recommend that the criterion for presence of CAPD be relatively lax, necessitating abnormal performance on one or more tests of central auditory function combined with significant educational and behavioral findings. The identification of CAPD, however, is only the first step in the overall interpretation process. To determine the relative impact of a given auditory processing disorder on a child's educational and behavioral functioning, as well as to develop a plan for management, the disorder must be described in functional, process-based terms, and the findings must be tied to the child's presenting educational and behavioral complaints.

Process-Based Interpretation

As previously mentioned, the ASHA Task Force on Central Auditory Processing defined auditory processing as the auditory system mechanisms and processes responsible for behavioral phenomena such as sound localization and lateralization, auditory discrimination, auditory pattern recognition, temporal aspects of audition, and auditory performance decrements with competing and degraded acoustic signals (ASHA, 1996). **Process-based interpretation refers to the assessment of these underlying processes with an eye toward the development of an individual auditory profile that will identify auditory strengths and weaknesses.** As discussed in the previous chapter, Schow et al. (2000) empirically identified four general auditory behaviors or processes that are tapped directly by commonly used measures of central auditory processing: Monaural Separation/Closure (MSC), Binaural Separation (BS), Binaural Integration (BI), and Auditory Pattern Temporal Ordering (APTO). Additional, more complex processes were also identified, including binaural interaction, temporal processing, and auditory discrimination. Here, we will describe how results of central auditory testing can illuminate functional difficulties in general auditory behaviors or processes that correspond to those factors identified by Schow and colleagues: auditory closure (analogous to MSC), binaural separation and integration (BS, BI), temporal patterning (analogous to APTO), binaural interaction, and other processes such as temporal resolution and auditory discrimination.

Again, readers should be aware that interpretation of central auditory tests is not without limitations and should be undertaken with caution. In addition, I do not wish to suggest that the processes discussed here are the only ones that may be assessed by tests of central auditory function, nor is the method discussed here the only manner in which tests of central auditory function may be interpreted. The information provided in this section will serve to provide clinicians with a starting point for approaching central auditory interpretation. Information regarding behavioral and academic characteristics will be provided in the section on subprofiles of auditory processing disorders, later in this chapter.

Auditory Closure

Auditory closure refers to the ability of the normal listener to utilize intrinsic and extrinsic redundancy to fill in missing or distorted portions of the auditory signal and recognize the whole message. A related ability is that of *monaural separation*, or the ability to listen to a target stimulus in the presence of another, competing signal delivered to the same ear. Both auditory closure and monaural separation play a part in listeners' ability to extrapolate the whole message from the individual components. Much of this ability relies on deciphering the components of an auditory signal, and then filling in the missing elements to construct a whole message. Therefore, auditory discrimination and decoding also play a role in this ability. Technically, monaural separation is rarely required in real-life listening situations, except perhaps for instances such as conducting a phone conversation with a very bad connection. Instead, most of our listening in competing backgrounds of noise occurs under binaural conditions, which will be discussed further in the section on binaural interaction. Therefore, this section will refer to the general act of deciphering and then filling in the missing components of an auditory message as auditory closure.

Auditory closure plays an important role in everyday listening activities. Rarely can our everyday listening environment be considered ideal. Instead, we must contend continually with background noise, regional dialects, conversation partners who speak with quiet voices or less than perfect diction, and other factors that make comprehension of auditory messages difficult. It is our ability to rely upon extrinsic and intrinsic redundancy of the signal that allows us to comprehend the overall message and engage in meaningful conversation.

Extrinsic factors that aid in our ability to achieve auditory closure include knowledge of the topic, familiarity with the vocabulary utilized, knowledge of phonemic aspects of speech, and familiarity with the rules of language, among others. Thus, if we are in a situation in which the topic of conversation is known, the speaker is using familiar vocabulary, syntax, and semantics, and the environment is acoustically adequate, then we will expend very little energy in following the conversation. If, on the other hand, one or more of these factors is missing, then we must rely upon the other factors, as well as upon the repeated representation of characteristics of the auditory signal throughout the CANS (intrinsic redundancy), in order to achieve auditory closure.

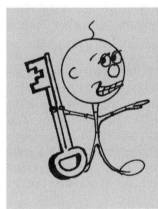

KEY CONCEPT

Extrinsic redundancy is provided by the characteristics of the auditory signal, whereas intrinsic redundancy refers to the repeated representation of that signal throughout the CANS.

For example, those of us in the field of speech and hearing often have been in the situation of conversing with a patient who exhibits an articulatory speech impairment. Depending on the degree of distortion in the acoustic signal, the phonemic aspects of the signal will be available to us in varying degrees. Therefore, we must rely upon knowledge of the conversational topic, vocabulary, and rules of language in order to understand what the speaker is saying. If any of these factors are taken away as well, then the listening task becomes much more difficult. Another familiar example would be the situation in which parents are attempting to decipher the requests of small children in whom spoken language is just beginning to emerge. The children's articulation may be distorted, and they may utilize immature language forms and word approximations. If the topic also is unknown, the parents may be rendered completely unable to comprehend the children's requests, resulting in frustration on both sides.

An individual with an auditory closure processing deficit exhibits a breakdown in the intrinsic redundancy of the CANS, thus reducing or eliminating the repeated representation of the incoming signal throughout the auditory pathways. Therefore, anything that reduces the extrinsic redundancy of the auditory signal may interfere with the individual's ability to achieve auditory closure. At its most basic level, an auditory closure deficit may arise from an inability to discriminate among or decode similar-sounding phonemes which, in turn, may be due to deficits in basic, fundamental temporal processing.

Auditory closure deficits may be much more apparent in listeners who exhibit inefficient top-down processing, such as those with attention- or language-related disorders. For example, a lack of familiarity with the vocabulary or syntax being used will certainly affect individuals' ability to fill in the missing pieces of the message, even if they exhibit only mild deficits in auditory discrimination or temporal processing. Similarly, listeners with auditory closure deficits may exhibit little or no difficulty understanding speech in ideal listening environments, but have great difficulty in extreme backgrounds of noise or with rapid or accented speakers. Attention, too, can play a role in auditory closure abilities in that distractibility may cause listeners to miss much more of a message than they would have if they had been able to sustain attention to the conversation. Language, attention, and related disorders may, in a sense, be thought of as "noise"—factors that reduce the extrinsic redundancy of the auditory signal and render bottom-up auditory closure deficits more disruptive.

On tests of central auditory function, individuals with auditory closure deficits will perform poorly on monaural low-redundancy speech tests, such as Low-Pass Filtered Speech or Time-Compressed Speech, as well as speech-in-noise tests. If the deficit is severe, word recognition skills in quiet may be affected.

Management of an auditory closure deficit would include methods of improving access to auditory information through environmental modifications, activities targeted at auditory closure from phonemic to sentence levels, preteaching of new concepts, and frequent repetition of key messages, among others. If phonemic decoding is affected, consonant or vowel discrimination training may be indicated. Strengthening top-down, compensatory mechanisms will also be important for individuals with auditory closure deficits. Therefore, strengthening vocabulary, using context to fill in missing or unfamiliar components of the message, and learning to attend actively to the speaker are useful management strategies. Specific management tech-

Table 7-1
Primary Characteristics of Deficits in Auditory Closure

Principal feature:	A breakdown in the intrinsic redundancy of the CANS
Behavioral characteristics:	Difficulty filling in the missing components when part of the auditory signal is inaccessible
Central test findings:	Poor performance on monaural low redundancy speech tasks
Suggestions for management:	Improve acoustic access to auditory information; preteach new concepts and vocabulary; implement auditory phoneme discrimination training (if indicated); teach compensatory strategies to strengthen top-down mechanisms, including vocabulary building, context-based auditory closure training, and principles of active listening

niques will be provided in Chapters 8 and 9. Table 7-1 provides an overview of the characteristics of a deficit in auditory closure.

Binaural Separation and Binaural Integration

Binaural separation refers to the ability to process an auditory message coming into one ear while ignoring a disparate message being presented to the opposite ear at the same time. A different, but related, ability is that of *binaural integration*, or the ability to process information being presented to both ears simultaneously, with the information presented to each ear being different. The terms *binaural separation* and *binaural integration* are not to be confused with the term *binaural interaction*, which is a brainstem function and will be discussed later in this section. Rather, the terms *binaural separation* and *binaural integration*, as used here, specifically refer to processes that are typically assessed through the use of dichotic speech tests.

Binaural separation and integration are processes that are critical to everyday listening, particularly in a school environment. Situations arise continually in which listeners are required to ignore linguistic information from one source while focusing attention on a primary message. Consider, for example, the situation in which a child is sitting quietly in a classroom, attempting to listen to the teacher provide instructions while, at the same time, a student next to the child is talking either to the child or to another student. For children to hear the information being presented by the teacher, they must be able to ignore the adjacent student's verbalizations, an activity that relies, in part, upon the process of binaural separation.

Binaural integration, likewise, comes into play in everyday listening situations. An example of a listening situation in which the process of binaural integration would be relied upon might be that of a mother who is attempting to carry on a phone conversation while simultaneously listening to the demands of her child, a situation that occurs frequently during the normal course of parenting. In this situation, the mother must be able to process information from both sources, thus utilizing the process of binaural integration.

Therefore, **dysfunction in the processes of binaural separation and integration may be expressed in the behavioral symptom of difficulty hearing in background noise or when more than one person is talking at the same time.** It should be noted that the behavioral characteristic of difficulty hearing in noise has been mentioned previously as a symptom of auditory closure deficit and will be mentioned again as a symptom of a deficit in binaural interaction. In fact, difficulty hearing in noise is one of the most common complaints of individuals with CAPD. Clinicians cannot automatically assume the cause of such a complaint, as **two children who present with the identical behavioral symptom may exhibit dysfunction in two entirely different underlying processes.** It is for this reason that careful, systematic assessment be undertaken in a test battery approach, so that identification of the underlying deficit may be attained in each case.

The child with binaural separation/integration dysfunction will perform poorly on dichotic speech tests. The determination of which underlying process is disordered (e.g., separation, integration, or a combination of both) may be made by the behavioral requirements of the tests themselves. For example, test tools such as Dichotic Digits and Dichotic Consonant-Vowels (CVs) require listeners to report all auditory information heard, thus tapping the process of binaural integration. Conversely, Competing Sentences requires listeners to ignore the information being presented to one ear while reporting the sentence heard in the target ear, thus assessing binaural separation abilities.

Approaches appropriate for management of binaural separation or integration dysfunction would include environmental adaptations that improve the listener's access to target auditory information while decreasing competing signals, and the teaching of compensatory

Table 7-2

Primary Characteristics of Deficits in Binaural Separation
and Binaural Integration

Principal features:	Difficulty in processing an auditory message in one ear while ignoring a competing message in the other (separation)
	Difficulty processing information presented to both ears simultaneously (integration)
Behavioral characteristics:	Difficulty hearing in background noise or when more than one person is talking at the same time
Central test findings:	Poor performance on dichotic speech tests
Suggestions for management:	Improve acoustic access to information in the environment; teach compensatory strategies re: directing attention; implement dichotic listening training (as indicated)

strategies to assist the listener in directing attention. Another treatment approach that may be useful is dichotic listening training in which the listener must either separate or integrate dichotically presented information under conditions of varying interaural intensity differences. Again, specific management strategies will be discussed in Chapters 8 and 9. Characteristics of a deficit in binaural separation or integration are presented in Table 7-2.

Temporal Patterning

The term *temporal patterning,* as used here, specifically refers to a listener's ability to recognize acoustic contours. Several auditory processes contribute to this ability, including discrimination of differences in auditory stimuli, sequencing of auditory stimuli, gestalt pattern perception, and trace memory (Musiek & Chermak, 1995; Musiek et al., 1980). As used here, temporal patterning is analogous to the auditory behavior identified by Schow et al. (2000) as Auditory Pattern Temporal Ordering (APTO). Of the tests of central auditory function discussed in Chapter 6, only Frequency Patterns and Duration Patterns may be considered tests of temporal patterning.

Being able to recognize the acoustic contour of a signal greatly contributes to a listener's ability to extract and utilize prosodic aspects of speech, such as rhythm, stress, and intonation. Relative differences in stress within a sentence allow listeners to identify the key words. Alterations in stressed words within a sentence may change the meaning of the sentence as a whole (e.g., *You* can't go with us versus You can't go with *us*), and changes in syllabic stress may alter the meaning of an individual word (e.g., *pro*ject vs. pro*ject*). Intonation provides clues regarding the intent of the message as well as the emotional status of the speaker (e.g., surprised, happy, angry, sad). Rhythm of speech may also affect the meaning of the utterance (e.g., He saw the *snowdrift* by the window versus He saw the *snow drift* by the window). In short, prosody provides a wealth of information that cannot be obtained from the words of a message alone.

Children with deficits in acoustic contour recognition and auditory temporal patterning may exhibit difficulty recognizing and using prosodic aspects of speech. They may have difficulty extracting key words from a spoken message and may be unable to discriminate subtle differences in meaning brought about by changes in relative stress and intonation. In addition, these children may, themselves, be "flat" readers or be somewhat monotonic in their own speech. Sequencing of critical elements within a message, as well as individual speech sounds within a word, may be an issue. These children tend to perform poorly on Frequency Patterns and Duration Patterns testing in both the linguistic labeling and humming response conditions.

Management approaches that may be useful for children with temporal patterning difficulty include prosody training and instruction in the extraction of key words from a message. If the child is unable to sequence intensity, pitch, or duration differences even in simple, nonverbal auditory stimuli, then training in this basic, fundamental skill may be required prior to moving on to prosody training, which requires the listener to recognize these subtle acoustic contours when they are embedded in conversational speech. In addition, reading aloud daily with specific emphasis on intonation, stress, and rhythm may help to enhance awareness of prosodic aspects of speech. Readers are referred to Chapters 8 and 9 for specific management suggestions. Table 7-3 summarizes the information presented in this section.

Binaural Interaction

As discussed in Chapter 2, auditory functions that rely upon binaural interaction include localization and lateralization of auditory stimuli, binaural release from masking, detection of signals in noise, and binaural fusion. Of these functions, **two are particularly important in**

Table 7-3

Primary Characteristics of Deficits in Temporal Patterning

Principal feature:	Difficulty recognizing acoustic contours
Behavioral characteristics:	Difficulty recognizing and using prosodic features of speech
Central test findings:	Poor performance on tests of temporal patterning in both the linguistic labeling and humming conditions
Suggestions for management:	Instruction in key word extraction; prosody training; temporal patterning training (in some cases); reading aloud with exaggerated prosodic features

everyday listening situations: localization of auditory stimuli and detection of signals in noise.

As shown earlier in this section, the ability to understand speech in noise is affected by the processes of auditory closure and binaural separation. However, to understand a signal in noise, the signal must first be detected. For this to occur, the listener must, at a preconscious level, be able to localize the sources of both the target and competing signal. The farther apart the target and competing signals are, the easier this task is. As the target and competing signals move closer together, it becomes more difficult to locate the sources of the stimuli. Therefore, detection of the target signal, likewise, becomes more difficult.

Localization and lateralization of an auditory stimulus is a function of binaural interaction, or the way in which the two ears work together. This ability may be significantly affected by peripheral hearing loss, particularly when the hearing loss is asymmetrical. In addition, an auditory processing disorder at the brainstem level may affect the listener's ability to localize auditory stimuli. **The primary behavioral characteristic of this type of processing disorder is the inability to detect speech in a noisy background.**

Tests of brainstem function, including the masking level difference (MLD), may be used to identify brainstem dysfunction that may affect localization and lateralization ability and, thus, the ability to detect speech in noise. Additional binaural interaction tests, such as Binaural Fusion and Rapidly Alternating Speech Perception, may be abnormal in some cases; however, as discussed in previous chapters, the sensitivity of these behavioral measures to anything other than very gross brainstem dysfunction is highly questionable. Furthermore, speech-in-noise tests, while not without significant limitations, may provide descriptive information regarding the listener's ability to recognize words in a background of noise.

Management of auditory processing disorders that affect the listener's ability to detect speech in noise should focus primarily on environmental adaptations that will improve access to the target signal while reducing the background competition. In addition, specific skills training in localization and lateralization of varied auditory stimuli, as well as selective attention training, may be useful. Children with binaural interaction and speech-in-noise deficits would also benefit from training in the use of context to achieve auditory closure and other top-down compensatory strategies. First and foremost, however, any clinical finding that suggests a possible deficit at the brainstem level—such as significantly asymmetrical findings on tests that are expected to yield relatively symmetrical findings (e.g., temporal patterning tasks, some tests of monaural low-redundancy speech, monaural separation tests such as the SSI-ICM, word recognition tests)—should result in follow-up to rule out retrocochlear pathology requiring medical follow-up. Information regarding binaural interaction deficits is summarized in Table 7-4.

Other Auditory Processes

Auditory abilities such as temporal processing and auditory discrimination are included in the ASHA (1996) definition of central auditory processes. Schow et al. (2000) suggested that these abilities, like that of binaural interaction, represent relatively complex mechanisms that may underlie auditory closure, temporal patterning, binaural separation, and binaural integration. As such, deficits in these basic areas may lead to dysfunction in those processes discussed in this section.

Temporal processing deficits may show up on tests of temporal resolution, such as gap detection testing. In addition, they may also result in poor performance on monaural low-redundancy speech tasks, especially those that involve time-compressed speech. Behaviorally, a child with a temporal processing deficit may exhibit the greatest difficulty with rapidly presented speech. Therefore, slowing down the speaking rate can improve these children's access to verbally presented information. As discussed in previous chapters, there is some controversy over whether temporal processing deficits in CAPD are auditory-modality specific and whether they can lead to

Table 7-4

Primary Characteristics of Deficits in Binaural Interaction

Principal feature:	A breakdown in the brainstem's ability to process binaural cues
Behavioral characteristics:	Difficulty localizing and lateralizing auditory information, leading to difficulty in detecting signals in noise
Central test findings:	Abnormally reduced masking level differences, abnormal findings on Auditory Brainstem Response, Binaural Fusion tests
Suggestions for management:	Improve acoustic access and signal-to-noise ratio in the environment; training in localization, lateralization, and selective attention (as indicated); recruitment of compensatory auditory closure strategies; referral for follow-up to rule out retrocochlear pathology

the types of learning, language, and communication difficulties that have been attributed to them (e.g., Cacace & McFarland, 1998). On the other hand, there is evidence that intensive therapy focusing on improving temporal processing results in concomitant improvement in language and auditory skills (e.g., Merzenich et al., 1996). More research is needed in the area of diagnosing temporal processing deficits and determining their functional impact and optimal means of treatment.

Auditory discrimination is a very general term used to refer to the ability to differentiate behaviorally between auditory stimuli of many types. This skill is also an important underlying ability subserving a vast array of auditory behaviors. Difficulties in speech-sound discrimination can affect word recognition and speech comprehension in quiet or in noise, auditory closure abilities, and performance on binaural separation, integration, or interaction tests. Deficits in nonverbal auditory discrimination can affect temporal patterning tasks that require the ability to discriminate between tonal patterns differing subtly in pitch or duration.

Children with auditory discrimination deficits may perform poorly on speech and language measures involving phonological awareness and similar tasks, as discussed in Chapter 4. In addition, evidence of a basic, fundamental discrimination deficit may be seen behaviorally using the Northwestern University PEST paradigm discussed in the previous chapter, or via the use of the mismatch negativity response (MMN); however, both of these procedures have drawbacks for current clinical use including availability of equipment (PEST) and difficulty obtaining and identifying reliable responses (MMN). Other psychophysical procedures involving just noticeable differences *jnd*s for frequency, intensity, and duration may illuminate basic discrimination difficulties in some listeners as well; however, these measures are not common in clinical use at the present time, and the functional ramifications of elevated *jnd*s for these stimuli have yet to be elucidated.

Children with auditory discrimination deficits will likely benefit from direct therapy involving minimal contrast speech or nonspeech pairs, environmental modifications to improve acoustic access to the speech signal, and recruitment of top-down auditory closure compensatory mechanisms.

Determination of Site of Dysfunction

The high degree of redundancy within the CANS makes absolute determination of site dysfunction difficult when tests of central auditory function are relied upon for this determination. However, it is possible to consider general trends in the central auditory test data and, in many circumstances, to determine the level of the CANS at which the dysfunction is occurring. This determination is important for a number of reasons, including identification of the need for a medical referral, as well as in monitoring effects of rehabilitative activities and tracking changes in the effects of lesions (Musiek & Lamb, 1994). Another value of site-of-dysfunction interpretation is in the confirmation of "logical" patterns across test findings that are consistent with one another in terms of underlying neurophysiology. That is, when results of central auditory tests suggest dysfunction in a particular brain region(s), this information can be compared with results of multidisciplinary speech, language, cognitive, learning, and related evaluations for indications of dysfunction in the same brain region(s). When test findings across disciplines agree in this regard, our confidence in our findings, impressions, and recommendations is strengthened, and our ability to create deficit-specific management programs is enhanced. This topic will be discussed further in the section on subprofiles of CAPD.

This section provides an overview of general trends of central auditory tests that are characteristic of dysfunction at the brainstem, cerebral, and interhemispheric levels of the CANS. It should be noted that if a neurological lesion or any condition requiring medical follow-up is suspected, clinicians should refer for follow-up immediately.

Brainstem Dysfunction

As previously mentioned, many of the behavioral tests of brainstem function have been criticized on the bases of poor sensitivity and specificity. Three behavioral measures of central auditory function have demonstrated relatively good sensitivity for brainstem lesions: the Synthetic Sentence Identification Test with Ipsilateral Competing Message (SSI-ICM; Jerger & Jerger, 1975), masking level difference (MLD; Olsen & Noffsinger, 1976), and Staggered Spondaic Words (SSW; Katz, 1977). In addition, Musiek and Guerkink (1982) reported that, while the sensitivity of procedures such as rapid alternating speech perception (RASP) and binaural fusion appeared questionable for identifying brainstem dysfunction, other tests of central auditory function did appear to be sensitive to both brainstem and cortical lesions, including Dichotic Digits, Competing Sentences, and Low-Pass Filtered Speech.

When undertaking brainstem assessment, clinicians should also keep in mind other tests of brainstem function, including acoustic reflex measures and speech audiometry. In addition, **the value of physiological measures, particularly auditory brainstem response (ABR) and acoustic reflex testing, in the assessment of brainstem function cannot be overemphasized.** Musiek, Gollegly, Kibbe, and Reeves (1985) reported that, when using a battery of seven central tests in listeners with multiple sclerosis, the combination of ABR along with either the MLD or Dichotic Digits test demonstrated the same sensitivity for brainstem dysfunction as did the use of the entire battery.

ABR results in cases of pontine brainstem lesions, in general, tend to be abnormal for the ear ipsilateral to the lesion (Chiappa, 1983). On the other hand, a large degree of variability in behavioral tests may be found, depending on the location, size, and type of the lesion, and abnormal findings may be contralateral, ipsilateral, or bilateral. As discussed in the section on binaural interaction, any test findings that suggest a possible brainstem site of dysfunction should be followed up immediately to rule out possible retrocochlear involvement requiring medical intervention.

When assessing central auditory function in children, it should be kept in mind that, although rare, space-occupying lesions and other neurological involvement of the brainstem can and do occur.

Therefore, we rely on the following rule of thumb: **if results of the behavioral test battery, along with acoustic reflex measures, suggest the possibility of brainstem involvement in a school-age child, the child should be referred for ABR and additional medical follow-up.**

Cerebral Dysfunction

The term *cerebral* is used to denote lesions that affect the gray or white matter of the brain. Musiek and Lamb (1994) used the terms *cortical* and *hemispheric* to differentiate between the two types of cerebral lesions. Cortical refers to the gray matter of the brain alone, whereas hemispheric refers to lesions that affect both the white and gray matter.

The specific pattern of central auditory test findings that result from cortical lesions will depend on both the auditory task and the region of the brain that is involved. In cases of left-hemisphere dysfunction, monaural low-redundancy speech tasks are often affected bilaterally; however, effects are typically more evident in the contralateral (i.e., right) ear. A similar pattern of findings is seen on dichotic listening tasks, particularly those that have some degree of linguistic loading. Tests of temporal patterning (i.e., Frequency and Duration Patterns) typically show a bilateral deficit in the ability to label tonal stimuli linguistically; however, the ability to hum the patterns heard is preserved. As will be seen, this finding is also indicative of dysfunction in the interhemispheric pathways, or corpus callosum. If the primary auditory cortex of the (usually) left hemisphere is involved, additional temporal processing and fundamental auditory discrimination deficits may be apparent on special tests of auditory function. Conversely, when there is involvement of the auditory association areas, such as occurs with receptive aphasia, we often find preserved auditory closure, temporal processing, and auditory discrimination abilities combined with left-hemisphere findings on tests of dichotic listening and temporal patterning.

Right-hemisphere cortical lesions typically yield a different pattern of findings from that of left-hemisphere dysfunction. With right-hemisphere involvement, a contralateral (left-ear) deficit on dichotic speech tasks is expected. Temporal patterning tasks show a deficit in *both* labeling and humming of tonal patterns; however, performance on tests of monaural low-redundancy speech, temporal processing, and auditory discrimination typically is not affected. The underlying mechanisms responsible for these differential hemispheric findings were discussed in some depth in Chapter 2.

Qualitatively, performance of listeners with temporal lobe lesions may differ from that of normal listeners or listeners with brainstem lesions. Thompson and Abel (1992a, b) reported that listeners with temporal lobe lesions generally demonstrated greater difficulty with temporal patterning and consonant discrimination tasks than did listeners with acoustic tumors and normal controls. In addition, listeners with temporal lobe lesions required a greater response time than did the other two groups. In all cases, listeners with lesions of the left temporal lobe tended to demonstrate greater performance deficits. These qualitative differences are likely the result of the dominance of the left hemisphere, particularly the primary auditory cortex, for speech processing and verbal labeling. As shown in Chapter 1, speech sounds requiring perception of rapid spectro-temporal acoustic changes are particularly vulnerable to disruption of the primary auditory cortex. However, vowel discrimination difficulties and deficits on tests using nonverbal auditory stimuli may be found in cases of right-hemisphere as well as thalamic dysfunction.

Interhemispheric Dysfunction

As shown in Chapter 1, the fibers of the corpus callosum, responsible for interhemispheric transfer of information, extend well into the cerebral hemispheres. Therefore, it is quite possible that a cortical lesion may affect fibers of the corpus callosum as well.

The classic pattern of central auditory test findings associated with interhemispheric dysfunction is a left-ear deficit on dichotic speech tasks *combined with* a deficit on temporal patterning tests (i.e., Frequency or Duration Patterns) in the *linguistic labeling condition only.* Often, the left-ear deficit will be more pronounced on dichotic speech tasks that are more linguistically loaded, possibly due to the additional processing required by callosal fibers for these types of stimuli. Tests of monaural low-redundancy speech are generally unaffected by interhemispheric dysfunction, as are most tests of temporal processing and auditory discrimination.

Because the corpus callosum is among the final portions of the CNS to attain maturation, young children will exhibit this same pattern of findings. It is critical, therefore, to have precise, age-appropriate normative data for all of these tasks. A significant left-ear deficit in an 8-year-old child may not be significant, whereas the same degree of deficit in a 10-year-old child may signal the presence of a disorder. In most cases, it is difficult to determine whether delayed maturation or actual disorder is responsible for the finding of interhemispheric dysfunction without longitudinal studies on the individual child. Therefore, I typically avoid using the term *delayed*, as this term implies that the child will catch up without specific intervention. Sequelae and intervention recommendations for children with interhemispheric dysfunction will be discussed in the section on subprofiles of CAPD and in Chapters 8 and 9.

Subprofiles of Central Auditory Processing Disorders

It has been emphasized again and again throughout this book that the whole child must be taken into account in order to assess the contribution of a given CAPD to academic, communicative, and associated difficulties. Myklebust (1954) stated that, when assessing children with auditory problems, a differential diagnosis is necessary because children having different types of auditory problems will vary greatly in their individual needs. To address these individual needs, we must first strive to define the underlying problem in as precise a manner as possible. In addition, we must realize that the act of listening involves both fundamental encoding and processing of acoustic signals along with higher-order cognitive, attention, language, and related abilities. Even if we consider CAPD to be primarily a bottom-up disorder, we must recognize that a large degree of interdependence exists in the CANS. Even subtle deficits in attention or memory, for example, may manifest themselves as "auditory attention" or "auditory memory" disorders if they are paired with—and impacted further by—a deficit in the bottom-up auditory system. This topic, and the related topic of differential diagnosis of CAPD from other nonauditory disorders, will be discussed at the end of this chapter.

Similarly, although general functions can be ascribed to specific brain regions, a great deal of interaction exists among different areas of the brain. Recent research using functional neuroimaging techniques indicates that even the simplest auditory task—such as passive listening—results in activation of many different brain areas, reflecting the incredible degree of integration and interdependency throughout the CNS. Our interpretation of central auditory findings and recommendations for management should reflect this interdependency. In other words, **a multidisciplinary approach that takes into account the individual child's auditory, language, learning, and associated characteristics is critical to appropriate interpretation and management** (Bellis, 1996, 1999, 2002; Bellis & Ferre, 1999; Ferre, 1994).

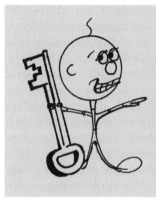

KEY CONCEPT

The interdependency of audition, language, and learning must be reflected in our approach to central auditory assessment and management.

In recent years, the use of subprofiles of central auditory processing deficits has begun to gain wider acceptance clinically (Bellis, 1996, 1999, 2002; Bellis & Ferre, 1999; Ferre, 1994; Katz, 1992; Katz, Stecker, & Masters, 1994; Musiek, Gollegly, & Ross, 1985). Each of these authors has approached subprofiling of CAPD from a slightly different perspective. For example, Katz et al. (1994) suggested that categories of CAPD be made up of skills that cluster with specific language and communication deficits. In their Buffalo Model, the authors separated CAPD and language/communication deficits into four categories: Phonemic Decoding, Tolerance-Fading Memory, Integration, and Organization.

The Bellis/Ferre model of categorizing CAPD (Bellis, 1996, 1999; Bellis & Ferre, 1999; Ferre, 1997) was developed in response to the need for a means of relating central auditory test findings to both their underlying neurophysiologic bases and their behavioral, cognitive, academic, and communicative sequelae. Although the initial version of this model included four primary subtypes, this model has been revised over the years and now consists of three primary and two secondary subtypes. The three primary subtypes—Auditory Decoding Deficit, Prosodic Deficit, and Integration Deficit—represent dysfunction in the left hemisphere (primary auditory cortex), right hemisphere, and interhemispheric pathways, respectively. The two secondary subtypes—Associative Deficit and Output-Organization Deficit—may be thought of as riding that fine, gray line between audition and higher-order abilities such as receptive language and executive function.

These revisions to our model arose from increased insight into and understanding of information processing and the effects of dysfunction in various brain regions, especially of the nondominant right hemisphere, on auditory processing. It should be emphasized that the

Bellis/Ferre model of CAPD is, at present, theoretical, and is not universally accepted. However, it does exhibit significant strengths not seen in other models of CAPD, especially in its ability to conform to the underlying science of how the CANS processes auditory information while, at the same time, bringing the auditory piece of the puzzle together with information from other disciplines so that a view of the whole child can be obtained. At the present time, preliminary data analysis from hundreds of children and adults is encouraging, and confirms the confluence of findings on auditory, cognitive, and language tests proposed by the Bellis/Ferre model. Still, however, much research needs to be completed before this model is empirically validated, and it may undergo yet more revisions as additional information is obtained.

This section provides a description of each of the subprofiles of the Bellis/Ferre model. It should be noted that the use of the subprofiles discussed herein is not intended to suggest that this is the only manner in which CAPD may be categorized. Rather, this method is delineated only so that it may provide clinicians with a useful way in which to view the interdependency of CAPD and education/communication, as well as assist in the development of a multidisciplinary approach to assessment and management. Finally, clinicians should be reminded that these subprofiles may exist singularly or in combination. However, the combination of subtypes should make sense from a neuroanatomical position in that brain regions typically involved are adjacent to one another. Thus, either left- or right-hemisphere-based CAPD may, and often does, coexist with interhemispheric-based deficit, because cerebral hemisphere dysfunction often also affects fibers of the corpus callosum. We would not, however, expect to see right- and left-hemisphere auditory processing deficits co-occurring in the same person. Similarly, findings that suggest dysfunction in both cerebral hemispheres as well as the corpus callosum would be indicative of global brain involvement. Therefore, failure on every single test of central auditory processing administered would not, as some would like to believe, signify a very severe auditory processing deficit. Rather, this pattern—or *lack* of pattern—of findings is highly suggestive of a higher-order cognitive, attention, or related deficit (or, possibly, a lack of motivation on the part of the listener during testing) that is not specific to the CANS. **It is the *pattern* of findings across measures of central auditory function and cognitive, language, and learning testing that will determine whether a CAPD exists, the specific type(s) of CAPD that is present, and the direction that management should take.**

Primary Subprofiles

The three primary CAPD subprofiles of the Bellis/Ferre model represent the auditory and related sequelae that arise from dysfunction in the left-, right-, and interhemispheric pathways. The key hallmarks of each of these subtypes will be described below but, first, it should be emphasized that very few children will exhibit *all* of the symptoms and sequelae of a given subtype. The way in which an auditory processing deficit manifests itself behaviorally will differ from person to person. Therefore, determining the functional impact of a given disorder, as well as making recommendations for management and intervention, should always be based on the presenting difficulties of the individual child.

Auditory Decoding Deficit

Auditory Decoding Deficit is the most auditory-modality-specific of the Bellis/Ferre subtypes and, as such, some might consider it to be the only true CAPD. Based on the specific auditory findings, which will be delineated below, along with the underlying neurophysiology of auditory signal encoding in the CANS, discussed in Part One of this book, the presumed site of dysfunction for Auditory Decoding Deficit is the primary auditory cortex in the language-dominant (usually left) hemisphere. Therefore, this deficit results in a decrease in the intrinsic redundancy of the auditory signal and will be much more pronounced in listening situations in which the external redundancy is also reduced, such as noisy environments. Although the following lists are designed to illuminate the most common findings in Auditory Decoding Deficit, it should again be emphasized that most children exhibit some, but not all, of these sequelae.

Auditory processes most likely to be impacted:

- Auditory closure
- Temporal processing
- Auditory discrimination (specifically, speech-sound discrimination)
- Binaural separation and/or integration

Typical findings on central auditory testing:

- Bilateral deficits on dichotic speech tests, often with right ear worse than left
- Deficits on tests of monaural low-redundancy speech, often with right ear worse than left and errors phonemically similar to target

- Elevated temporal gap detection thresholds and other temporal processing deficits
- Elevated *jnds* for speech-sound discrimination, especially those that involve rapid spectro-temporal acoustic changes (e.g., stop consonants)
- Electrophysiology may show decreased responses over left hemisphere and/or absent MMN to speech contrasts involving rapid spectro-temporal acoustic change
- Performance on tests of temporal patterning, binaural interaction, and discrimination for slowly changing speech sounds (such as vowels, glides, liquids) is typically normal

Primary auditory complaints:

- Difficulty hearing in noise or with speakers who do not enunciate clearly, resulting in frequent requests for repetition
- Frequent "mishearing" and subsequent misunderstanding similar to what is seen in peripheral hearing loss
- Feeling as if a hearing loss is present, even if peripheral hearing sensitivity is well within the normal range
- Auditory fatigue or overload due to extra energy required for listening
- Faring far better in quiet listening environments or when visual or multimodality cues are added

Related sequelae:

- Poor phonological awareness abilities, including difficulty with sound blending, phonological manipulation, and similar tasks
- Possible presence of phonological production errors that are not developmental in nature and are consistent with possible auditory confusions (e.g., substituting "b" for "d" in speech)
- Vocabulary and syntax may be affected
- Good pragmatic communication abilities
- Poor word-attack abilities during reading and spelling, combined with good sight-word abilities
- Verbal IQ lower than Performance IQ
- Good performance in nonverbal tasks such as mathematics calculation, art, music

Management and intervention strategies (Note: specific treatment methods will be discussed in Chapters 8 and 9):

- Improve acoustic access to information
- Preteach new vocabulary and concepts
- Augment with visual and/or multimodality cues
- Repeat, rather than rephrase, messages (repetition allows for the filling in of the missing components, whereas rephrasing provides a whole new message with new "holes" to be filled)
- Phoneme training, focusing on discrimination of minimal contrast pairs and speech-to-print skills
- Compensatory strategies training to include principles of active listening, auditory closure skills, and vocabulary enhancement activities
- Speech and language therapy may be indicated to address phonological and language deficits

It should be noted that the presentation and management of Auditory Decoding Deficit is very similar to that seen in children with peripheral hearing impairment. Therefore, strategies and interventions that are useful for children with hearing loss will likely be of benefit to children with Auditory Decoding Deficit. Finally, although difficulty hearing speech in noise is a hallmark symptom of Auditory Decoding Deficit, this complaint is also common in a variety of other types of CAPD as well as in nonauditory disorders. Therefore, the presence of poor speech-in-noise skills should not, alone, constitute evidence of a CAPD.

Prosodic Deficit

Although the previous subtype of CAPD may be thought of by some as the only "true" auditory-specific processing deficit, **we should not discount the importance of brain regions other than the primary auditory cortex to auditory processing.** Historically, the majority of research into the neurophysiology of auditory and language processing has focused on the functions of the language-dominant, or left, hemisphere. However, as seen in Part One of this book, the right hemisphere subserves a vast array of auditory abilities that are important for communication. The recent upsurge in interest in right-hemisphere communication disorders has illuminated the contribution of this brain region to communication and related abilities. It should be noted, however, that the functions of the right hemisphere are somewhat less circumscribed than are those of the left hemisphere. In other words, there is a great deal of multitask and multimodality integration that occurs throughout the right hemisphere. As such, although right-hemisphere-based CAPD can often significantly impact communication, it may be just one portion of a more global right-hemisphere deficit that results in far more pervasive and severe nonauditory difficulties. **When present, these other associated symptoms of right-hemisphere involvement should not be considered to arise from the CAPD,** but rather should be thought of as comorbid conditions. Therefore, Prosodic Deficit is often just the auditory piece of a larger, general central processing deficit arising from dysfunction in the right hemisphere. Following are the typical central auditory test findings and related sequelae indicative of Prosodic Deficit:

Auditory processes most likely to be impacted:

- Temporal patterning
- Auditory discrimination of nonspeech stimuli (e.g., frequency, intensity, or duration discrimination); vowel discrimination difficulties are possible
- Binaural separation and/or integration

Typical findings on central auditory testing:

- Left-ear deficit on dichotic speech tasks
- Deficits on temporal patterning tasks in *both* the linguistic labeling and humming conditions, indicating difficulty with perception of the acoustic contour itself
- Electrophysiology may show decreased responses over right hemisphere; MMN are typically present to consonant-vowel contrasts, but may be absent to tonal stimuli
- Performance on tests of binaural interaction, temporal processing, monaural low-redundancy speech, and speech-sound (especially consonant) discrimination is typically normal; however, some difficulty with vowel discrimination may be present

Primary auditory complaints:

- Difficulty comprehending the *intent* (rather than the content) of communications
- Frequent misunderstandings, complaints of hurt feelings, and perceptions of others' communication as abrupt, rude, sarcastic, or negative in some other way
- Difficulty perceiving jokes, sarcasm, and other messages that rely on subtle prosodic cues

- Possible difficulty understanding messages in which subtle changes in stress alter the meaning (e.g., "Look out the window" versus "Look out! The window!")
- Difficulty comprehending overly abstract communicative exchanges or topics
- Auditory complaints are typically not dependent on acoustic environment

Related sequelae:

- Poor pragmatic and social communication abilities
- Poor sight-word reading and spelling abilities, combined with good word-attack or phonological decoding skills
- Performance IQ often lower than Verbal IQ
- Significant difficulty with nonverbal tasks such as mathematics calculation, art, and music
- Poor visual-spatial abilities
- Poor gestalt patterning abilities
- May be at risk for depressive disorder secondary to right-hemisphere dysfunction
- May meet diagnostic criteria for nonverbal learning disability; alternatively, presentation may be very subtle and performance across academic areas may be loosely within the normal range
- Performs far better with concrete, rather than abstract, information
- May have difficulty staying on topic during conversation
- Phonological awareness abilities, vocabulary, and syntax are usually intact

Management and intervention strategies (Note: specific treatment methods will be discussed in Chapters 8 and 9):

- Placement with "animated" teachers who make generous use of prosodic cues and multimodality augmentation
- Avoid hints; spell out precisely what is meant
- Temporal patterning and prosody training
- Reading aloud with exaggerated prosodic features
- Compensatory strategies training to include social communication and judgment, role-playing, comprehension of underlying intent, topic maintenance, and communication repair strategies

- Psychological counseling often critical in addressing social concerns and depressive symptoms
- Intervention by other professionals (e.g., vision therapy, mathematics tutoring, pragmatic therapy) may be indicated

For children with Prosodic Deficit, the auditory complaints may be the least severe of their difficulties. Instead, social concerns, depression, difficulty with allocation of attention and topic maintenance, and visual-spatial difficulties may be far more pervasive. Therefore, although this book is concerned with auditory processing deficits, we should always keep in mind that the auditory system does not exist in a vacuum, and the whole child must be taken into account when developing meaningful intervention programs. Furthermore, we should never assume that the higher-order social and cognitive difficulties associated with Prosodic Deficit arise from an underlying auditory-based cause. For example, in my experience, clinical central auditory findings consistent with Prosodic Deficit are often found in disorders such as Asperger's syndrome, for which a right-hemisphere site of dysfunction is suspected. We cannot attribute Asperger's syndrome to an underlying auditory deficit. Rather, we must acknowledge that the auditory processing manifestations are merely symptoms of the larger, more global cognitive entity.

Integration Deficit

Just as integrity of both the left and right cerebral hemispheres is important for processing auditory information, several auditory skills are reliant on efficient communication between the two hemispheres. Integration Deficit is characterized by difficulty in tasks that require interhemispheric transfer. Symptoms of Integration Deficit may be primarily within a single modality, or may be multimodal in nature. This is because the corpus callosum is a multimodal structure, and dysfunction in the callosal pathways may give rise to a host of seemingly unrelated symptoms. Therefore, the child with Integration Deficit may present with a wide variety of behavioral auditory complaints, many of which are difficult to pin down precisely. Once again, as with Prosodic Deficit, **the auditory symptoms of Integration Deficit may be the primary presenting factors, or may be just one manifestation of more far-reaching multimodality difficulties arising from inefficient interhemispheric integration.** Key findings and sequelae of Integration Deficit may include:

Auditory processes most likely to be impacted:

- Temporal patterning
- Binaural separation and/or integration

Typical findings on central auditory testing:

- Left-ear deficit on dichotic speech tasks, which may be more pronounced with linguistically loaded material
- Deficits on temporal patterning tasks in the linguistic labeling condition only, indicating intact perception of the acoustic contour itself but inefficient transfer to the left hemisphere for verbal output
- Electrophysiology may show a lack of typical hemispheric asymmetry patterns to speech stimuli
- Performance on tests of binaural interaction, temporal processing, monaural low-redundancy speech, and auditory discrimination is typically normal

Primary auditory complaints:

- Significant difficulty hearing in noise
- Difficulty linking the linguistic content with the prosodic intent, leading to possible misunderstandings of the overall message, especially for sarcasm and similar communications in which the content and prosody differ (e.g., "Oh sure, I'd really like to date *him*," spoken in a sarcastic tone of voice)
- Difficulty with localizing and tracking a moving sound source, especially if it crosses midline
- Feeling as if the right ear is "better," or preference for monaural (right-ear) amplification over binaural hearing aids

Related sequelae:

- Difficulty with any task in which interaction between the two hemispheres of the brain is required
- Difficulty associating the visual symbol on the page with the sound, affecting both sight-word and word-attack skills, reading speed, and reading fluency
- Performance IQ and Verbal IQ usually relatively evenly developed, with scatter *within* scales depending on task demands
- Poor bimanual or bipedal coordination abilities
- Musical difficulties such as playing an instrument that requires significant bimanual coordination (e.g., piano),

hearing the lyrics of songs, or singing in time to a melody
- Greater difficulty when multimodality cues are added
- Significant difficulty taking dictation or notes
- Difficulty drawing a picture from verbal or written descriptions or instructions
- Auditory and related symptoms vary widely

Management and intervention strategies (Note: specific treatment methods will be discussed in Chapters 8 and 9):

- Improve acoustic access to information in the classroom
- Avoid multimodality cues; present information via one modality at a time
- Some aspects of prosody training may be indicated to assist in integrating content with intent, including reading of body language cues
- Directed therapy to target interhemispheric activities and binaural separation/integration training
- Compensatory strategies training to include principles of active listening, and recruitment of stronger, top-down language and cognitive functions
- Occupational therapy, tutoring in specific academic areas, and other intervention may be indicated, depending on type and degree of associated sequelae

Again, it should be emphasized that the nonauditory, related sequelae often seen in Integration Deficit cannot be considered to *arise* from an underlying auditory cause. Rather, they coexist with the auditory difficulties as the result of corpus callosum dysfunction. Many functions have been attributed to the corpus callosum and, theoretically, any combination of them can be affected by interhemispheric involvement. Therefore, as with Prosodic Deficit, Integration Deficit may be considered just the auditory piece of interhemispheric dysfunction. Finally, I should mention that many of the symptoms and sequelae of Integration Deficit may be found in sensory integration (SI) disorders as well. Indeed, it may well be that the two disorders are not independent diagnostic entities. However, in my experience, children with SI typically have far greater difficulties with the multimodal, sensory, and motor aspects of their disorder, which can result in an overall delay across all areas, extreme sensitivity to sensory input, and similar complaints. In contrast, children with Integration Deficit typically report the auditory symptoms as primary, with the other sequelae being of far less concern. However, this differentiation between the two has yet to be examined fully, and may ultimately prove to be an artificial distinction. In any case, our primary objective is to determine the degree to which the child is exhibiting auditory difficulties and address those in a deficit-specific manner.

Secondary Subprofiles

As we saw in Chapter 2, it is very difficult to determine precisely where auditory processing leaves off and language begins. Furthermore, other top-down factors, including executive function, play a significant role in children's ability to process and respond to auditory information. The two secondary subprofiles of the Bellis/Ferre model represent those disorders that reside in the gray areas between auditory processing and language, and auditory processing and efferent/executive function. Although their inclusion in a model of auditory processing disorders may be somewhat controversial, they are identified as secondary subprofiles for two main reasons: (1) each of them yields a specific pattern of findings on tests of central auditory function, and (2) their behavioral symptoms are significantly more (and sometimes solely) evident in the auditory modality. Nevertheless, there is an inherent danger in including these types of deficits under the "CAPD umbrella," in that some may consider this a reason to attribute any and all language, executive function, or related disorders to an underlying auditory cause which, as we have seen throughout this book, cannot and should not be encouraged. It is for this reason that the subprofiles discussed in this section are considered secondary profiles: they tend to manifest themselves primarily as language disorders, and direct therapy for these deficits often consists of traditional receptive and expressive language intervention.

Associative Deficit

The primary feature of Associative Deficit is an underlying inability to apply the rules of language to incoming acoustic information. For example, children with Associative Deficit often exhibit difficulty with sentences presented in the passive voice (e.g., The ball was thrown by the girl), compound sentences, and other linguistically complex messages. At its most severe, Associative Deficit can manifest itself in the inability to attach linguistic meaning to phonemic units of speech. This disorder was, at one time, called "receptive childhood aphasia"; however, that term has fallen into disuse in recent years. Nevertheless, the symptoms associated with pure receptive aphasia for spoken language have been shown to arise from lesions or dysfunction in the auditory association cortical areas. Therefore, the use of the term *auditory processing disorder* may well be appropriate for these types of "language" disorders.

On tests of central auditory function, children with Associative Deficit will demonstrate bilateral deficits on dichotic listening tasks, often with the right ear worse than the left. This finding is clear evidence of left-hemisphere auditory involvement, and is also seen in adults with receptive aphasia following stroke or trauma. Performance on tests of monaural low-redundancy speech (using appropriate vocabulary), temporal processing, temporal patterning, and binaural interaction is often good, indicating intact function of the primary auditory cortex, corpus callosum, and right hemisphere. Speech-sound discrimination typically is quite good; however, word recognition itself may be poor depending on the child's receptive vocabulary abilities. Electrophysiology may show decreased response amplitudes over the left hemisphere.

Behaviorally, the child with Associative Deficit may exhibit receptive language deficits in vocabulary, semantics, and syntax. For many of these children, early academic achievement appears to be age-appropriate. However, as the linguistic demands within the classroom begin to increase, often around the third grade, general academic difficulties may begin to become apparent.

Management approaches indicated in cases of Associative Deficit likely will contain elements of language intervention, and speech-language services are often a key component of remediation. Metacognitive techniques designed to strengthen the memory trace and aid in item recall are helpful. These would include training the child to utilize verbal rehearsal, chunking, tag words (e.g., first, second, before, after), and other organizational aids. Classroom management strategies useful in cases of Associative Deficit would include preteaching of new information and imposition of external organization within the classroom. These children often have difficulty with independent work, whole-language approaches, and other classroom techniques that require self-monitoring of learning behavior.

Children with Associative Deficit often are able to repeat verbatim instructions they have been given. This behavior can be deceptive, as the ability to repeat an instruction does not necessarily imply comprehension of the instruction. Therefore, repetition as a clarification strategy is rarely effective for children with Associative Deficit. Instead, instructions or other verbal messages should be rephrased using simpler language. Comprehension should be checked by asking these children to paraphrase or demonstrate what is expected of them, rather than requesting simple repetition of the instruction.

Output-Organization Deficit

Output-Organization Deficit is, in my mind, the least understood and least defined of the five subprofiles. Because its symptoms can overlap with those of many other disorders, it is important that evidence of auditory involvement be confirmed before its diagnosis can be enabled. As its name implies, Output-Organization Deficit is an inability to sequence, plan, and organize responses *to auditory information or instructions*. Children with this deficit typically do far better if the instructions are provided in written form. In Output-Organization Deficit, receptive auditory skills are good; however, the difficulty lies in the ability to act upon incoming auditory information. Children with Output-Organization Deficit often demonstrate poor performance on any task that requires report of more than two critical elements. Therefore, performance on low-pass filtered or time-compressed speech tasks will remain unaffected, as the child is required simply to repeat one word at a time. In contrast, performance on speech-in-noise tests may be significantly impacted because of the extreme auditory figure/ground difficulties seen in Output-Organization Deficit. Performance on tests such as Frequency and Duration Patterns, Dichotic Digits, Competing Sentences, and SSW will also be poor, because all of these tests require the child to report multiple elements. The deficit found on these tests is not due to difficulty in auditory input skills, but rather to the inability to formulate and sequence the appropriate response. Physiologic indicators of Output-Organization Deficit often include abnormal contralateral acoustic reflexes or absence of contralateral suppression during otoacoustic emissions (OAE) testing.

Behaviorally, children with Output-Organization Deficit complain of significant difficulty hearing in noise. They may also demonstrate poor organizational skills, difficulty following directions, reversals, and poor recall and word retrieval abilities. It is important to note, however, that these symptoms are either much more pervasive, or present only, to auditory input. Furthermore, the ability to follow routines that are already learned typically is intact, and difficulty is apparent primarily with novel instructions or directions. Expressive speech errors often consist of perseverative responses in which the target is substituted by a previously heard word. Sequencing errors and sound blending difficulties are not uncommon. Academically, children with Output-Organization Deficit may demonstrate good reading comprehension; however, spelling and writing skills may be poor, especially when attempting to write from dictation or take notes during class.

As previously discussed in Associative Deficit, children with Output-Organization Deficit will benefit from management strategies designed to aid in organization, including imposition of external organization (including written reminders and checklists) within the classroom and use of metacognitive techniques to draw upon higher-order strengths and enhance the memory trace. Because of the expressive language component in this profile, speech-language services will likely be an important component in the overall management of the child. Finally, both repetition and rephrasing of critical messages and instructions may be useful for the child with Output-Organization Deficit, but only if the message and required response is broken down into smaller linguistic units of no more than two critical elements.

The precise site of dysfunction for Output-Organization Deficit is not certain at this time. However, it is possible that Output-Organization Deficit is the behavioral manifestation of impaired temporal-to-frontal-lobe transfer and/or efferent function. Further details regarding the management suggestions made in this section will be provided in Chapters 8 and 9.

Differential Diagnosis of CAPD

In recent years, much attention has been given to the differential diagnosis of CAPD and other disorders that can coexist with or mimic CAPD. Perhaps the most familiar example is that of AD/HD. Because CAPD and AD/HD share many common behavioral symptoms, such as distractibility in noise, and often coexist, the ability to differentiate between the two is critical for management and treatment purposes. Behavioral tests of central auditory function can easily be confounded by attention, memory, or related deficits. Because of these potential confounds, the sensitivity and specificity of these test have been criticized in recent years. Some have even asserted that, because of their objectivity, electrophysiologic measures of central auditory function are far more valid indicators of central auditory disorder than are behavioral measures. As discussed in the previous chapter, however, there are significant limitations to the use of electrophysiologic measures in CAPD diagnosis and, as such, behavioral tests remain indispensable tools for both quantifying and describing CAPD, as well as for directing management efforts.

Nevertheless, it is true that attention, memory, low cognitive ability, very young chronological age, and even lack of motivation can cause children to perform poorly on behavioral tests of central auditory function. Therefore, it is critical that we be able to separate the effects of these other, often coexisting conditions, from those of the underlying auditory deficit. General guidelines for how such differential diagnosis can be accomplished will be provided in this section.

Attention

There is no doubt that difficulties in attention will, in a top-down fashion, affect the ability to process auditory information. However, what is not always clear is which deficit is preeminent—the attention disorder or the auditory disorder. Chermak and Musiek (1997) provided an excellent overview of the separate and overlapping characteristics of CAPD and AD/HD. Further, they set forth a compelling argument, based on the neurobiologic bases of the two disorders, that supports the concept that AD/HD represents a higher-order, more global cognitive attention or motivational deficit that is not sensory-modality-specific. In contrast, CAPD represents a disorder in the auditory system that, in turn, can impact the ability to attend selectively to auditory information in the presence of distractors. As such, CAPD and AD/HD are two distinct entities, each with its own underlying neurobiologic origins and diagnostic findings.

The ability to diagnose AD/HD and CAPD differentially is dependent on one's familiarity with the diagnostic indicators of the two disorders. When we consider the diagnostic criteria for AD/HD set forth in the DSM-IV-TR (2000), it is apparent that, although some of the criteria listed are commonly found in CAPD, others are not. For example, the hyperactivity and impulsivity components required to enable a diagnosis of attention deficit, hyperactive-impulsive type or combined (inattentive and hyperactive-impulsive) type are not considered hallmarks of CAPD. It is more difficult, however, to differentiate CAPD and attention deficit, inattentive type, because some of the behavioral symptoms do, indeed, present themselves in both disorders, such as distractibility, not seeming to "listen" when spoken to, and perhaps avoidance or dislike of difficult tasks that require sustained effort (e.g., homework). However, the majority of key diagnostic indicators of attention deficit, inattentive type are not considered to be consistent with CAPD, including frequent forgetfulness (including forgetting during daily, routine activities and losing items, such as school supplies, frequently), lack of attention to detail and abundance of careless mistakes in schoolwork and related activities, difficulty with *sustained* attention, and difficulty with organization and self-control. In addition, the diagnostic criteria for the inattention that occurs in AD/HD specifically state that, although children with AD/HD often do not follow through on instructions and directions, this behavior is *not due to an inability to understand the directions* as would occur with CAPD. Clearly, if examined closely, the diagnostic criteria specified for AD/HD do not describe the child with CAPD.

On behavioral and electrophysiologic tests of central auditory function, AD/HD and CAPD result in different findings as well. For the most part, auditory electrophysiologic measures will be normal in cases of AD/HD. They are, however, also normal in many cases of CAPD as well, as discussed in the previous chapter. Therefore, the finding of normal auditory electrophysiologic responses does not, in and of itself, rule out CAPD as a diagnosis.

I have emphasized throughout this chapter that **CAPD is a heterogeneous disorder that yields specific patterns of test findings of behavioral central auditory tests. It is this concept of *patterns* that is important when attempting to differentiate CAPD from AD/HD.** Children with AD/HD typically do not show patterns of performance on behavioral tests of central auditory function that are consistent with dysfunction in an underlying CANS region (or adjacent CANS regions) or that suggest a particular subprofile. Instead, my experience has been that children with AD/HD most often either do poorly on all tests administered or, conversely, perform normally on behavioral central auditory test batteries. When poor performance on one or two tests does occur, no *logical* pattern is evident in the findings. Thus, this lack of a pattern of performance consistent with CAPD tends to be the most common finding in AD/HD.

When considering other areas of function (e.g., cognitive, speech/language, academic, and behavior) the search for patterns consistent with CAPD can also assist in differentiating attention and auditory deficits. For example, whereas the child with AD/HD typically has difficulty with sustained attention, children with CAPD most often demonstrate deficits in the ability to attend selectively to auditory signals in the presence of background noise or when information is presented dichotically. Similarly, AD/HD typically manifests itself across sensory modalities; that is, it is apparent that AD/HD impacts rule-governed behavior, maintenance of attention, and self-control during activities that are auditory, visual, motor, and any combination thereof. CAPD, in contrast, is viewed as a disorder that is either restricted to, or significantly more evident in, the auditory modality. Moreover, the presence of behaviors that cannot reasonably be attributed to an underlying auditory deficit, such as poor turn-taking skills, inability (or unwillingness) to follow rules and routines, excessive talking or interrupting, "dreaminess," or off-task behavior, argues strongly against CAPD as a primary disorder.

One common clinical practice that may confuse the issue further is the frequent mention of "auditory attention" in CAPD diagnostic reports and even some diagnostic tests of auditory function. It should be noted that the attentional system is a supramodal one—that is, it is not restricted to a single sense modality. True attention disorders, or disorders affecting rule-governed behavior, such as AD/HD, are apparent across sensory modalities, as discussed above. In contrast, the auditory "attention" difficulties that arise from CAPD tend to be related specifically to the ability to hear in noise (auditory closure and binaural separation abilities), unilateral—usually left-ear—deficits on dichotic speech tasks (binaural separation or integration abilities), and similar, auditory-specific complaints. As such, it may not be appropriate to refer to these difficulties as "attentional" at all. For this reason, **I tend to avoid the use of the terms *attention, selective attention*, or *auditory attention* when referring to children with CAPD and, instead, use the proper process-based terminology that more accurately describes the specific auditory deficit(s) a given child exhibits.**

The previous discussion has centered on the differential diagnosis of CAPD and AD/HD when each exists alone, but what of those situations in which the two co-occur in a child? The comorbidity of CAPD and AD/HD is well recognized and, although precise prevalence data are scarce, evidence exists to suggest that auditory areas of the brain, including the planum temporale, insula, and corpus callosum, are smaller in some children with AD/HD (e.g., Hynd, Semrud-Clikeman, Lorys, Novey, & Eliopulos, 1990). Therefore, although CAPD and AD/HD are distinct diagnostic entities, they may arise from common underlying neurobiologic bases in some cases. It is important, therefore, for clinicians to be able to separate the effects of the attention deficit from the auditory deficit for purposes of diagnosis and management.

First, as discussed extensively in Chapter 4, it is imperative that attention deficits be diagnosed and treated prior to entering into central auditory assessment. Because the presence of attentional confounds will most often affect performance on tests of central auditory function, all steps must be taken to remove this confound when possible. When children who are taking medication for AD/HD are referred to me for possible CAPD, I always recommend that their medication be taken as usual prior to testing. I also make all attempts to conduct my diagnostic assessment during the morning hours, when the medication is at full effectiveness, particularly for those children who are not on time-release forms of medication. My goal is to try to separate the auditory component from the attention-related component, and this can best be done when interventions are in place to reduce or eliminate the attentional confound.

In those cases in which medication either is not indicated or not effective, the task of separating auditory from attention effects becomes more complicated. Again, however, the emphasis should be placed on looking for patterns of performance across test measures. Thus, a child with AD/HD who also exhibits CAPD may perform poorly across all test measures; however, a pattern may emerge in which relatively greater difficulty is seen in some measures that suggests a deficit in specific auditory processes or a particular subtype of CAPD. For example, left-ear performance may be affected more than right on dichotic speech tasks, performance on linguistic labeling of temporal patterns may be poorer than humming, and so forth. These findings, combined with careful, multidisciplinary analysis of a child's presenting behaviors and complaints, can help us to determine the relative impact of an auditory deficit and recommend auditory-specific directions for management in a child with comorbid AD/HD and CAPD. For an excellent overview of diagnostic indicators and neurobiologic bases of AD/HD, as well as the conceptualization of AD/HD as a disorder of self-control rather than of attention, per se, readers are referred to Barkley (1999).

Memory

Although it is not within the scope of this book to describe memory disorders in depth, the frequent mention of "auditory memory" disturbances in many writings on the topic of CAPD deserves some discussion. It is important to understand that there is no evidence at present to support modality-specific memory. Although different types of memory—memory for recent events, memory for procedures and routines, memory for new information—have been shown to have distinct neurophysiologic substrates, these memory categories are delineated on the basis of *type* of information, not whether the information is presented visually, auditorily, or through another modality. Moreover, although the presence of selective memory deficits that affect certain categories of words or visual input—such as nouns, verbs, face recognition, object recognition—while leaving other categories untouched has been documented, again, these types of memory deficits are not typically considered sensory modality specific. **As such, one must question whether "auditory memory" is an appropriate term to describe the difficulties some children with CAPD exhibit. Indeed,** one must question whether auditory memory, as a distinct entity, exists at all.

Memory is best conceptualized as a higher-order, supramodal cognitive skill that interacts with incoming sensory input to affect retention of information. As such, the "auditory memory" deficits exhibited by some children with CAPD can be explained by allocation of effort. That is, when a deficit exists in the processing of the incoming auditory input, so much effort is expended in hearing and understanding the information that very little energy may be left over for remembering it. Moreover, because decoding the auditory input may be a slow, laborious process for some children, information presented at the beginning of the communication may no longer be held in working memory by the time the latter portion of the message is processed. Thus, the entire message may be "forgotten," or not understood completely.

As with attention, I typically avoid the use of the term *auditory memory* when describing the deficits exhibited by children with CAPD. Instead, I focus on the specific auditory process(es) affected in a given child and direct my interventions toward those processes. I do, however, include compensatory strategies that strengthen the memory trace and assist in decreasing the effort required for retention of information in the overall management process, as will be discussed in Chapter 8. For an excellent overview of memory and learning, readers are referred to Kandel and Hawkins (1999).

Cognition

The differential diagnosis of CAPD and cognitive disorders, such as mental retardation, autism, pervasive developmental delay, and similar disabilities that may be considered to fall under the general "cognitive umbrella" is relatively straightforward. Cognitive disorders are conceptualized as higher-order, supramodal disorders that affect function across sensory modalities. **Therefore, the presence of relatively equally developed skills across language, auditory, visual, motor, and related areas would argue against CAPD as a primary diagnosis,** as discussed in Chapter 4. Nevertheless, I frequently encounter parents of children diagnosed with these disorders who are convinced that misdiagnoses have occurred and that CAPD is the true, underlying deficit responsible for their children's difficulties.

This topic was discussed in some depth in Chapter 4; however, it bears mentioning again. When significant delays or deficits across most or all sensory and motor modalities are present, or when a child tends to adhere to stereotypical "scripts" and routines or engages in self-stimulating behavior such as rocking or hand-flapping, a diagnosis of primary CAPD is not defensible. Although the presence of a higher-order cognitive deficit will certainly affect a child's ability to process auditory information in a top-down fashion, **it is important that parents and other professionals understand that CAPD does not underlie these more pervasive, higher-order disorders. Instead, the auditory difficulties should be considered a symptom, rather than a cause, of the cognitive deficit.**

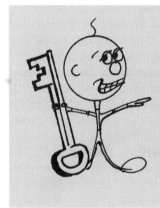

KEY CONCEPT

CAPD does not *cause* higher-order disorders such as AD/HD and autism. Rather, the auditory difficulties seen in these disorders should be considered associated symptoms, NOT CAPD.

Nevertheless, there are some cases in which specific auditory processing deficits do occur in children with cognitive delays, autistic spectrum disorders, or related disabilities that require deficit-specific intervention. I am often asked whether I require that children exhibit normal cognitive function—normal IQs—before I will consider central auditory assessment. Although some audiologists do have such criteria, I do not. Instead, I require that children be able to understand the directions and perform the tasks required of them rather than relying on a pre-set, arbitrary IQ number or other cognitive criterion. I also require that some evidence exist that these children exhibit relatively greater difficulty with auditory abilities than would be expected on the basis of their primary diagnosis, as described fully in Chapter 4. Therefore, I do occasionally test children with cognitive delays or high-functioning autism. In some of these cases, I am able to uncover an underlying auditory process, such as binaural separation or integration, that is dysfunctional to a degree that is out of proportion to the child's other difficulties. Although I make it very clear to the parents and referral source that this auditory deficit cannot account for the wide range of symptoms evident in the child, I acknowledge that the presence of the deficit can interact in a bottom-up fashion with the higher-order, top-down disorder, resulting in greater difficulties than either disorder would have if present in isolation. As such, I have found that directed, deficit-specific treatment of the auditory deficit can help in alleviating some of the burden imposed by the overlying, top-down disorder.

Once again, the importance of being familiar with the diagnostic criteria for these disorders and of approaching CAPD from a multidisciplinary perspective cannot be overemphasized. It is also important that, when cognitive disorders coexist with CAPD, parents and others are counseled regarding which behaviors and difficulties can be attributed to the auditory deficit, and which cannot. All too often, children are simultaneously diagnosed with auditory processing, visual processing, sensory integration, motor, and related disorders, and yet the overriding developmental, neurologic, or cognitive disorder—the true diagnosis—is ignored or goes undetected. In my experience, this is a common occurrence when specialists practice in a vacuum, focusing on their own small pieces of the puzzle in isolation and failing to consider the child as a whole. This practice not only does a disservice to the children we serve, but also to the parents, who often come away misinformed and then communicate that misinformation to other parents of children with similar difficulties.

Chronological Age

As we have seen, there are few behavioral tests of central auditory function that are appropriate for use with children younger than approximately age 7. Even if a child is able to participate in the procedure and understand the task, the inherent variability in brain function at very young ages precludes our ability to interpret the results of such testing with accuracy. Although some auditory electrophysiologic measures may confirm the presence of CAPD in very young children, this is not always the case. Therefore, differential diagnosis of CAPD in toddlers, preschoolers, and very young elementary school-age children may not always be possible.

Yet, the importance of early intervention for auditory disorders is clear. Therefore, we cannot simply wait until the child is of testable age before addressing potential CAPD. Instead, we must attempt to estimate, as accurately as possible, the type or types of auditory deficit that may be present in a given child and, on the basis of that information, design an early intervention plan that is as deficit-specific as possible.

To accomplish this goal, I approach the issue of CAPD in very young children via the screening approach described in Chapter 4. The input from others on the multidisciplinary team regarding the child's areas of strengths and weaknesses, coupled with the information presented in this chapter on patterns of behavioral signs and symptoms characteristic of various types of CAPD, allows me to rule out one or more subprofiles or deficit areas and to make a best-guess hypothesis as to the type(s) of CAPD most likely present. **I can then design a management plan that includes direct treatment for those deficit areas while, at the same time, emphasizing that CAPD has *not* been diagnosed definitively, but has been judged likely on the basis of available evidence.**

Hearing Loss

A final topic of concern that frequently arises in the clinical community is that of differential diagnosis of CAPD in children who also have hearing loss. Several issues render this a most difficult topic to address. First, we know that peripheral hearing dysfunction changes the input that is provided to the CANS for processing. Second, we know that structural and functional reorganization of central auditory pathways occurs at the subcortical and cortical levels secondary to hearing impairment. Finally, although some measures of central auditory function are relatively unaffected by mild to moderate degrees of hearing loss, the vast majority of them are not.

All of this leads to difficulty in appropriately diagnosing CAPD in children with hearing loss. Nevertheless, there appears to be a general consensus that CAPD can and does coexist with hearing loss in some children, and certainly in aging adults. Moreover, some of the most pervasive central auditory disorders, such as "central deafness" and auditory neuropathy, manifest themselves as a hearing loss accompanied by severe speech perception deficits. Yet, in both cases, cochlear function is intact when measured by OAEs, but electrophysiologic abnormalities are present in the ABR (auditory neuropathy) and cortical potentials (central deafness). These findings clearly demonstrate that the hearing loss seen in these pathologies is due to physiologic factors central to the cochlea.

The presence of central auditory dysfunction that cannot be attributed to peripheral factors has also been demonstrated in adults with hearing loss (e.g., Bellis & Wilber, 2001). However, the topic of comorbidity of hearing loss and CAPD in children is an area of much needed future research. There is a certain logic to the theory that the presence of speech perception and related difficulties of a far greater degree than would be expected on the basis of an audiogram may be due to central auditory factors. Similarly, it is entirely possible that differences in the integrity of central auditory function may explain why one child can achieve outstanding success with amplification while another child with the same audiometric configuration, age of onset, and intervention plan does not. However, these and related topics have yet to be explored fully.

In my practice, I do see children with hearing loss for central auditory evaluation. To evaluate, I must choose from those tests that have been shown to be relatively unaffected by peripheral hearing dysfunction. Therefore, tests of monaural low-redundancy speech, temporal processing, and many dichotic measures are not available to me. In children (or adults) with no more than a mild to moderate degree of hearing loss that is symmetrical between ears, and who possess the speech perceptual skills to repeat words and sentences, I can administer dichotic tests such as Digits and Competing Sentences. The presence of a significant left-ear deficit on these tests in the face of symmetrical hearing sensitivity may signal the presence of a concomitant CAPD. Similarly, I can administer tests of temporal patterning, such as Frequency or Duration Patterns, in cases of unilateral or bilateral hearing loss, as long as the stimuli are audible to the listener. However, I always approach interpretation of my test results with caution, and acknowledge that CAPD can occur secondary to peripheral hearing loss in some cases. If specific auditory processing deficits are found in a child with comorbid hearing loss, we can include auditory training activities that are directed specifically at those deficient, bottom-up areas in our aural rehabilitative efforts.

Summary

This chapter has described a variety of ways in which results of a comprehensive central auditory assessment may be interpreted. No one method of interpretation is considered to be the only correct method. Rather, I encourage clinicians to look at the assessment data from as many different perspectives as possible so that the full value of the information may be realized.

Based on central auditory test findings, clinicians should be able to make a determination regarding presence or absence of disorder. I recommend that the identification of CAPD be based on abnormal findings on one or more test tools, combined with significant educational and behavioral findings.

In addition to identifying the presence of the disorder, all attempts should be made to identify the underlying process or processes that are dysfunctional in order to develop a deficit-specific management plan. If possible, information regarding site of dysfunction within the CANS should also be obtained, most importantly to determine whether further medical follow-up is warranted.

Finally, results of central auditory tests should be related to the academic, communicative, and behavioral characteristics of the individual child so that a multidisciplinary management program that will address the child's functional difficulties may be developed. To this end, the use of subprofiles or categories of CAPD may be useful. This chapter has described the Bellis/Ferre model of CAPD, which consists of three primary subtypes (Auditory Decoding Deficit, Prosodic Deficit, and Integration Deficit) and two secondary subtypes (Associative Deficit and Output-Organization Deficit). These subprofiles are useful in relating results of central auditory tests to both the underlying neurophysiologic site of dysfunction as well as to the language, learning, and communication difficulties exhibited by children with CAPD. The topic of differential diagnosis of CAPD and attention, cognitive, and related disorders was also addressed. At all times, the importance of looking for logical patterns of performance across test measures in diagnosing and describing CAPD was emphasized. Readers are referred to Chapters 8 and 9 for specific management strategies.

Review Questions

1. Identify four questions that may be answered by the results of central auditory testing.

2. Differentiate between strict and lax criteria for the interpretation of test results.

3. What two components are recommended to be present in order for identifying the presence of a CAPD?

4. Define process-based interpretation.

5. Identify the behavioral auditory characteristics of dysfunction in the following underlying auditory processes:

    Auditory Closure   Binaural Separation and Integration

Temporal Patterning   Binaural Interaction
Temporal Processing   Auditory Discrimination

6. What findings would be expected on tests of central auditory function for dysfunction in each of the processes listed above?

7. What management approaches may be appropriate for deficits in each of the processes listed above?

8. What is the clinical utility of determining the site of dysfunction?

9. What central auditory test findings are indicative of dysfunction in the following areas of the CANS?

brainstem   cerebral
interhemispheric

10. List the behavioral, academic, and central auditory test characteristics of each of the following Bellis/Ferre subprofiles of CAPD:

Auditory Decoding Deficit   Integration Deficit
Prosodic Deficit   Output-Organization
Associative Deficit   Deficit

11. What management approaches might be appropriate for each of the CAPD subprofiles listed above?

12. What is the most important findings-related factor to look for when attempting to differentially diagnose CAPD and AD/HD, cognitive disorders, or hearing loss, or when determining the likelihood of CAPD being present in a very young child?

13. Why might the terms *auditory attention* and *auditory memory* not be appropriate when discussing CAPD?

CAPD Management and Service Delivery

CHAPTER

EIGHT

General Principles of CAPD Management

There is a paucity of empirical data regarding the efficacy of management approaches to CAPD. In fact, it would not be unreasonable to suggest that treatment efficacy may be the area of greatest need for further research within the field of auditory processing disorders. However, recent research in neuroplasticity, as discussed in Chapter 3, suggests that neuroplasticity and neuromaturation are dependent, at least in part, on stimulation. Therefore, a comprehensive approach to management of CAPD, including auditory stimulation designed to bring about functional change within the CANS, should be undertaken in all cases of CAPD (Chermak & Musiek, 1995).

While further data are sorely needed within this area, logic tells us that the decision regarding what should be included in a comprehensive management program is one that should be based on the child's individual presenting profile and should be as deficit-specific as possible. In other words, all attempts should be made to remediate auditory areas that have been shown to be dysfunctional, while building upon the child's auditory strengths. In addition, the management program also should address behavioral, educational, and communicative sequelae so that maximum functional benefit may be achieved. Therefore, **management of CAPD, like assessment, should be multi-**

disciplinary in nature. Speech-language pathologists, psychologists, audiologists, neuropsychologists, learning disabilities specialists, social workers, teachers, parents, and others may all be involved in the child's overall care. The extent of each team member's contribution will depend on the nature and functional manifestations of the disorder, and the degree to which the problem may be medically treatable.

This chapter provides readers with an overview of general management strategies appropriate for children with CAPD. Included in this chapter will be a description of the three components of any comprehensive CAPD management and intervention program, as well as an in-depth discussion of environmental modifications and compensatory strategies designed to help children with CAPD function more efficiently in real-world listening and learning situations. Deficit-specific remediation techniques will be discussed in Chapter 9, as will developing management programs for hard-to-test, including very young, children for whom CAPD is suspected but cannot be diagnosed. Finally, the topic of determining treatment efficacy using statistical analysis and outcomes data will be addressed in Chapter 11.

Throughout this chapter and the next, emphasis will be placed on the need for deficit-specific management and intervention. As such, although a variety of activities and techniques for managing CAPD will be described, readers are cautioned not to assume that each suggestion is equally appropriate or beneficial for all children with CAPD. The relative efficacy of any management or remediation technique will depend on the underlying auditory deficit and how that deficit affects the specific child in question.

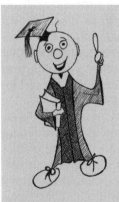

Learning Objectives

After studying this chapter, the reader should be able to:

1. Discuss the general principles of CAPD management.
2. List the three components of any CAPD management program.

3. Delineate several environmental modifications appropriate for children with CAPD.
4. Discuss the purpose of compensatory strategies training and provide specific examples of the types of skills that fall into this category of CAPD management.

Overview of Central Auditory Processing Disorders Management

CAPD management in the educational setting may be divided into three main categories: (1) environmental modifications and teaching suggestions designed to improve children's access to auditory information; (2) remediation techniques designed to enhance discrimination, interhemispheric transfer of information, and associated neuroauditory functions; and (3) provision of compensatory strategies designed to teach children how to overcome residual dysfunction and maximize use of auditory information. In other words, **management of CAPD should focus on changing the environment, remediating the disorder, and improving learning and listening skills.** Every management program should include components from each of these three categories; however, the overall management plan should be individualized based on the child's specific presenting profile and sequelae.

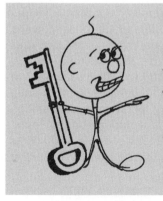

KEY CONCEPT

CAPD management may be viewed as a tripod: without all three "legs" (environmental modifications, remediation activities, and compensatory strategies), the tripod cannot stand.

As a clinician who works with CAPD on a daily basis, I am frequently asked for general recommendations appropriate for all children with CAPD. It may surprise readers to find that, in truth, very few management recommendations apply to CAPD in general. Let us take, for example, the situation in which the teacher is instructed to augment auditory information with visual and other cues. This seemingly innocuous recommendation, while appropriate for some listeners, may actually confuse children for whom the ability to integrate auditory and visual information is dysfunctional. Likewise, it is commonly suggested that teachers repeat or rephrase information. However, whether repetition or rephrasing of auditory information will be effective will depend upon the specific presenting deficit as well as the manner in which the repeating or rephrasing is accomplished.

On the other hand, the use of an auditory trainer or other assistive listening device is routinely recommended for children with CAPD. While this recommendation may be appropriate for some, it may not be for others. This is not to say that improving the acoustic environment is not beneficial. It is universally accepted that all children (and adults) perform better in environments that are listener-friendly. The Technical Committee on Architectural Acoustics of the Acoustical Society of America (2000) discussed a variety of methods to improve signal-to-noise (S/N) ratios in the classroom by reducing reverberation, decreasing sources of internal and external noise, and installing sound reinforcement (or sound-field assistive listening systems). These interventions would likely benefit all children in any learning environment. In an ideal world, all classrooms would be rendered listener-friendly with desirable S/N ratios.

However, this is not an ideal world. Many of today's schools are of older construction, have undesirable acoustic characteristics (e.g., reflective surfaces, radiator or other mechanical noise, or open designs in which walls are not flush to the ceiling or temporary "walls" have been erected), and could not even remotely be considered ideal listening environments. Yet, money to improve these conditions may be scarce in many districts or areas. Although I will discuss some low-cost interventions to improve classroom acoustics later in this chapter, they will not have the same effect that a personal or sound-field frequency modulated (FM) or infrared system would. Installing sound-field systems may be out of the question for many schools or districts, and there may be a paucity of funds for personal assistive listening devices for individual children.

In these cases, it becomes an issue of paramount importance to determine specifically *which* children are *most* likely to benefit from a personal FM system or similar device. Although conventional wisdom might suggest that such individual devices would be indicated for any child with an auditory-based deficit—thus leading to the recommendation for FM or similar systems for all children with CAPD—logic (and practical experience) based on the nature of the underlying deficit(s) dictates that this would not be the case.

For example, children with Auditory Decoding Deficit, for whom auditory closure, performance with degraded or competing acoustic signals, speech-sound discrimination, and similar skills are deficient, rely heavily on acoustic clarity in the listening environment. Because the internal redundancy of the signal is reduced by the auditory deficit, external redundancy and clarity become of paramount importance. Thus, these children are likely to benefit significantly from the use of personal assistive listening devices. A similar rationale holds true for children with Integration Deficit, for whom binaural separation and integration likely are areas of difficulty.

On the other hand, children with Prosodic Deficit typically perform like all other children under conditions of degraded or competing acoustic signals because of intact auditory closure, speech-sound discrimination, and related abilities. Their difficulty, instead, arises from a deficit in perceiving subtle rhythm, stress, and intonation aspects of the message that leads to comprehension of communicative *intent* rather than *content*. Because their difficulties persist even in ideal listening situations, improving the S/N ratio through the use of an assistive listening device is unlikely to result in an increase in salience of these suprasegmental aspects of speech. Similarly, for children with more language-based deficits, such as Associative Deficit, acoustic clarity of the signal is not the issue. Therefore, the use of personal assistive listening devices for these children would not be expected to improve listening and learning any more than it would for any other child in the classroom. From a simple cost/benefit analysis perspective, if sound-field systems are not feasible, it is incumbent upon clinicians to determine where best to spend the available funds for personal assistive listening devices, rather than merely recommending such devices for all children with CAPD. A similar logic applies to virtually all of the acoustic- and teacher-related environmental modifications that will be discussed in this chapter.

Therefore, **I urge clinicians entering the CAPD arena not to surrender to the urge to make general recommendations to classroom teachers and others regarding management of CAPD and to avoid at all costs preprinted lists of "general" suggestions without first analyzing the list to ensure that each suggestion contained therein is, in fact, appropriate for the specific child in question.**

That having been said, a few recommendations may be generalized as being useful, not only for all children with CAPD, but for listeners in general. These recommendations may be referred to as Smart Listening suggestions, and would include reduction in or elimination of obvious adverse noise sources within the listening environment, education of educators and other significant individuals regarding listening and the nature of auditory disorders, and optimization of the learning environment based on the individual child's needs.

For children with CAPD, **the primary goal is to increase the child's ability to use information presented in the auditory mode.** Therefore, management suggestions for classroom use should focus on environmental modifications and the child's use of *compensatory strategies* to increase the redundancy of the learning environment, thereby improving access to and use of new information.

In contrast, remediation techniques for CAPD are designed to provide direct intervention for specific deficit areas. In order to do this, the remediation environment should be challenging and varied, so that adequate auditory stimulation occurs and the child has ample opportunity to practice new skills that will ultimately be used in everyday listening situations. Therefore, the only effective management approach for a child with CAPD is to combine a highly redundant learning environment with a highly challenging, low-redundancy therapy environment.

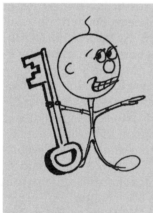

KEY CONCEPT

Environmental modifications and compensatory strategies are designed to improve children's access to and use of auditory information. In contrast, remediation activities are designed to provide direct intervention for deficit areas.

Finally, the child's own internal motivation often will need to be addressed. Many children with CAPD are considered to be passive listeners, or listeners who do not take an active part in their own comprehension. By the time children are identified as having CAPD, they may have experienced failure in listening situations for so long that a prevailing attitude exists in which they feel that they are stupid and nothing can be done to remedy the situation. To the extent that chil-

learned helplessness

dren can be helped to understand the nature of the disorder, and helped to analyze difficult listening situations, a sense of control may be achieved. Children will need to be taught to be active participants in their own listening and learning experience to maximize the efficacy of the overall management program and enhance their sense of motivation and control.

Environmental Modifications and Classroom-Based Strategies

This segment of CAPD management is the one that is probably most familiar to clinicians. In my experience, I have found that most clinicians are able to provide good suggestions for classroom-based management of CAPD; however, it is in the area of direct remediation activities that the need for outside guidance arises. Therefore, this section will briefly discuss measures that may be taken to improve children's access to auditory information within the learning environment.

It should again be emphasized that **the learning environment needs to be a highly redundant one.** By this, I mean that children should be required to expend as little extra energy as possible in order to obtain critical information presented in the classroom. To accomplish this, classroom teachers and other involved individuals may need to be reminded that it is the ultimate desired outcome that is important, rather than the manner in which that outcome is achieved. In other words, the goal is to see that children learn and understand the information presented. The method through which the information is learned, and the way in which comprehension of the information is demonstrated, is of much lesser concern.

For example, beginning in the later elementary school years and continuing through college, information begins to be presented via lecture format, and notetaking often becomes a requirement. Tests, usually written, are often developed from lecture notes. Children with CAPD are often poor writers, and exhibit difficulties with listening. The division of attention that ensues from attempting to listen to a message, write the message in a coherent manner, and return attention to the speaker may be detrimental for a child with CAPD. The writing often lags behind the spoken message, with the result that the next piece of information is simply missed. In addition, the inability to direct full attention toward the spoken message and invoke listening strategies virtually ensures that much of the spoken message will not be understood. The final result, of course, will be that the child does not learn the critical information presented.

In this situation, classroom teachers will need to realize that, although lecture format and notetaking may be a standard requirement for the class, accommodations may need to be made for children with CAPD to be able to demonstrate the desired learning outcomes. Provision of lecture notes prior to the class presentation may be helpful, as children can become familiar with the lecture content prior to class time and can use the notes for studying at a later date. If teacher-made lecture notes are not available, a notetaker may be provided. This could be accomplished simply by providing carbon paper to another student in the class, but teachers should take pains to check the chosen student's notes and ensure that the critical information is reflected accurately. Whatever the method or combination of methods chosen, the goal is to allow children with CAPD to focus all attention on the speaker during lecture time, thus avoiding the division of attention and loss of information that occurs during notetaking.

A second concern in the classroom is acoustic access to and clarity of the spoken message. Children with deficits in the areas of auditory closure, phonemic decoding, binaural separation or integration, and binaural interaction characteristically demonstrate difficulty hearing in noise. Although, as discussed in the previous chapter, the mechanism by which this difficulty occurs is different in each of these disorders, the final result is the same. Even if notes are provided so that a child can focus all attention on the speaker, comprehension of the spoken message will be adversely affected if the acoustic signal is contaminated by competing noise or lack of clarity. Therefore, **measures should be taken that improve the child's access to target information, while simultaneously decreasing background noise.**

One frequent recommendation for children with auditory disorders, including CAPD, is **preferential seating.** Many clinicians and teachers may assume that preferential seating simply means placing the child in the front row of the classroom. However, depending on the proximity of the teacher to the students, arrangement of desks in the room, room lighting, use of overhead projectors or other potentially noisy equipment, and similar issues, the front row may be the *least* beneficial placement for a child with CAPD.

In some smaller classrooms with a large number of students, teachers may be so close to the students when speaking that children in the center of the front row are forced to look upward and are afforded a good view of only the teacher's chin or nostrils. Similarly, children at the sides of the front row may only be able to view the teacher's profile. Neither of these viewing conditions allows for desirable addition of speaker-related visual cues. In addition, overhead projectors or other mechanical teaching aids are most likely to be placed near the teacher for convenient access. This equipment may generate noise that is quite audible to children in the front rows, and that interferes with their ability to hear what is being said. Similarly, if the room is arranged so that teachers are backlit by windows or other light sources, children are unlikely to be able to use speechreading cues that assist in access to the message. Thus, **preferential seating should be thought of as placement in the classroom where the teacher's face is clearly visible at no more than a 45 degree angle and away from competing noise sources** (Bellis & Ferre, 1999). The distance from teachers in terms of rows is far less important than is the visibility of their facial features.

To complicate matters further, not all classrooms are arranged in the typical row-by-row format that was so prevalent many years ago. Today, alternative desk placements are common, particularly in lower elementary school grades when children are learning the very bases for all subsequent skills and abilities. In many of these classrooms, desks are arranged in "pods" in which approximately four students are grouped together facing one another. These pods are arranged artfully throughout the room, allowing students to work together in groups and teachers to move freely throughout the room. In a situation such as this, what constitutes preferential seating will differ, depending on the specific classroom and teacher characteristics. Therefore, it is critical that clinicians visit the classrooms of children with CAPD to determine the best way to improve access to visual cues that is tailored to the individual room, child, and teacher.

We should also keep in mind that **not all children benefit from the addition of visual cues. Children with Integration Deficit, in particular, may do better if placed in an area of the classroom in which visual cues are *less* accessible.** I often see children with Integration Deficit close their eyes or stare at their desks when being given spoken instructions or information. Although we may be tempted to admonish them to "look at us when we're speaking," this behavior may be a clear signal that they are trying to reduce visual input (and the necessity for multimodality integration) and focus attention fully on the auditory signal. Often, these same children will turn their attention toward any visual augmentations, such as pictures or overheads, only after the auditory message has been given. Once it is determined that these children are not merely "tuning out" and that their strategy is designed to enhance comprehension of the spoken message (a determination that often is made easily simply by asking the children why they are closing their eyes, a question that is often answered by, "Because it helps me concentrate"), placement in a location with a significantly reduced amount of visual distractions should be sought.

In any classroom, special attention should be given to overall classroom acoustics. Although it might not be possible to renovate the room completely or to install a sound-field listening system, there are many low-cost ways of reducing sound reflection and enhancing the S/N ratio. First, it is important to determine the amount of background noise and reverberation that is present in the room when it is unoccupied. According to Crandell and Smaldino (2001), ASHA recommends that the unoccupied background noise not exceed 30 dB (A-weighted) and reverberation be less than 0.4 sec. These recommendations are slightly less than those suggested by the American National Standards Institute (ANSI). The S/N ratio needs to be at least +15 dB.

If the acoustic characteristics of the room do not conform to these recommendations, several steps can be undertaken. Reflective surfaces can be minimized by the addition of sound-absorbing material. Optimally, highly rated sound absorbing material such as acoustic tiles can be installed. However, even carpet squares on the walls, throw rugs on the floor, and decorated cardboard egg cartons on the ceiling (making sure not to cover smoke detectors or sprinkler systems) can do much for reducing reverberation in a low-cost, colorful manner. Sources of mechanical noise, including fluorescent light bulbs, overhead projectors, fish tanks, and the like, should be identified and such noise kept to a minimum or eliminated. Other mechanical noise arising from heating or air conditioning systems may be more expensive to correct; however, all attempts should be made to do so whenever possible. Additional information regarding measuring classroom acoustics and suggestions for improving S/N ratios can be found in the report by the Technical Committee on Architectural Acoustics of the Acoustical Society of America (2000).

Once children with CAPD are placed in the classroom in a location that appears, visually, to be preferential for them, sound level meter readings should be taken at their desks to ensure that they are receiving information at an appropriate S/N ratio during class time. If the S/N ratio is not desirable, or if children require additional S/N enhancement, personal assistive listening devices should be considered. However, as previously discussed, personal devices are not indicated for all children with CAPD.

The fitting of assistive listening devices should never be undertaken lightly. I recommend that use of assistive listening devices begins with a trial period in order to evaluate effectiveness. The trial period should begin with baseline information regarding listening and comprehension behaviors, as well as a baseline audiogram obtained prior to fitting. The decision to use the device on a regular basis should be made only after post-trial data indicate benefit. Serial audiograms should be obtained on a regular basis during equipment use to monitor for possible adverse effects on peripheral hearing sensitivity. **It must be emphasized once again that under no circumstances should an auditory trainer or other assistive listening device be provided simply on the basis of a diagnosis of CAPD, without further corroborating evidence of need and careful, ongoing documentation of efficacy.** Even when personal or sound-field assistive listening devices are used properly, children should be given frequent opportunities throughout the day to listen in real-world environments. A great deal of learning occurs vicariously, through overhearing adjacent conversations and discussions. In addition, it has been my clinical experience that some children with CAPD or hearing loss begin, over time, to rely heavily on the ideal listening conditions afforded them by the use of FM or related technology and essentially lose the ability to listen in a background of noise or to localize sound sources. This is especially true for children who have used assistive listening devices for the majority of the time they spend in environments that require "listening," such as on an all-day basis at school, for many years. For some of the children with whom I have worked, this has been significantly detrimental to their daily function outside school or when they become more involved in extracurricular activities and social events during their teenage or young adult years.

Research on auditory neuroplasticity, which was reviewed in Chapter 3, clearly shows that sensory deprivation can result in undesirable changes in central auditory pathways and concomitant functional skills. In one sense, the use of an FM or similar assistive listening device can be thought of as a form of sensory deprivation of sound localization and auditory figure/ground cues. Thus, it is possible that consistent use of such devices over extended periods of time for many years may actually result in CANS alterations that reduce the ability to process such cues.

Furthermore, because assistive devices require listeners to put forth less effort to listen, some children may gradually lose the motivation to expend extra effort in real-world listening situations. I have worked with many children who have adopted the habit of "listening" only when wearing their personal assistive devices, but who "tune out" on other occasions. I suspect that some of these children have come to rely heavily on the crutch afforded them by their assistive devices, and have come to expect that, if the information is important, it will be imparted directly to their ears.

Although this is a highly controversial issue, I feel that we must consider the potential drawbacks to consistent use of FM or related technology for children with auditory disorders. It is important that children in content-based academic classes learn the information presented in class—that is their purpose for being in school in the first place. However, it is equally important that these children be able to function independently in the real world. The real world is not wired for sound, and S/N ratios are often undesirable. We may do a real disservice to children if we do not teach them how to listen outside the classroom.

Therefore, I usually recommend that assistive listening technology be limited to content-based academic classes in which important information is being imparted. During other times, such as at recess and lunch, and during art, music, physical education, and group discussions, I encourage children with CAPD to go without their devices, relying instead on their auditory figure/ground and related abilities to understand spoken language. I also include auditory figure/ground training in remediation activities when necessary.

In conclusion, although the enhancement of S/N ratios through the use of technology is advantageous for improving the listening and learning environment, it is my opinion that immediate and extensive research is needed into the potential deleterious effects of consistent use of such technology over long periods of time. In addition, steps should be taken to ensure that children retain those skills that are reliant on binaural stimulation, including sound localization and auditory figure/ground abilities. Our ultimate goal is to ensure that all children learn in the classroom. However, it is equally important that we assist children in real-world functioning. As a profession, audiologists need to address and investigate any possible drawbacks to the usually beneficial interventions we employ, including the use of assistive listening technology, even if such drawbacks seem to fly in the face of conventional wisdom.

Not all environmental modifications address classroom acoustics. Many important classroom management techniques for CAPD rely on teacher- or speaker-based activities. Teachers should be encouraged to **make frequent checks for understanding** after giving instructions. These checks may be visual, watching to see if the child in question follows the instructions, or they may be verbal. However, simply asking a child to repeat the instruction is rarely effective, because many children with CAPD are able to repeat verbatim what was said without actually understanding the content of the message. Therefore, the child should be asked to paraphrase the instruction or to demonstrate the action requested. If it is clear that the instruction was not understood, **repetition or rephrasing** may be necessary. However, the decision regarding whether to repeat or rephrase should depend on the underlying deficit. Repetition means that the same message is presented again, perhaps with enhanced enunciation or slower, clearer speech, as speaking rate can influence comprehension of the spoken message significantly. This strategy is good for children who have missed a portion of the message the first time it was presented and who have difficulty filling in the missing components to achieve auditory closure, such as children with Auditory Decoding Deficit or, perhaps, Integration Deficit. On the other hand, children with one of the more language- or executive-function-based secondary CAPD profiles are unlikely to benefit from simple repetition, even if the second presentation is acoustically clearer than the first. Instead, rephrasing the message using smaller linguistic units and simpler speech will be far more effective. For children with Prosodic Deficit, repetition may be useful, but only if the intonational aspects of the message are exaggerated to enhance their perceptual salience. **Thus, the relative efficacy of repetition or rephrasing as a clarification strategy is highly dependent on the nature of the underlying deficit.**

Likewise, the use of **multimodality cues and hands-on demonstrations** may be effective aids to understanding, but only if utilized correctly. The multimodality cues should match precisely, in content and timing, the spoken information. For example, if, during a discussion about transportation, the teacher is describing types of cars and a slide is presented showing a truck, confusion may result from the lack of agreement between the spoken and visual messages. Also, it should be emphasized that not all children with CAPD will benefit from a multimodality approach. As we have seen, children with Integration Deficit may be confused by the addition of visual or multimodality cues, even though such augmentations will be beneficial for the vast majority of children with auditory, language, or learning difficulties. **If children seem confused by multimodality cues, or are observed to close their eyes in an effort to block out competing visual stimuli, information should be presented via one modality at a time.** That is, the instructions can be given orally, *then* demonstrated visually. If there is a practical component to the exercise, such as occurs when leading children through science laboratory experiments or similar activities, children with Integration Deficit should be allowed to listen to the directions, watch the demonstration, and then perform the task prior to moving on to the next step in the process. Because of their difficulty planning and organizing behavior in response to auditory directions, children with Output-Organization Deficit may also benefit from this type of instruction. Similarly, children with Associative Deficit may also need to have instructions compartmentalized in this manner, particularly if the instructions are linguistically complex; however, they are far more likely to benefit from the provision of simultaneous visual or tactile cues.

A classroom-based management approach that is often effective for children with CAPD is **preteaching of new information and new vocabulary.** Teachers should be encouraged to provide introductory information and new vocabulary before presenting the subject in the classroom. Doing this helps to ensure that the subject to be discussed will be familiar, thus inceasing the external redundancy of the information. When children are familiar with the vocabulary or subject matter prior to its introduction in the classroom, they are much more likely to be able to fill in any portions of the message that might be missed and achieve auditory closure. Therefore, preteaching of new information or vocabulary is most beneficial for children with Auditory Decoding Deficit. However, it is a useful tool for many students, including college students, both with and without CAPD. If students have read the material and reviewed the vocabulary prior to class, they are much more likely to follow and comprehend the information that is presented in the accompanying lecture.

As previously mentioned, many children with CAPD will benefit from the **provision of a notetaker.** Because taking notes inherently involves a division of attention between listening and writing, children with auditory deficits often find that both their listening comprehension and the quality of their notes suffer when writing during lectures. For children with Auditory Decoding Deficit, this may arise because the act of writing and spelling (likely areas of difficulty for them) leaves little energy for "hearing" the spoken message. For children with Integration Deficit, taking notes involves multimodality integration—the very area with which they have difficulties. For children with Prosodic Deficit, extracting the key words from the message may be difficult, because key words are usually heralded by the subtle changes in stress or intonation that they are unable to perceive. Therefore, these children's notes may be poorly organized, lacking in key points and elements, and include many unstressed (and unimportant) verbiage such as conjunctions (e.g., "and") and articles (e.g., "the") that are not usually included in lecture notes. The purpose of notetaking is to reinforce the information presented verbally and provide a study guide for later review; however, it serves neither of these purposes for most children with CAPD.

On the other hand, **recoding the information into a picture** that conveys the key concept, rather than writing in words and phrases, may be a useful reinforcement strategy for some children with CAPD, particularly those with Auditory Decoding Deficit or the two secondary subtypes, Associative and Output-Organization Deficit. This is often especially helpful for children who exhibit very good visualization skills. However, even this strategy is unlikely to aid children with

Integration or Prosodic Deficit because it requires both multimodality skills and the ability to grasp the gestalt meaning and transfer it to a right-hemisphere-based pictorial art form.

For all children with CAPD (and others as well), **gaining attention prior to speaking** is the first step in ensuring active involvement in the listening process. Similarly, **positive reinforcement** should be used generously to keep the children motivated throughout the day, and all attempts should be made to avoid drawing negative attention to any child through public admonishment or in any other way. Finally, the academic day should be organized so that children have **regularly planned "listening breaks,"** or periods of time during which listening is kept to a minimum, to avoid auditory fatigue. Although this suggestion may be most useful for children with Auditory Decoding Deficit, who are at the greatest risk for significant auditory fatigue, it is important for all children with auditory disorders.

If all else fails and it is determined that a particular classroom setting is not beneficial for a child with CAPD, despite all attempts to incorporate environmental modifications, clinicians and teachers should **consider the possibility of alternative placements.** For children with Prosodic Deficit, placement with an animated teacher who makes more use of prosodic and body-language cues is often indicated. Children with Auditory Decoding and Integration Deficit, as well as those with Output-Organization Deficit, will be most reliant on the acoustic characteristics of the classroom and the clarity of the spoken message. Thus, if their present setting continues to be noisy despite acoustic interventions, movement to a quieter classroom that affords a better S/N ratio should be considered. Finally, children with Associative and Output-Organization Deficit will benefit most from a teacher who is able to speak at their level, breaking messages into smaller linguistic units and allowing for action upon each step before providing the next task in a sequence.

Perhaps the most critical factor in ensuring efficacy and follow-through of classroom-based management approaches to CAPD is obtaining teacher support and cooperation. Teachers who are unconvinced about the need for classroom modifications, or who feel that such modifications may be "unfair" to the other students, are unlikely to implement management suggestions on a daily basis. Therefore, classroom teachers should be included in all aspects of assessment and management of CAPD, and every effort should be made to educate teachers and other professionals regarding the nature of the disorder and the underlying theoretical bases for suggested management approaches. The more these individuals understand, the more likely they will be to cooperate with any recommendations made.

Suggestions regarding methods of imparting information to teachers and other significant individuals are provided in Chapter 10.

Finally, it should be recognized that not all sources of classroom-based difficulties will be readily apparent by the differential diagnosis. Therefore, it is helpful for clinicians to visit the classroom and analyze the listening environment in order to make better classroom-specific suggestions. Through classroom observation, issues that had previously gone unnoticed may surface. For example, it may be discovered that the teacher speaks very rapidly or in a very soft tone of voice. It may be found that, due to the unique characteristics of a specific classroom, preferential seating actually means seating toward the back, rather than the front, of the classroom. Unnoticed sources of external noise may be identified and eliminated. A myriad of issues may become apparent simply through the act of observing a child in the classroom.

In conclusion, a variety of classroom-based management suggestions may be made for children with CAPD. However, not all suggestions will be appropriate for every child. **Therefore, it is critical that clinicians approach the management of each child from an individualized perspective and that teachers be involved in the decision-making process.** By working closely with teachers, clinicians can help to ensure that the learning environment is a highly redundant one, thus improving access to information and opportunity for success.

Finally, this section did not discuss all possible recommendations for classroom management. Clinicians are encouraged to gather as much information as possible and to use common sense combined with knowledge of the underlying auditory deficit when providing guidance to classroom teachers. To summarize the information presented in this section, the primary goal of environmental modifications for CAPD is to render the learning or listening environment highly redundant so that children are able to access the information presented. These modifications may be both acoustic- and teacher-based, and include:

- **Acoustic interventions to reduce reverberation or noise and enhance S/N ratio.** *Most important for:* All children.
- **Use of assistive listening devices**. *Most important for:* Children with Auditory Decoding Deficit. *May also be important for:* Children with Integration Deficit, Output-Organization Deficit. *May not be appropriate for:* Children with Prosodic Deficit, Associative Deficit.
- **Preferential seating with good visual access to the teacher at an angle of no greater than 45 degrees.** *Most important*

for: Children with Auditory Decoding Deficit. *May also be important for:* Children with Prosodic Deficit, Associative Deficit, Output-Organization Deficit. *May not be appropriate for:* Children with Integration Deficit.

- **Frequent checks for comprehension of instructions or directions.** *Most important for:* All children.
- **Employment of multimodality cues and hands-on demonstrations to augment verbally presented information.** *Most important for:* Children with Auditory Decoding Deficit, Associative Deficit. *May also be important for:* Children with Prosodic Deficit, Output-Organization Deficit. *May not be appropriate for:* Children with Integration Deficit.
- **Repetition.** *Most important for:* Children with Auditory Decoding Deficit. *May also be important for:* Children with Integration Deficit, Prosodic Deficit (if prosodic cues are rendered more salient via exaggeration during repetition). *May not be appropriate for:* Children with Associative Deficit, Output-Organization Deficit.
- **Rephrasing.** *Most important for:* Children with Associative Deficit, Output-Organization Deficit. *May also be appropriate for:* Children with Prosodic Deficit (if prosodic cues are rendered more salient via exaggeration during rephrasing). *May not be appropriate for:* Children with Auditory Decoding Deficit, Integration Deficit.
- **Preteaching new information or new vocabulary.** *Most important for:* Most children.
- **Provision of a notetaker.** *Most important for:* Most children.
- **Recoding information into pictorial form.** *Most important for:* Children with Auditory Decoding Deficit. *May also be important for:* Children with Associative Deficit, Output-Organization Deficit. *May not be appropriate for:* Children with Integration Deficit, Prosodic Deficit.
- **Gaining children's attention prior to speaking.** *Most important for:* All children.
- **Generous use of positive reinforcement.** *Most important for:* All children.
- **Avoidance of auditory fatigue.** *Most important for:* Children with Auditory Decoding Deficit. *May also be important for:* All children.
- **Placement with an "animated" teacher.** *Most important for:* Children with Prosodic Deficit. *May also be important for:* All children.

- **Alternative classroom placement.** *May be important for:* Any child for whom current environmental modifications are insufficient or ineffective.

Compensatory Strategies

Perhaps one of the most important components of any CAPD management program is that of teaching children to become active rather than passive listeners. Children must learn to accept responsibility for their listening comprehension and to invoke strategies for determining and retaining the content and meaning of each message.

In Part One of this book, top-down influences on auditory processing were discussed. As we have seen, children's linguistic competence, cognitive capacity, motivation to put forth effort, and other factors can greatly affect how they comprehend spoken language and can even alter the sensory percept at the fundamental auditory input level. Training in compensatory strategies will not only help children to strengthen these important top-down skills, ensuring that more effort is left over for the difficult task of auditory processing. It will also render any bottom-up remediation activities more effective by enhancing children's active participation in such activities. Finally, teaching children compensatory strategies will also help children with CAPD to live with the residual effects of their disorders, and to succeed in spite of them.

Much of our current theory regarding compensatory strategies training for children with CAPD comes from the research of Chermak and Musiek (1995, 1997; Chermak, 1992, 1998; Musiek, 1999). In addition, Bellis and Ferre (1999; Bellis, 1996, 1999, 2002) provided a framework for integrating compensatory strategies training into the overall CAPD management program. These authors have outlined several strategies for effective listening that children with CAPD may be trained to utilize. The strategies include *linguistic, metalinguistic*, and *metacognitive abilities*, and are intended to aid children in actively monitoring and self-regulating their own message comprehension abilities, as well as in developing general problem-solving skills.

Principles of Active Listening

The first, and arguably most important, compensatory skill that children with CAPD must learn is how to be active listeners. Active listening requires, first, taking responsibility for one's own listening success or failure by recognizing that many elements of the listening or learning environment are directly under one's own control. Second, active listening requires the use of physical, effortful listening behaviors to enhance access to the message. Finally, active listening involves becoming a participant in listening and learning by taking overt steps to avoid or correct potential pitfalls in the communicative environment that can interfere with auditory processing and spoken language comprehension.

All too often, teaching is thought of as an active process and learning as passive. Teachers are expected to somehow "fill children's brains" with all of the information they are expected to learn in school with little or no participation on the part of the learners. Although passive learning behaviors may be seen in students of all ages and capabilities (including college students), they may be much more prevalent in children with disorders, including CAPD. There are many reasons for this. It may be that, because children are afforded special education and related services through the implementation of individualized education plans (IEPs), some children become over-reliant on the support provided by those services and feel helpless without them. This perspective may be unintentionally propagated by well-meaning parents who emphasize the sometimes accurate, but unfortunately one-sided, view that "The school is there to teach our children. If our children are not learning, it is the fault of educational system." This viewpoint places the responsibility for learning squarely on the shoulders of educators, and does not recognize the reciprocity that is inherent in the teacher/learner partnership.

A second factor resulting in passive listening and learning behaviors in children with CAPD is lack of motivation. Although many of these children enter the educational system eager to learn, repeated failures, misunderstandings, and embarrassments may, over time, dampen their enthusiasm and lead to secondary motivational deficits. They may withdraw from the listening and learning situation altogether instead of continuing to put forth effort to participate in classroom discussions and activities, fearful of further failure and embarrassment. In time, these children may feel that they are helpless in the face of their disorders and simply give up. The fact that most of the special education and related interventions delineated in IEPs typically focus on those services that will be provided *to* children, rather than skills that will empower children to seek out solutions on their own, may unintentionally reinforce feelings of helplessness. Thus, children with CAPD may be completely unaware of steps that they can take to effect changes in their own listening and learning accomplishments.

Finally, many children with CAPD develop maladaptive strategies to cope with ongoing communicative and learning failures. They may begin to rebel, or to engage intentionally in off-task behaviors in an effort to exercise some control over their situations and gain some type of attention, even if it is only of the negative variety. These acting-out behaviors, unfortunately, will interfere further with their ability to listen and learn and to benefit from any intervention techniques directed toward their specific deficit areas. Therefore, before educators and clinicians can expect to see significant gains from management and remediation activities for children with CAPD, the children must be taught to re-engage in the listening and learning process actively.

The first step in this process is *attribution training*, or teaching children to attribute listening failures to factors under their immediate control (Chermak, 1998; Chermak & Musiek, 1997). Specifically, attribution training requires children to acknowledge that a listening or communication failure (e.g., misunderstanding orally presented instructions for a class assignment) was due, at least in part, to insufficient effort. At the same time, the effort and hard work that *was* put forth is acknowledged. Therefore, children are both rewarded for previous effort and encouraged to put forth greater effort in the future to reap even greater rewards. The success they experience from working harder then, in a cyclical fashion, leads to even more motivation, higher self-esteem, and greater effort. In addition, children learn not to attribute every communicative or related failure to their disorders but, instead, learn to work harder to overcome the limitations imposed by their disorders.

A related component of becoming an active listener involves teaching children specific strategies to enhance effortful listening and learning. Many of these strategies are purely physical in nature, and are surprisingly easy to learn and apply in any communicative setting. Yet they set the foundation for virtually all of the principles of active listening discussed in this section. I refer to these strategies as **whole-body listening techniques** (Bellis, 2002), and they include (1) placing the body in an alert posture by straightening the spine, (2) inclining the upper body and head toward the speaker, (3) keeping the eyes firmly on the speaker, and (4) avoiding any activity that can detract attention from the speaker, such as excess movement or fidgeting. In addition, children are taught to reinvoke these strategies forcefully and actively whenever they realize that their attention has wandered. Although these are merely external, physical behaviors, children quickly find that it is difficult *not* to attend to the speaker when their bodies are actively engaged in this manner. As a result, these easy-to-implement techniques provide a tangible starting point for children to learn how to put forth more listening effort.

Finally, children must learn to analyze their listening and learning environments and to take proactive steps to correct any impediments to their success instead of waiting for others to act on their behalf. This requires both the recognition and identification of possible adverse listening conditions and the development and implementation of solutions to the problem. For example, if a child has difficulty hearing the teacher, there may be an extraneous sound source located nearby (e.g., an overhead projector fan, another student rustling papers or whispering). The child must learn to identify the source of the competing noise independently, and then determine how best to correct the situation (e.g., request to be moved to another place in the classroom, politely ask the other student to be quiet). Additional problem-solving strategies will be addressed in a subsequent section of this chapter.

The principles of active listening discussed in this section are important for any child with CAPD, especially those who exhibit secondary motivational deficits. However, different aspects of active listening may be emphasized, depending on the nature of the underlying auditory deficit(s). For example, children with Auditory Decoding Deficit, who are reliant on acoustic clarity and visual cues, will benefit significantly from whole-body listening techniques that also emphasize speechreading as visual augmentation to the auditory message. Children with Prosodic Deficit may also benefit from these techniques, but likely will experience more success if they are encouraged to pay special attention to nonverbal body-language and facial expression cues that provide additional insight into the speaker's communicative intent. Children with Associative or Output-Organization Deficit may do best if also encouraged to avoid potential miscommunications by requesting that instructions be rephrased using smaller linguistic units, or by paraphrasing the instructions themselves and checking with the teacher for accuracy. Finally, children with Integration Deficit may find that the whole-body listening techniques described herein actually impede their comprehension, and that they do far better by closing their eyes and focusing their attention solely on the speaker's voice. Therefore, like all other aspects of CAPD management and intervention, the determination of which active listening strategies will be most effective and how such strategies should be organized and implemented will depend upon the specific difficulties exhibited by the individual child.

Metacognitive Strategies

Metacognitive strategies are designed to assist listeners in thinking about and planning methods of enhancing spoken language comprehension. Specifically, these strategies focus on self-regulation behaviors and require knowledge-driven development of specific goals, systematic plans to achieve those goals, and self-monitoring of the outcomes of strategy implementation (Chermak, 1998; Chermak & Musiek, 1997). The principles of active listening discussed in the previous section may be thought of as metacognitive strategies. Others involve a variety of cognitive behavioral modification and problem-solving techniques that assist listeners in understanding task demands and determining specific methods of enhancing task performance.

One particularly useful metacognitive strategy for children with CAPD is **self-instruction and step-by-step reauditorization.** This strategy begins with clinician or teacher modeling, during which the chosen task is demonstrated while simultaneously "talking out" the procedural steps as they occur. Then, clinicians verbalize the steps as the children engage in performing them. Next, children are taught to self-instruct—or "talk out"—the steps of the procedure during their own performance of the task. This self-instruction first occurs aloud, then progresses gradually to whispering and, ultimately, silent self-instruction. In this manner, children learn to "coach" themselves through particularly demanding tasks and listening/learning situations.

An integral component of task performance and success is **self-regulation and problem solving.** Children with CAPD need to be taught to anticipate difficult listening or learning situations and to develop plans for avoiding or alleviating them. Self-regulation and problem-solving strategies require (1) an understanding of the nature of the problem (e.g., inability to hear clearly, lack of comprehension of spoken instructions), (2) the determination of possible causes for the problem (e.g., adverse S/N ratio because of extraneous noise source, incomplete information re: key elements of the task), (3) the generation of possible solutions (e.g., move to another location, ask for repetition or clarification of instructions), (4) implementation of the most appropriate solution, (5) evaluation of the effectiveness of the solution, and (6) self-reinforcement if the solution was successful or reanalysis of the problem if the solution was unsuccessful. These steps can be undertaken when the problem arises, or prior to difficult listening tasks through **anticipation and problem-solving planning** in advance. Finally, **self-reflection** after the event during which children are taught to review (and possibly write down in a journal kept for that specific purpose) the characteristics of the communicative problem and the effectiveness of solutions to the problem can assist them in planning for future potential communication breakdowns and difficult listening situations.

A final skill area that is important, particularly for children who have difficulty remembering auditory information, is that of **metamemory strategies.** In Chapter 2, the topic of "auditory memory" was discussed and it was emphasized that, although evidence to support modality-specific auditory memory deficits is lacking, many children with CAPD may expend so much effort just trying to comprehend the message in the first place that very little energy may be left over for remembering what was said. These children may, thus, appear to have secondary "auditory memory" disorders, and any intervention designed to help them remember better with less effort will benefit them significantly.

Several metamemory strategies designed to enhance the memory trace and aid in retention of information are available for use with children, and most of them can be effective memory tools for anyone of any age. They include mnemonic techniques such as **chunking**, which involves breaking down long messages or lists into smaller components and grouping similar concepts or objects together, and **elaboration** through the use of analogies and acronyms.

Another metacognitive strategy that may be of use for children with CAPD who exhibit good visualization and art skills is that of **recoding the information into a pictorial representation.** Although this technique was discussed under the section on environmental modifications, it bears mentioning again. Musiek (1999) described a particularly helpful recoding strategy he termed *auditory memory enhancement.* This strategy involves reducing the overall message into one picture that illustrates the main concept and then drawing that picture on a notepad. It is important that the picture accurately reflects the main idea of the message and that a time limit be enforced so that children are required to perform this task in as little time as possible. The nature of this task renders it a good multisensory reinforcement strategy for many children with CAPD. However, it is likely to be ineffective or too difficult for children with Integration Deficit because of the multimodality integration component. It is also likely to be inappropriate for children with Prosodic Deficit because of the art-based difficulties often associated with this type of CAPD, as well as the fact that children with Prosodic Deficit often have difficulty grasping the gestalt message in the first place. Therefore, recoding the information in pictorial form is unlikely to enhance memory for children with these latter two types of CAPD, and will probably require them to put forth even more effort than they would otherwise expend to remember verbally presented information.

A final memory enhancement technique that I have found useful, especially for young children, is to **set the steps of a task to music or motion.** Often, we remember best when words are accompanied by a catchy tune or by illustrative hand movements. Furthermore, the **verbal rehearsal and reauditorization** involved in having children repeat the message over and over again in this way serves to reinforce the memory trace. However, incorporating rhythm, tunes, or motion to words in this manner would, again, probably not be an effective strategy for children with Integration or Prosodic Deficit because of the multimodality, musical nature of this activity.

Metacognitive, including metamemory, strategies can aid children with CAPD in planning, remembering, and carrying out responses to verbal input. Such strategies can be used to strengthen these top-down skill areas for children in whom secondary metacognitive or motivational deficits have arisen. Alternatively, they can be beneficial for those children who exhibit very strong cognitive and related abilities by teaching them to recruit their strength areas as a means of compensating for weaknesses in bottom-up auditory processing. In either circumstance, however, the specific strategies chosen and the ways in which they are taught and implemented should be individualized for each child. For a detailed discussion of metacognitive and metamemory strategies, readers are directed to Chermak and Musiek (1997) and Chermak (1998).

Linguistic and Metalinguistic Strategies

One of the primary functional ramifications of CAPD is difficulty understanding spoken language. As such, anything that can be done to strengthen top-down linguistic and metalinguistic skills likely will have a significant effect on children's daily functioning in listening, learning, and communicative environments.

For some children, **training in the rules of language** may be necessary. Children may benefit from specific training in the use and meaning of tag words that help them to order or sequence steps of a task (e.g., first, last, next, before, after), adversative terms (e.g., but, however, although), and other terms that imply relationships among parts of a message. Chermak and Musiek (1997; Chermak, 1998) referred to these types of linguistic forms that connect portions of complex messages as **discourse cohesion devices.** Other discourse cohesion devices include but are not limited to referents (e.g., pronouns), additives (e.g., and), and causal terms (e.g., because, therefore). Once children have become adept at identifying and interpreting these terms, they will be more able to separate the message into smaller linguistic units independently without relying on the speaker to simplify the communication.

Children who have difficulty applying the rules of language to incoming auditory messages or breaking down tasks into their constituent parts, such as those with Associative or Output-Organization Deficit, will most likely benefit from training directed toward recognizing and interpreting discourse cohesion devices. However, this strategy may also be appropriate for many other types of auditory deficits as well. It should be noted that children with Prosodic Deficit may exhibit particular difficulty with these tasks, as extracting key elements from a message is often difficult for these children.

Training in recognizing and interpreting discourse cohesion devices will also help children with **formal schema induction.** The linguistic markers discussed above serve to organize information and to predict relationships among elements of a message. As such, they provide a means for listeners to narrow the list of possibilities and to make predictions on the basis of expectations (Chermak, 1998; Chermak & Musiek, 1997). For example, if a speaker says during a lecture, "The first point I'd like to make is . . ." then this would imply that at least one or more additional points will follow. When the speaker says, "In conclusion . . ." then we assume that all of the salient points have now been covered, and what will follow will review those points or bring them together into one, cohesive, take-home message. "However . . ." indicates that an exception or caveat to information provided previously is about to occur. Learning to be on the lookout for formal schemata such as these will assist children in organizing and comprehending complex messages.

An additional type of schema induction involves the use of **content (or contextual) schemata.** These are scripts based on context and experience that assist in interpreting messages. For example, when we enter a restaurant and are greeted by the maitre d', there are certain communications that we could expect based on experience with the restaurant environment. If he were to say, "How many, please?" or "Do you have a reservation?" this would conform to our expectations. If, however, he were to say, "I have an extra golf ball in my pocket," this would probably lead us to believe that we must have misheard him, as such an utterance would not conform to our expectations of acceptable messages for restaurants. Therefore, we would immediately request a repetition of the message.

Content schemata allow us to make predictions about the likelihood that certain types of messages will occur and help us to achieve auditory closure when we miss portions of the spoken communication. They also allow us to draw inferences about the speaker and situation based on the message's congruence with expectations. For example, if the maitre d' *did* actually greet us at the door of a restaurant with the statement, "I have an extra golf ball in my pocket," we might certainly draw a very different conclusion about his character and possible mental state than we would if he were to utter the very same statement while on a weekend outing to a golf course. Again, although training in content schema induction may be beneficial for many children, it is likely to be most important for those with difficulty achieving auditory closure, such as occurs with Auditory Decoding Deficit. In addition, children with Prosodic Deficit may also benefit significantly from content schema induction techniques, as becoming aware of expected "scripts" in various communicative situations may help these children with the social communication difficulties that often accompany right-hemisphere-based auditory processing deficits.

This has been just a brief overview of the types of skills that might be addressed when training linguistic and metalinguistic strategies. For further detail, as well as valuable suggestions for implementing such strategies training in the clinical arena, readers are referred to Chermak and Musiek (1997).

Specific Compensatory Skills Training

The preceding discussion has focused on those general, more global compensatory strategies that most of us employ automatically and that assist all of us in comprehending, organizing, making predictions about, and responding to information. Many children with CAPD may already be utilizing these skills; however, those that are not would likely benefit from training in their use.

Because of the specific nature of their deficits, however, some children with CAPD may lack the fundamental underlying skills that allow for the employment of these more general compensatory strategies. For example, as discussed previously, children with Prosodic Deficit may have greater difficulty recognizing and interpreting discourse cohesion devices because of a fundamental difficulty in extraction of key words from an ongoing spoken message. These same children may also exhibit difficulty with content schema induction if they also demonstrate social communication difficulties that interfere with their ability to judge what is expected and appropriate in social communication situations. Similarly, children with Auditory Decoding Deficit may continue to have significant difficulty achieving auditory closure, even when relying on metacognitive and metalinguistic strategies, simply because they grasp very little of the message from a bottom-up perspective. Poor vocabulary, a common finding in children with Auditory Decoding Deficit, may further hamper their effort. In addition, until they are able to fill in the missing pieces of the message, they have little need for metamemory strategies, for they are not yet sure precisely what it is they are supposed to remember. Therefore, depending on the child, specific training in these underlying skill areas may be necessary if they are to take full advantage of higher-order compensatory strategies training.

In the next chapter, specific auditory skills training and deficit-specific remediation will be addressed. Included in this discussion will be principles of training auditory closure, vocabulary, recognition of prosodic elements of speech, key word extraction, and other auditory skills that provide a bridge between the incoming message at a purely acoustic, bottom-up level and the higher-level compensatory strategies that have been addressed in the current chapter. Only when the problem is attacked at each processing level will children with CAPD be able to take full advantage of all of the information available to arrive at an accurate, complete understanding of the message.

In summary, compensatory strategies serve to strengthen top-down processing abilities so that more effort can be allocated to decoding and perceiving the incoming message. Strategies discussed in this chapter include, but are not limited to:

- **Attribution training.** *Most important for:* Any child with secondary motivational deficits or concerns.
- **Whole-body listening techniques.** *Most important for:* Any child with secondary motivational or attention concerns, especially children with Auditory Decoding Deficit, Prosodic Deficit (especially if also encouraged to pay attention to facial expression and body-language cues). *May also be appropriate for:* Children with Associative Deficit, Output-Organization Deficit (if rephrasing using smaller linguistic units is also requested). *May not be appropriate for:* Children with Integration Deficit.
- **Self-instruction and step-by-step reauditorization.** *Most important for:* Any child who has difficulty organizing and carrying out particularly demanding tasks that involve listening.
- **Self-regulation and cognitive problem solving.** *Most impor-*

tant for: Any child who has difficulty analyzing difficult listening or communicative situations and independently arriving at a solution.

- **Self-reflection and journaling.** *Most important for:* Any child who has difficulty analyzing difficult listening or communicative situations and independently arriving at a solution. *May be too difficult for:* Very young children.
- **Mnemonic devices to assist memory.** *Most important for:* Any child with secondary "auditory memory" difficulties.
- **Recoding information into pictorial form.** *Most important for:* Any child with secondary "auditory memory" difficulties who also exhibits good visualization and art skills, especially children with Auditory Decoding Deficit. *May also be appropriate for:* Children with Associative Deficit. *May be overly difficult for:* Children with Integration Deficit, Prosodic Deficit, Output-Organization Deficit.
- **Setting steps to music or motion.** *Most important for:* Any child with secondary "auditory memory" difficulties who also exhibits good music, especially children with Auditory Decoding Deficit. *May also be appropriate for:* Children with Associative Deficit, Output-Organization Deficit. *May be overly difficult for:* Children with Prosodic Deficit, Integration Deficit.
- **Discourse cohesion devices and formal schema induction.** *Most important for:* Most children with CAPD, particularly those who are not automatically employing this strategy. *May be particularly difficult for:* Children with Prosodic Deficit due to the need for key-word extraction.
- **Content schema induction.** *Most important for:* Most children with CAPD, particularly those who are not automatically employing this strategy, especially those with Auditory Decoding Deficit. *May be particularly difficult for:* Children with Prosodic Deficit due to the need for comprehension of social communication conventions and scripts.

Summary

This chapter has addressed general principles of CAPD management. Clinicians should remember that the management program should be individualized and should be as deficit-specific as possible. Further, it should be emphasized that although environmental modifications and compensatory strategies can improve access to and use of auditory information, they are only two of the three necessary components of a comprehensive CAPD intervention plan. The final component, which will be discussed in the following chapter, is direct remediation or deficit-specific auditory skills training. All three components are necessary to ensure access to auditory information, strengthen top-down cognitive and related skills, and improve or ameliorate fundamental auditory input skills. Therefore, this three-pronged approach to intervention will significantly enhance the probability of success for children with CAPD. If any of these three components is missing, the management program cannot be considered to be comprehensive.

Review Questions

1. What are the three main categories of CAPD management in the educational setting, and what is the goal of each?

2. What general recommendations for management may be made for all children with CAPD?

3. List three classroom-based management recommendations that may be appropriate for children with each of the following CAPD profiles:

   Auditory Decoding Deficit   Associative Deficit
   Prosodic Deficit   Output-Organization Deficit
   Integration Deficit

4. List at least five compensatory strategies that may be of use for children with CAPD.

5. Discuss the role of the child's internal motivation in the success or failure of a CAPD management program.

CHAPTER

NINE

Deficit-Specific Intervention for Auditory Processing Disorders

In the previous chapter, the topics of environmental modifications and compensatory strategies were examined in some depth. It was repeatedly emphasized that the nature of the management and intervention effort should be driven logically by the nature of the underlying auditory processing deficit. Thus, some environmental modifications and compensatory strategies are likely to be more appropriate or helpful for certain types of CAPD than others. Conversely, certain management techniques (e.g., multimodality cuing) may actually exacerbate the auditory disorder in some cases, resulting in a decrease in the ability to understand spoken language in listening or learning environments.

Nevertheless, it can be concluded that virtually all children with CAPD will benefit from some form of intervention designed to ensure access to the message and improve control and use of top-down central resources such as language and cognition, regardless of the nature of the deficit (ASHA, 1996). Likewise, direct auditory stimulation and training should be included in the intervention plans for all children with CAPD to address their auditory deficit(s) at the fundamental, bottom-up input level. Because neuroplasticity is reliant upon stimulation, this auditory training should be frequent, challenging, and intense, and should take place in a low-redundancy therapy environment so as to achieve maximum results as quickly as possible.

That having been said, it should be emphasized that the precise meaning of "frequent, challenging, and intense" is unknown at present. As we will see later in this chapter, there has been a recent upsurge of auditory and language stimulation programs—many of them computer-based—that advocate the need for at least an hour of daily stimulation, five times per week, for a period of several weeks. But it should be recognized that this prescription for frequency and intensity of stimulation is based on the fundamental concept that "more is better," and enjoys little empirical support at the present time. It is entirely possible that virtually identical results can be obtained from such stimulation and direct remediation programs in less than half the time. For example, Tremblay and colleagues (Tremblay, Kraus, Carrell, & McGee, 1997) demonstrated significant improvement in both phoneme discrimination skills and neurophysiologic representation of the same phoneme stimuli in just two weeks of training. It is, however, unknown whether the improvements noted in their study represented the maximum improvement that could have been obtained for their subjects. Therefore, the minimum time and frequency required to achieve maximum improvement is an area requiring further research, and may well depend on the individual child's characteristics and the type and severity of deficit exhibited. Elucidation of this matter deserves attention because therapy can be costly in terms of both money and time.

A second fundamental principle guiding direct remediation and therapy for CAPD is that children must be actively engaged in the therapy process. That is, most of the remediation activities currently recommended for children with CAPD require not just frequent and intense auditory stimulation, but they also require children to make responses to what they hear. This serves both to enhance clinicians' ability to track progress and improvement and to engage the "input-output" loop so that auditory skills are learned and can be demonstrated behaviorally. Although this seems logical, and certainly appears to increase the likelihood that skills learned can be generalized to auditory performance in novel environments outside the therapy room, it remains possible that auditory stimulation alone—without the need for active response on the part of listeners—may effect similar changes in auditory function. In fact, a few therapy programs that have been advocated for use with CAPD and related disorders are, indeed, simple stimulation programs requiring little or no involvement on the part of listeners other than that they listen for an extended period daily. Although data supporting the therapeutic efficacy of these programs are either lacking or are unconvincing at present, the possibility still remains that stimulation alone may lead to desirable alterations in function of the CANS.

Despite these unknowns, however, simple logic (as well as available research on neurophysiology, neuroplasticity, and information processing) dictates that the most effective direct therapy techniques will be those that (1) are frequent, intense, and challenging; (2) require active engagement and participation on the part of listeners; and (3) target the specific auditory deficit(s) present. Furthermore, the teaching of deficit-specific compensatory skills that focus on the *use* of these fundamental auditory processes in spoken language comprehension will help to bridge the gap between bottom-up and top-down processing levels and enhance generalization of skills learned to real-world listening environments.

Therefore, this chapter will delineate several direct remediation or auditory training activities that are either intended to ameliorate the auditory deficit at the fundamental, bottom-up processing level, or to teach compensatory skills that improve the use of auditory information in spoken language comprehension. Customizing CAPD intervention plans according to specific deficit profiles, the use of currently popular computer-based therapy approaches to CAPD intervention, and CAPD management in very young children in whom diagnosis cannot yet be obtained will also be addressed. Readers are cautioned that empirical data to support the treatment efficacy of many of the approaches that will be discussed herein are lacking at the present time. Therefore, the information presented in this chapter is intended to be a theory-based, practically applied approach to CAPD intervention rather than an exhaustive, prescriptive list of tried-and-true therapies. As such, the need for further research to document treatment efficacy and determine precisely who will benefit most from which type of intervention is more pressing than ever.

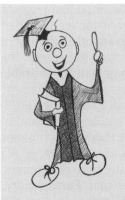

Learning Objectives

After studying this chapter,
the reader should be able to:

1. Discuss the rationale underlying deficit-specific auditory skills training for CAPD.
2. Delineate several remediation activities that can be employed for children with CAPD.
3. Discuss methods of customizing CAPD intervention for children with various functional deficit profiles.
4. Identify several areas of research needed in the field of deficit-specific CAPD intervention.
5. Give examples of management approaches appropriate for very young children for whom definitive diagnostic central testing is not possible.

Rationale Underlying Deficit-Specific Auditory Skills Training

Bellis (in press) identified three fundamental assumptions that are critical to the utility of deficit-specific intervention for CAPD. First is the assumption that fundamental auditory mechanisms and processes underlie and are important to more complex listening, learning, and communication behaviors. These auditory processes and mechanisms have been identified by ASHA (1996) and include those that our diagnostic tests of CAPD are designed to assess, as discussed in Chapters 6 and 7. Our interpretation of behavioral central auditory tests is based, in large part, on the theoretical construct set forth by ASHA (1996). However, it should be noted that the causal relationship between deficits at fundamental auditory input levels and higher-order language, learning, or related disturbances has been questioned by a number of researchers (e.g., Cacace & McFarland, 1998; McFarland & Cacace, 1995; Rees, 1973). Moreoever, higher-order language and learning disorders can be caused by factors that are not related to auditory processing whatsoever, and the presence of these disorders can interfere with our ability to evaluate central auditory function. Further complicating the picture is the fact that some of these higher-order, more global disorders can mimic CAPD in many of their presenting characteristics. Therefore, the need for future research into the linkage between auditory input deficits and communication/learning disorders is clear.

A second assumption underlying the rationale for deficit-specific auditory skills training for CAPD—and one that is, at least in part, reliant on the verification of the first assumption—is that we are able, at present, to isolate and identify precisely those auditory mechanisms or processes that are dysfunctional in a child (Bellis, in press). Chapters 6 and 7 provided an in-depth discussion of how we can use our current tests of central auditory function to achieve this goal. In those chapters, the need for a test battery approach was emphasized in which several tests that assess different auditory processes are employed to look for deficit patterns that are representative of dysfunction in CANS regions. Still, however, the topic of central auditory test development and validity remains to be elucidated fully, as does the issue of possible concomitant multimodality or pan-sensory deficits in children with "auditory" processing disorders.

Finally, the utility of deficit-specific CAPD intervention is reliant upon the assumption that improvement in fundamental auditory processes will lead to improvement in functional listening skills in daily life (Bellis, in press). That is, the ultimate goal of deficit-specific auditory training is to improve children's ability to comprehend spoken language through amelioration of the underlying causal disorder. This assumption is, of course, dependent upon the veracity of both of the previous assumptions. As such, treatment outcomes research that addresses not just degree of improvement in testable auditory processing areas, but also concomitant improvement in functional language, learning, and communication abilities, is sorely needed. Furthermore, the importance of both bottom-up and top-down processing to spoken language comprehension must be acknowledged. The relative efficacy of auditory skills training alone versus a combined approach in which higher-order top-down and environmental factors are also addressed remains an area of needed study. However, logic and science dictate that the most ecologically valid approach to

CAPD intervention would be one in which deficit-specific auditory skills training is accompanied by intervention and management strategies that focus on the deployment of those auditory skills in real-world listening and learning environments.

A great deal of research is still needed to verify the utility of deficit-specific intervention for CAPD in general. In fact, there are some preliminary data to suggest that the deficit-specific nature of the auditory activities included in a therapy program may not be as important to overall functional outcomes as the intensity and frequency of auditory stimulation. For example, Gillam and colleagues (Gillam, Crofford, Gale, & Hoffman, 2001; Gillam, Loeb, & Friel-Patti, 2001) reported that two very different auditory/language computer-based stimulation programs resulted in surprisingly similar functional language outcomes in a group of children with language impairments. It is entirely possible that the duration, frequency, intensity, and interactive nature of the remediation activities are more critical to ultimate functional outcomes than are the specific auditory skills trained. However, again, only a great deal of additional research will illuminate this issue.

In the meantime, I advocate the use of a deficit-specific approach to CAPD intervention that is based largely on medical models in which both the underlying (presumed) "cause" of the disorder is treated directly through targeted auditory training. At the same time, functional "symptoms"—or secondary language, learning, and related deficits—are addressed through the use of environmental modifications and compensatory strategies, as discussed in the previous chapter. At present, this appears to be the most efficacious approach to CAPD intervention, and decreases the potential time and money that can be wasted when shotgun approaches to remediation and management are employed. Nevertheless, readers are cautioned once again that a significant amount of further research is needed to verify the efficacy of the treatment methods presented herein.

Direct Remediation Activities

A primary purpose of direct remediation is to attempt to alleviate the disorder through specific therapeutic activities, either by training the recipient how to perform a specific auditory task, or by stimulating the auditory system in hopes of facilitating a structural, and concomitant functional, change. The degree to which the dysfunction will be ameliorated through these activities varies and, indeed, cannot be estimated a priori for any given child. In fact, many of the activities that will be discussed here are based primarily on what is currently known about how the brain and auditory system function and have little documented efficacy at this time.

As was seen in Chapter 3, recent research in neuroplasticity has shown us that, **just as lack of stimulation may result in structural and functional neurophysiological alterations within the CANS, increased stimulation may, likewise, result in structural changes and functional improvement.** Just as an unused muscle will atrophy and wither, a muscle that is exercised regularly in a challenging manner will grow in size and strength. So it may be with structures within the brain, if recent findings in neuroplasticity are any indication. It should be remembered, however, that the degree to which any remediation technique will serve to remedy the dysfunction will depend on the individual child, and efficacy of treatment activities awaits further research and validation.

As with all of the information contained in this book, the presentation of the following remediation activities is not intended to suggest that these are the only techniques that may be utilized, nor that the activities discussed are equal in effectiveness. In addition, it should be remembered that therapeutic techniques typically utilized by speech-language pathologists and associated professionals may also be useful for children with CAPD, particularly if they exhibit a language-based disorder. These activities are presented in order to provide clinicians with a starting point for therapeutic intervention once a diagnosis of CAPD has been made.

Finally, it is important for readers to understand the purposes of the types of activities that will be discussed in this chapter. Direct remediation activities seek to train fundamental auditory mechanisms and processes such as auditory discrimination, localization, and temporal processing that underlie more complex auditory behaviors. A second purpose of direct remediation activities is to teach specific compensatory skills that focus on deploying auditory processes in listening and learning environments. For example, auditory closure training and vocabulary building—two of the direct remediation activities that will be discussed in this chapter—teach children how to use context (either spoken or written) to fill in missing components of a message so that the meaning of the overall communication is understood. By employing activities at both the auditory input and compensatory skills levels, we are able to bridge the gap between bottom-up and top-down processing and help to ensure that generalization to environments outside the therapy room will take place.

The training activities discussed herein may be overseen by audiologists, speech-language pathologists, or a variety of other professionals. I have found it most helpful to try to integrate auditory skills training into ongoing management programs both to facilitate generalization further and render auditory skills training more applicable to an individual child's presenting language and learning difficulties and streamline the therapy process. Therefore, it is possible that a reading specialist may incorporate phoneme training and speech-to-print skills in the reading therapy program. Speech-language pathologists may focus on prosody training in addition to intervention for pragmatics. Activities involving music or multimodality activities may be incorporated into the home or extracurricular environment in a fun manner. By analyzing children's current management programs and goals, these auditory activities may be included in such a way as to make them meaningful to a specific child while, at the same time, maintaining opportunities to address functional academic or communication difficulties. Alternatively, these activities may be done on a pull-out, one-on-one basis by audiologists, speech-language pathologists, or others. The decision as to how an auditory skills training program can be implemented best is, like all aspects of CAPD intervention, one that should be based on the presenting circumstances of each child.

In Chapter 7, process-based interpretation of central auditory test results was discussed. Here, I provide suggestions for activities that target those specific processes that are found to be areas of deficit during diagnostic testing. In a later section of this chapter, methods of programming intervention plans on the basis of functional deficit profiles will be addressed.

Remediation Activities for Auditory Closure Deficits

As discussed in Chapter 7, children with deficits in auditory closure tend to perform poorly on tests of monaural low-redundancy speech, such as band-pass filtered or time-compressed speech. Because the intrinsic redundancy of the auditory signal is reduced, any extraneous factor that renders the message less clear or more difficult to hear will significantly impact spoken language comprehension. Training in top-down compensatory skills that aid in context-derived prediction of missing elements will help compensate for the inevitable misunderstandings that can ensue from decreases in intrinsic signal redundancy. Two such activities will be described in this section: auditory closure activities and vocabulary building.

Auditory Closure Activities

The purpose of auditory closure activities is to assist children in learning to fill in the missing parts in order to perceive a meaningful whole. As such, context plays an important role in auditory closure, because prediction of the complete word or message often depends on the surrounding context. The activities discussed herein are presented in sequential fashion, from least to most difficult. Children in question should demonstrate mastery of one level before moving on to the next.

Missing Word Exercises

These exercises are designed to teach children to use context to fill in the missing word in a message. It is best to begin with very familiar subject matter and then move to new information. For example, when working with very young children, clinicians may wish to begin with familiar songs or nursery rhymes in order to familiarize them with the task of listening to the whole in order to predict the missing part. For example, the following rhymes may be used:

> Twinkle, twinkle, little _____. (star)
> Little Jack Horner sat in the _____. (corner)
> Hey diddle diddle, the cat and the _____. (fiddle)

In these examples, the children's task would be to fill in the missing word. It may surprise some clinicians to find that, even with a great amount of external redundancy due to familiarity of the message, some children will exhibit difficulty with even this simple task. In this case, and at all stages of auditory closure activities, children

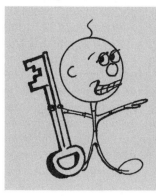

KEY CONCEPT

Auditory closure activities focus on contextual derivation for the purpose of teaching children to fill in the missing elements of a message in order to perceive a meaningful whole.

should be talked through the process and prompted with questions such as, "What is the sentence talking about? What word comes next when you sing the song? What word would rhyme with 'Horner' and make sense in this sentence?"

A slightly higher-level activity might be prediction of rhyming words. For example, clinicians may ask, "Can you name an animal that rhymes with house?" If children are unable to perform the task, prompts should be given that guide them in solving the puzzle. For example, they may be instructed to begin at the beginning of the alphabet and substitute the initial consonant of the word with different letters until the correct consonant is reached (aouse, bouse, couse, douse, etc). If they are demonstrating difficulty with the concept of rhyming, the initial consonant of the target word, in this case m, may be provided, requiring the children to add it to the remainder of the word *ouse* to derive the whole *mouse*. A third method of *prompting,* useful when children correctly choose an initial consonant and combine it with the remainder of the word to derive a meaningful, but incorrect, word (e.g., *douse*), may be to draw the children's attention to the key word or words in the clue. In this situation, clinicians would remind them that, while *douse* is, indeed, a word that rhymes with *house,* what is wanted here is an animal. Some examples of stimuli that may be used in this activity are as follows:

> Color that rhymes with bed. (red)
> Family member that rhymes with other. (brother or mother)
> Fruit that rhymes with beach. (peach)

Once mastery of these steps has been demonstrated, clinicians may move to new, unfamiliar messages in which children must utilize the context of the phrase, sentence, or paragraph in order to predict the missing component. When using this approach, clinicians should begin with simple sentences (e.g., When I'm hungry, I _____), then move to more complex material, such as paragraphs in textbooks or popular novels. In addition, clinicians should progress from omitting the subject or object of the sentence or phrase (e.g., Jill hit the _____ with a bat), to omissions of verbs, adjectives, and other portions of the message (e.g., Jill _____ the ball with a bat; The water was so _____, it took his breath away). Children should be prompted continually to use context in order to predict missing components, as well as to derive meaning from the whole message. In addition, materials appropriate for this exercise can be taken from classes in which children are demonstrating difficulty, in order to assist them in further understanding of the class material.

Missing Syllable Exercises

Once children have demonstrated that they can predict missing words based on context, clinicians may move to omission of syllables. As with missing words, missing syllable exercises should be presented in a progression from least to most difficult. Initially, the context should be familiar so that children are best able to fill in the missing components of the target word. Clinicians may find that, even if children are able to predict an entire missing word from a sentence easily, they may have great difficulty when only a portion of the target word is omitted. In addition, achieving closure for words in which the initial syllable is omitted is a more difficult task than for words in which the final syllable is omitted. Therefore, clinicians should begin by omitting the final syllable of the target word and, once mastery is achieved, move to omission of medial and initial syllables.

Clinicians may begin with sentences in which the target word is embedded (e.g., There are twenty-six letters in the al-pha-_____), and then gradually move to single words in which the only contextual cue may be a category designation (e.g., Sports: base_____, soc_____, ten_____). Through repeated drills such as these, children learn to become less dependent on hearing and decoding every component of the target word and more aware of the need for contextual derivation when the complete acoustic signal is inaccessible.

Missing Phoneme Exercises

Exercises in which specific phonemes are omitted may be carried out in a fashion similar to the missing syllable exercises. Again, it is best to use a progression of least to most difficult, moving to the next stage only when children have demonstrated mastery of the previous stage. Therefore, children should be able to supply the missing phonemes in words with contextual cues (e.g., I like to (w)atch (t)ele(v)ision), before moving on to isolated words. With these exercises, tape-recording the target sentences or words may be useful, as it may be difficult to perform the necessary phonemic omissions using a live-voice approach. With specialized equipment, phonemes can be electronically edited from isolated words or running speech, thus preserving the coarticulation characteristics of the surrounding phonemes—a situation that will most closely resemble real-life speech. Some of the computer-assisted auditory skills training programs currently available commercially already include such phoneme deletion auditory closure activities. The use of computer-based programs will be discussed later in this chapter. Again, when focusing on isolated words, it is helpful to provide general categories as a contextual cue (e.g., Animals: ti(g)er, (m)on(k)ey), and to require mastery with final phonemes prior to moving on to medial and initial phonemes.

Speech-in-Noise Training

Virtually any method whereby the external redundancy of the acoustic signal is reduced may be utilized to train auditory closure skills. Therefore, auditory closure activities such as those discussed in the previous sections may be undertaken in distracting or noisy situations to increase the difficulty of the task further. In addition, variations in speakers, such as the introduction of regional dialects, misarticulations, and other speaker-related characteristics may be utilized to help train children to use context to achieve auditory closure.

It should be noted that, as discussed in the previous chapter, difficulty understanding speech in noise may be due to any number of factors. Dysfunction at any level of the CANS from brainstem through cortex may result in speech-in-noise difficulties. Regardless of the underlying dysfunctional region, however, deficient speech-in-noise skills render auditory closure much more difficult to achieve. Furthermore, it is difficult to predict precisely which components of the message will be obscured by competing noise. Therefore, once children have attained success at predicting and filling in missing components of a message in ideal listening environments, their ability to use context to arrive at meaning should be taxed further by the introduction of competing noise or other methods of degrading the auditory signal. It is best, however, to progress to this step only after children are successful at the same activity in quiet listening environments to avoid frustration and facilitate generalization of auditory closure strategies to classroom and other listening environments.

Vocabulary Building

A final activity useful for children with auditory closure deficits is vocabulary building (Chermak & Musiek, 1997; Musiek, 1999). Just as a word may be indecipherable due to missing syllables or phonemes, requiring the listener to use context to predict the word, a word may be indecipherable due to lack of familiarity with the word or subject itself. As in all of the other auditory closure activities discussed in this section, the ability to derive or predict word meaning for an unfamiliar term depends on the ability to utilize context effectively. As discussed in Chapter 2, top-down linguistic factors have a significant impact on sensory processing at the fundamental, bottom-up input area. Familiarity with the subject matter and vocabulary, therefore, will greatly enhance auditory closure abilities, which is why preteaching of new information is a beneficial teacher-based environmental modification for many children with CAPD. Just as a jigsaw puzzle is much easier to complete when we have a picture of what the final assembly should represent, putting together disjointed elements of a message is easier when we know the topic and vocabulary. However, many children with CAPD also exhibit poor vocabularies, a difficulty that exacerbates their auditory closure deficits further and renders them more disabling in listening and learning situations. The use of context-derived vocabulary building, as discussed in this section, serves both to aid children in determining the meaning of unfamiliar or missed elements of a message and to build better vocabulary skills.

Miller and Gildea (1987) delineated several important points in describing how children learn new vocabulary. First, children must be able to associate the sound of the word with its meaning. Later, many new vocabulary words are encountered and learned through reading. Most important, children must be exposed to the new word in several different contexts in order to internalize the meaning of the word fully. Musiek (1999) emphasized that **the most effective vehicle for learning the meaning of new vocabulary is through contextual derivation, or utilizing the surrounding context to predict meaning of the unfamiliar term.**

Therefore, when approaching vocabulary building from an auditory closure perspective, it is important that children learn to use the context in which the word appears to deduce its meaning. First, children should learn to say the word aloud a few times, a technique known as *reauditorization*, so that the sight and sound of the word becomes familiar. Then, they should be encouraged to *attempt a definition* of the new word based on the context in which it appears.

Next, *the actual definition of the word should be provided.* It should be noted that although dictionary skills are encouraged in academic pursuits, the goal of vocabulary building is to help children achieve closure. This can occur only if the context is kept in the forefront of their minds and motivation to learn the meaning of the word remains high. **Therefore, immediate problem solving in the form of providing the definition, rather than telling the child to look it up in the dictionary, is necessary.**

Finally, children should be encouraged to *define the new word in their own way*, thus assuring that comprehension of the provided definition has been achieved. By following this process, children learn to recognize the new word visually and auditorily, utilize contextual cues to achieve closure, and also add a new word to their internal vocabulary stores.

Materials for vocabulary building should be interesting and encourage maintenance of a high level of motivation. Therefore, popular novels and stories are often good choices for this activity. In addition, because vocabulary is frequently a weak area for children with CAPD, it may be useful to utilize new vocabulary from students' specific academic classes so that they are able to become familiar with the new terminology prior to its introduction in the classroom setting.

Finally, although vocabulary building is a beneficial activity in and of itself, in the context described here it serves as a vehicle for emphasizing the skills learned in all auditory closure activities—namely, the use of context to predict missing or unfamiliar components of the whole. Therefore, the use of contextual cues to deduce word meaning is an appropriate addition to a comprehensive CAPD management plan (Chermak & Musiek, 1992, 1997; Musiek, 1999), particularly when children exhibit a deficit in the area of auditory closure.

The auditory closure activities discussed in this section are summarized in Table 9-1.

Remediation Activities for Binaural Separation/Integration Deficits

Children with deficits in the processes of binaural separation or binaural integration exhibit difficulty processing auditory input in the presence of competing signals. Thus, performance on dichotic listening tasks typically is poor, with either ear-specific effects (e.g., left-ear deficit) or bilateral effects noted. Although most children will demonstrate dichotic listening deficits regardless of whether separation or integration is required, some children with CAPD may exhibit selective deficits in just one process. In my clinical experience with those cases in which such isolated deficits are found, children tend to have greater difficulty with binaural separation (the ability to attend to and process the target signal while ignoring a competing signal delivered to the opposite ear) than with binaural integration (the ability to attend to and process the signals delivered to both ears).

Furthermore, some children (e.g., those with Prosodic or Associative Deficit) may exhibit poor performance on dichotic listening tasks but have little or no functional difficulty in binaural listening environments. In these cases, the dichotic listening findings appear to

Table 9-1

Summary of Auditory Closure Activities

- Missing word exercises
    - familiar songs or rhymes
    - prediction of rhyming words
    - new, unfamiliar messages in which context is used to fill in the missing word
- Missing syllable exercises
    - sentences in which the target word is embedded
    - single words
- Missing phoneme exercises
    - sentences in which the target word is embedded
    - single words
- Repeating above activities in noisy or distracting situations
- Vocabulary building
    - reauditorization
    - contextual derivation of word meaning
    - immediate provision of definition
    - reinforcement of definition

be the diagnostic manifestations of cortical dysfunction but, because of intact auditory closure and related skills, they may pose little or no barrier to listening in noisy or competing environments. Therefore, it is important that clinicians analyze the presenting difficulties of children who perform poorly on tests of dichotic listening to determine precisely what, if any, intervention is indicated in the areas of binaural separation and/or integration. Two types of remediation activities for binaural separation/integration deficits will be discussed in this section: dichotic listening training and localization training.

Dichotic Listening Training

In dichotic listening training, the relative intensity of signals presented to each of the two ears is varied systematically while children are instructed either to attend to both ears (integration) or attend to the target ear only (separation). Because of the acoustic control necessary for this task, equipment capable of recording channel-specific information is required. In my experience, local radio stations can be extremely instrumental in providing assistance with digitizing channel-specific stimuli. Alternatively, many acoustics laboratories also have such equipment available onsite; however, most clinics do not. Although dichotic listening tests themselves may be used for training purposes, I have found that they are usually not interesting enough to engage children's attention and maintain motivation over long periods of time. Furthermore, the use of diagnostic test material for training purposes carries an inherent danger of "training-to-the-test." That is, improvements noted in dichotic listening tests post-training may be isolated only to the stimuli trained, and may not generalize to other, less structured environments requiring binaural listening skills.

The type of material used for dichotic listening training should be targeted toward the interests of the children undergoing the training. Thus, for example, I have used live-voice recordings of children's literature (e.g., the Harry Potter series) for the target stimuli in binaural separation activities. The competing signal can be virtually anything, but should also hold some inherent interest for the child (e.g., descriptors of animals and insects from popular encyclopedias). The time involved in recording the material can be extensive; however, if the material is selected carefully to appeal to most children of a general age group, the same tapes can be duplicated and used over and over again with many children in the same age group. The steps of my binaural separation dichotic training paradigm are as follows:

1. **Determination of beginning target-to-competition intensity ratio.** It is important to begin this exercise on a note of success, both to encourage children to participate willingly in the activity and to engage them in the story plot. Therefore, the initial ratio chosen should be one that allows the children to hear the target messages clearly while, at the same time, being aware of the competing message to the opposite ear. For some children, the competing message will need to be barely audible whereas others may begin at a more challenging target-to-competition ratio. The target message should be delivered to the weaker (usually left) ear while the competing message is delivered to the stronger (usually right) ear. Children are instructed to listen to the story presented in the target ear and told that they will be asked to summarize the story plot after the activity is completed.

2. **Manipulation of target-to-competition ratio.** Once children are engaged in the task and interested in the story line, the intensity of the competing signal is gradually increased to render the directed listening task more challenging. This increase usually takes place over several sessions, and the rapidity with which such increases can be implemented will differ from child to child. The goal is to increase the difficulty of the listening task while, at the same time, maintaining interest, motivation, and success on the part of the listeners.

3. **Readjustment of target-to-competition ratio as needed.** If children begin to exhibit significant frustration with the task or are unable to summarize the plot after each session, the intensity of the competing signal should be decreased to a manageable level for one or more sessions before increasing it once again. It should be noted that difficulty summarizing the plot may also occur if the language level of the material is too challenging for a child. Therefore, the choice of target material should be made with the specific child's language abilities in mind. For some children, novels can be used so that they are provided with the target message in the form of daily installments of an ongoing plot line. For others, however, short children's books that are written at elementary language levels and can be completed in a single sitting may be a more appropriate choice.

This activity should be engaged in as often as possible. I recommend that children undergoing binaural separation dichotic listening training listen to stories under controlled competing signal conditions for a minimum of twenty to thirty minutes daily. Because this can pose a hardship to families if therapy is conducted in a clinical environment, necessitating scheduling and travel on a daily basis, I have found it beneficial to adapt this activity to home use. With the use of a portable cassette tape player or "boom box" that has a left/right balance control knob and stereo headphones, the target-to-competition ratio can be gradually adjusted over time and the activity can take place at home as a bedtime storytelling activity. In my experience, children begin to look forward to the nightly listening session just as any child looks forward to hearing the next installment read from a favorite book. Their motivation, combined with their improving binaural separation abilities, renders them better able to cope with the gradual increase in the competing signal and more likely to continue to put forth effort as the listening task becomes more and more challenging. Comprehension of the main points of the target message can be assessed simply by having parents ask, "So what happened in the story tonight?" Most children are quite happy to share the details of the characters' adventures with a willing parent or sibling.

If this activity is done on a home basis where the actual intensity of the dichotic signals cannot be ascertained, children should be carefully monitored to ensure that the relative right/left loudness ratios are sufficiently and increasingly challenging. In addition, dichotic testing should be readministered after a few weeks to determine whether an improvement in binaural separation abilities can be documented. Finally, concomitant improvement in daily listening skills in real-world listening environments should also be monitored and documented carefully. Through the use of this activity, I have found that many children with deficits in binaural separation exhibit significantly improved performance on tests such as Competing Sentences within five to six weeks. Specifically, the degree of left-ear deficit typically decreases dramatically, sometimes improving to the normal range. This is accompanied by enhanced ability to listen in the classroom, on the playground, and in other noisy or competing situations. However, additional research is needed to investigate further the efficacy of this dichotic listening training approach.

Binaural integration skills can also be trained in a similar manner. However, because of the need for attention to messages delivered to both ears, the signals should be equally interesting and far simpler than ongoing story material. As such, I have found it more difficult to engage children's attention, interest, and motivation in binaural integration tasks. Furthermore, because children rarely need to listen to two competing signals simultaneously in their daily environments, binaural integration training may have far less ecological application than would training in binaural separation skills.

Localization Training

As discussed in previous chapters, sound source localization is fundamental to binaural hearing, including speech-in-noise, abilities. If children demonstrate little or no progress during speech-in-noise or dichotic listening training, or minimal carryover of binaural separation or integration skills to real-world listening situations, it may be necessary to train basic localization skills. This can be accomplished in a variety of ways. In the clinical environment, stimuli (either speech or nonspeech) can be delivered through multiple speakers set at various vertical and horizontal planes. Signals can be delivered either in isolation or in the presence of competing noise or multitalker babble. The child's task is simply to point to the speaker from which the target signal came.

Once again, because motivation and interest is critical to the success of any remediation activity, I have found that any way in which this task can be made fun and stimulating for the child enhances the opportunity for success. For example, I have allowed children to use laser pointers to "zap" the target speaker once the sound source is localized. I have also incorporated the use of a swivel stool in the center of the room for this activity, allowing children to change positions in a fun manner both to locate the sound source and to change the direction and S/N ratios of the localization cues.

Table 9-2

Summary of Binaural Separation/Integration Activities

- Dichotic listening training
- Establish beginning target-to-competition ratio
- Reduce target-to-competition ratio over time
- Readjust target-to-competition ratio as needed
- Localization training
- Sound room activities with speakers at various horizontal and vertical planes
- Children's games such as "Blind Man's Bluff" and "Marco Polo"

Several common children's games also train sound localization abilities. Chief among these are "Blind Man's Bluff" and "Marco Polo," both of which involve blindfolding listeners and having them locate the other participants through voice cues alone. These games can provide an excellent opportunity for generalization of localization abilities to real-world listening environments in a fun, entertaining manner, especially for young children. Localization training may be indicated for any child with speech-in-noise or binaural separation, integration, or interaction deficits.

The activities discussed in this section are summarized in Table 9-2.

Remediation Activities for Temporal Patterning Deficits

Deficits in auditory temporal pattern recognition are apparent diagnostically by poor performance on Frequency and/or Duration Patterns testing in both the labeling and humming conditions. As discussed in Chapter 7, children with temporal patterning deficits may have difficulty perceiving subtle rhythm, stress, and other intonational (or suprasegmental) cues in spoken language that provide illumination of the *intent* underlying the communication. As such, prosody training may be indicated for many of these children. Further, some children with temporal patterning deficits also exhibit difficulty in the perception and sequencing of basic sequential auditory patterns or contours, a skill that is fundamental to perception and use of prosody. For these children, training in sequencing basic rhythmic patterns may be indicated before specific training in the deployment of suprasegmental speech patterns for prosodic purposes can be undertaken. Therefore, this section describes two types of remediation activities for temporal patterning deficits: prosody training and basic temporal patterning training.

Prosody Training

Children with deficits in APTO who exhibit difficulty on the Frequency or Duration Patterns Tests may also exhibit difficulty recognizing acoustic contours. Therefore, **specific training in recognition and use of prosodic aspects of speech, such as rhythm, stress, and intonation, may be indicated** (Musiek & Chermak, 1995, 1997; Musiek, 1999).

Prosody training may begin with words in which changes in the syllabic stress patterns change the meaning of the words (e.g., con*vict* versus *con*vict, re*cord* versus *re*cord, sub*ject* versus *sub*ject). Each version of the word should be introduced and, if the word is unfamiliar, the steps delineated in vocabulary building should be utilized to familiarize children with the sight, sound, and meaning of the new word. The change in meaning brought about by relative syllabic stress should be pointed out clearly. Once children are able to define both versions of the word in isolation, the word may be embedded in a sentence, so that they must listen for relative stress within the word as well as use contextual cues to determine which meaning of the word is appropriate.

Following work with words, training may focus on sentences in which subtle differences in stress, temporal cueing, or other prosodic features alter the meaning of the entire sentence (e.g., Don't touch that *book* versus Don't touch *that* book. He saw the *snowdrift* by the window versus He saw the *snow drift* by the window). At first, the stress and rhythm characteristics of each sentence will need to be exaggerated; however, once children become familiar with the task, the activities may be undertaken in a more normal tone of voice. Children should be led, step by step, through analyzing the sentences for meaning depending on relative stress and rhythm characteristics. For example, in the sentence "Don't touch that *book*," the implication is that the listener is not to touch books, although he or she may be permitted to touch other items. Conversely, in the sentence "Don't touch *that* book," it is clear that the listener is not to touch one book in particular, although other books may be allowed.

Another example of a sentence in which changes in prosodic cues may alter the general meaning is "You can't go to the movies with *us*," versus "*You* can't go to the movies with us." In this example, emphasis on the word *us* implies that, while the listener is welcome to go to the movies, he or she cannot join the speaker's group. Emphasis on the word *you* implies a rejection of the listener; although others may be invited to go to the movies with the group, the listener will not.

It is interesting that many children with deficits in APTO often misunderstand or misconstrue what they hear, resulting in hurt feelings as they jump to often erroneous conclusions about the intent of the message. This may be attributed to the difficulty these children experience in extracting and using prosodic features of speech correctly, which contribute not only to meaning, but to emotion and intent as well. For these children, prosody training may help in determining intent of a message, as well as understanding the overall meaning of the message.

In addition, many of these children exhibit difficulty in sequencing and following directions, understanding complex messages, and so forth. If, in fact, children's perception of prosodic features is dysfunctional, they may well hear messages simply as strings of equally stressed words, so that remembering the message for dictation or follow-through purposes becomes a task of memory rather than comprehension. Many of these children, when taking dictation, tend to write down sentences that make little or no sense, and articles and other filler words may be transcribed accurately, while key words in the message are left out.

For these children, training in *key words extraction* from a message is very helpful. Children may need to be taught to listen specifically for subjects, verbs, and objects, while placing less emphasis on articles, conjunctions, and other less important words. After being given a complex direction, clinicians may prompt the children with questions such as, "What was the action word? Who or what are you supposed to do it to? When?" and so on. Training in key word extraction, a component of prosody training, may greatly help children to remember and understand complex directions or messages.

Finally, many children with CAPD are described as flat or monotonic readers. This may be due to their lack of awareness of prosodic features of speech. **Reading aloud daily, with special emphasis on animation, is a good task for these children that may be done at home or school. Reading aloud serves not only to increase reading aptitude but also to reauditorize and reinforce the use of rhythm, stress, and intonation in expressive language.**

Temporal Patterning Training

Temporal patterning training is an activity that is closely related to prosody training, but is more basic in nature. If children have significant difficulty discriminating subtle changes in stress or rhythm or are unable to sequence information, these activities may be indicated.

As in all training activities, temporal patterning training should be organized so that the least difficult activity is mastered before going on to analysis and imitation of rhythm patterns. Virtually any auditory stimulus may be used for temporal patterning training, but it is recommended that nonverbal stimuli be utilized first and linguistic stimuli be added only after children have demonstrated success.

The goal of temporal patterning training is for children to analyze and imitate rhythmic patterns of auditory stimuli. Clinicians may begin with short (no more than three elements) patterns that may be clapped, tapped on the table, or done in any manner that will hold a child's attention. The patterns may be presented in pairs, requiring children to report if the two patterns are the same or different, or they may be required to imitate the pattern exactly. The patterns should be altered in terms of speed (by increasing or decreasing the inter-tap interval), relative loudness (by placing more emphasis on one or more taps than the others), and rhythm (by including silent intervals). In addition, the rhythms may be made gradually more complex by adding more elements, up to seven or eight.

Once children master analysis and imitation of nonverbal rhythmic stimuli, clinicians may move on to word sequences. The children's task may be to determine which of three words was different (e.g., tick, tick, *tick*). Clinicians should begin with words that are easiest to discriminate, then move to more difficult stimuli (e.g., pen, pin, pen).

Next, clinicians may introduce sentences of three or four elements in which one word is stressed more than the others. At this point, the task is not to derive relative meaning from the sentences, but merely to indicate which of the four words was emphasized. The same sentence may be used over and over again, each time stressing a different word (e.g., *You* are going home. You are going *home*. You *are* going home. You are *going* home). Once children have demonstrated that they can detect relative stress within a sentence, clinicians may move on to prosody training, discussed previously, in order to attach meaning to relative differences in stress.

It should be noted that not all children with deficits in APTO will need to undergo training in this area before moving on to prosody training. These activities may be quite simple for many children, whereas recognition of very subtle prosodic features of speech is a much more difficult task. However, if a child is unable to discriminate relative stress in a sentence, even when the stress features are exaggerated, clinicians may wish to backtrack and work on temporal patterning skills before returning to the more challenging task. Prosody training and temporal patterning activities are summarized in Table 9-3.

Remediation Activities for Auditory Discrimination and Temporal Processing Deficits

Children with CAPD may demonstrate deficits in auditory discrimination of speech or nonspeech signals. Certainly, the presence of discrimination deficits will affect many of the more complex auditory processes discussed in this and previous chapters. For example, phoneme discrimination is an important skill for achieving auditory closure in degraded or competing listening environments. A significant phoneme discrimination deficit will reduce the intrinsic redundancy of the signal, leading to greater reliance on external signal clarity. Similarly, the ability to discriminate between nonspeech sounds that differ in duration, frequency, or intensity is a prerequisite skill for the temporal patterning activities discussed in the previous section.

Temporal processing, as discussed in Chapters 2 and 7, is an even more basic auditory skill. Indeed, it has been hypothesized that auditory-based learning or language deficits may arise in some children because of a fundamental underlying deficit in the ability to process rapidly changing acoustic stimuli (e.g., Kraus et al., 1996; Tallal et al., 1996; Wright et al., 1997). Therefore, temporal processing training may be indicated for some children with CAPD, and many of the computer-assisted intervention programs that will be discussed later in this chapter are based largely on training children to process rapid acoustic stimuli.

Because both auditory discrimination and temporal processing are important to a wide variety of more complex auditory mechanisms and processes, they may need to be addressed either prior to or along with intervention focusing on skills such as auditory closure and temporal patterning. Although further research is needed in this area, it appears logical that children with such deficits would be served most efficaciously if direct remediation is directed toward these fundamental, basic underlying skill areas when needed, and that improvement in these areas will facilitate improvements in behaviors and skills that are reliant on auditory discrimination and temporal processing. Because discrimination and temporal processing are inextricably

---

Table 9-3
Summary of Temporal Patterning Activities

- Prosody training
  - Words in which change in syllabic stress alters meaning (e.g., con*vict* versus *convict*)
  - Sentences in which change in stress alters meaning (e.g., He saw the *snowdrift* by the window versus He saw the *snow drift* by the window)—exaggerated prosodic features
  - Sentences as above—normal intonation
  - Reading aloud with exaggerated prosodic features
  - Key word extraction
  - Role playing or charades games focusing on prosodic and nonverbal expression of emotion
- Basic temporal patterning training
  - Same/different judgments of nonspeech or speech patterns differing in
    - Pitch
    - Stress
    - Loudness
    - Interstimulus interval
  - Imitation of nonspeech or speech patterns differing in
    - Pitch
    - Stress
    - Loudness
    - Interstimulus interval
  - Identification of stressed words within sentences (or stressed elements within a nonspeech pattern)

---

intertwined, they will be discussed together in this section. Two types of remediation activities will be described: nonspeech discrimination activities and phoneme discrimination training activities.

Nonspeech Discrimination Activities

Nonspeech discrimination activities can take the form of simple same/different judgments of frequency, intensity, or duration differences accompanied by feedback. For example, children can be presented with two tones of the same duration and frequency, but that differ in intensity. The children's task is to report whether the two tones are the same or different. Positive reinforcement is provided following correct responses, and the intensity difference is decreased. Negative (or no) reinforcement is provided following incorrect responses, and the intensity difference is increased. Thus, over time, the children's ability to perceive small differences in intensity improves. The same task can be accomplished using differences in frequency or duration of the signal as well. Some children will be able to discriminate relatively small differences in frequency, intensity, or duration. Others—particularly those with significant right-hemisphere-based findings on central auditory testing—may require a great deal of difference between stimuli before they are able to make a "difference" judgment. In addition, I have found that many children with difficulties discriminating minute difference in frequency, duration, and intensity often exhibit concomitant vowel discrimination deficits. Thus, training in these nonspeech discrimination skills may be indicated for children with difficulties discriminating among the vowel sounds of speech as well as in those for whom right-hemisphere-based skills such as prosody perception and auditory pattern recognition are areas of weakness.

It should be noted that the ability to generate the stimuli required for many of these tasks may not be available through standard equipment found in most clinics. Furthermore, these activities can prove difficult and relatively uninteresting to many children, necessitating a means of engaging their attention and providing rewarding reinforcement. Therefore, I have found that the use of signal generation software that allows for exquisite acoustic control of the signals' acoustic parameters, provides the ability to program a built-in algorithm that automatically adjusts the degree of difference following correct and incorrect responses using a two-alternative forced-choice paradigm, and reinforces correct responses through visually engaging computer-generated graphics is most effective for this type of activity. There are countless acoustic signal software programs available today that can be used (either singularly or in combination) to create these types of tasks. Two commercial companies that I have found particularly helpful in this regard are NeuroScan (Stim) and Tucker-Davis Technologies (SigGen). Readers should be aware, however, that many of these programs are expensive and require additional signal generation and computer hardware to implement. An additional program that is easy to use (although somewhat less flexible) and less expensive while, at the same time, allowing for the generation of a wide variety of stimuli is SuperLab Experimental Laboratory Software (Cedrus Corporation, 1997).

The list of nonspeech auditory discrimination tasks that can be implemented is almost endless. Thus, for example, activities can be created that require children to discriminate the direction of tone glides (either rising or falling in frequency or intensity), stimuli differing in size of temporal gaps (either within- or between-channel, as discussed in Chapter 2), and steady-state versus interrupted noise—a condition known as flutter fusion (Chermak & Musiek, 1997). More complex tasks can also be developed using nonspeech stimuli, including backward masking paradigms (e.g., Wright et al., 1997) and two-tone ordering (Chermak & Musiek, 1997).

The utility and efficacy of auditory training activities directed toward these types of skills is unclear at the present time. However, because speech-sound discrimination and spoken language comprehension are dependent, at least in part, on the ability to perceive time-based intensity, duration, and frequency contrasts between consecutive phonemes, it can be hypothesized that these activities may lead to improved phonological awareness abilities in some children with CAPD (Chermak & Musiek, 1997). Nevertheless, a great deal of research is still needed into the ecological validity of nonspeech auditory discrimination and related training tasks. Further, because of the difficulty inherent in creating and implementing these types of activities under controlled acoustic conditions, many clinics may be unable to engage in them at present. Therefore, greater focus may be placed on phoneme discrimination training, to be discussed in the next section, and on the auditory discrimination and temporal processing tasks available in commercial computer-assisted auditory training programs, to be discussed later in this chapter.

Phoneme Discrimination Training and Speech-to-Print Skills

The purpose of phoneme discrimination training is to help children learn to develop accurate phonemic representation and to improve speech-to-print skills.

Sloan (1995) detailed a comprehensive program for phoneme training. In her program, she emphasized that the most important feature of this type of therapy is not only to teach children to discriminate speech sounds correctly, but, even more crucial, to help them know when they have perceived a sound incorrectly or are unsure. In these situations, children can put to use additional strategies they have learned throughout the course of therapy in order to resolve the uncertainty, resulting in an improvement in confidence and self-esteem.

Sloan's program, which focuses primarily on consonant discrimination skills, involves the presentation of minimal contrast phoneme pairs, or phoneme pairs that are very similar (e.g., /t/ versus /d/). Phonemes are presented in isolation, and children must demonstrate mastery of minimal contrast pair discrimination, in terms of both accuracy and promptness of response, before adding new pairs.

Following discrimination of phonemes presented in isolation, activities move to discrimination of minimal contrast pairs of phonemes in consonant-vowel and vowel-consonant syllables, and then to words of increasing complexity. The final portion of Sloan's program focuses on *speech-to-print skills*, and involves demonstrating the connection between the phoneme segments previously trained auditorily with their corresponding printed letter symbols. Thus, the word attack difficulty often exhibited by children with Auditory Decoding Deficit is addressed as well.

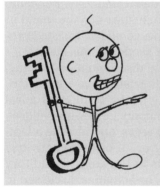

KEY CONCEPT

The most important function of phoneme training is to teach children to know when they have perceived a sound incorrectly, and to take action to clarify what was heard.

It should be noted that although Sloan's program deals primarily with consonant discrimination, the need for vowel training should not be overlooked. As in consonant discrimination activities, vowel discrimination can be facilitated through the presentation of contrast pairs in isolation, followed by syllables and words. The speech-to-print activities previously discussed may also be used effectively with vowels.

Another more recent CAPD intervention program is Processing Power (Ferre, 1997). This program targets phoneme discrimination training along with a variety of additional auditory and language skills, including rhyming, word associations, speech in noise, and speechreading. The program consists of a manual that clearly explains the goals of and rationale underlying CAPD management, and a game that incorporates the target activities into a fun format for children. An advantage to this program is that it, like Sloan's, is performed in traditional therapy format via live-voice and without the need for computers or other technology and, therefore, can be implemented anywhere by anyone. Similarly, many therapy activities that fall under the general umbrella of "phonological awareness," including phonemic synthesis, sound blending, phonological manipulation, and similar tasks can help to train phoneme discrimination and related skills.

Computer-assisted phoneme discrimination and phonological awareness activities allow for manipulation of very subtle characteristics of the auditory signal to enhance perceptual and discrimination abilities. For example, the amplitude and duration of formant transitions in consonant-vowel syllables can be enhanced, then gradually reduced as children become more and more adept at discrimination. Evidence suggests that targeted stimulation involving acoustically modified speech may significantly improve auditory, language, and related skills (e.g., Gillam et al., 2001a, b; Merzenich et al., 1996; Tallal et al., 1996; Tremblay et al., 1997); however, the efficacy and ecological validity of these approaches have yet to be delineated fully. Phoneme discrimination, speech-to-print, and related activities may be found in many currently popular commercially available computer-assisted programs, a topic that will be discussed in a later section of this chapter.

In conclusion, when considering phoneme discrimination training, speech-to-print skills, and related abilities, clinicians have a wide variety of options from which to choose. Many of the traditional aural (re)habilitation programs and activities commonly used with children with hearing impairment focus on these skill areas, and may be adapted for children with CAPD quite easily. Any or all of these activities may be appropriate for children with deficits in the areas of auditory discrimination and/or temporal processing. The activities discussed in this section are summarized in Table 9-4.

Interhemispheric Exercises

In Part One, the importance of the integrity of the interhemispheric pathways (i.e., corpus callosum) to a variety of auditory, language, and related abilities was discussed. Corpus callosum dysfunction can manifest itself behaviorally through difficulty in virtually any task, whether auditory or not, for which cross-hemisphere transfer or integration is required. On tests of behavioral central auditory function, interhemispheric dysfunction results in a predictable pattern of left-ear deficit on dichotic speech tasks combined with a deficit on temporal patterning tasks in the verbal (or linguistic labeling) report condition only. Therefore, although interhemispheric transfer of information is not one of the auditory behavioral phenomena identified in the ASHA (1996) definition of central auditory processes, direct remediation targeting

Table 9-4

Summary of Auditory Discrimination and Temporal Processing Activities

- Nonspeech discrimination activities
  - Duration, frequency, or intensity difference limens
  - Discrimination of direction of tonal glides
  - Temporal gap detection
  - Flutter fusion
  - Backward masking
  - Two-tone ordering
- Phoneme discrimination and speech-to-print skills
  - Minimal contrast pairs discrimination—consonants or vowels, live-voice
  - Computer-assisted acoustically modified speech-sound discrimination
  - Phonological awareness activities (sound blending, segmentation, manipulation)
  - Sound-symbol association

cross-hemisphere integration may be indicated for those children exhibiting diagnostic and behavioral indicators of corpus callosum dysfunction (Chermak & Musiek, 1997). **Exercises need not always be linguistic in nature. Rather, the key factors in these activities are that a single or double transfer across the corpus callosum must occur, and the exercises must provide enough opportunity for repetition so as to stimulate the corpus callosum efficiently.** Even the simple act of throwing a ball from hand to hand meets these criteria.

Interhemispheric exercises are particularly appropriate for home-based therapy activities and lend themselves easily to parent or sibling involvement. Verbal-to-motor transfers may be utilized, in which children are instructed to find a particular object or shape with the left hand from a grab bag or behind a screen, where they cannot see the objects. A motor-to-verbal transfer occurs when this process is reversed: Children find objects with the left hand and are instructed to label them verbally in terms of shape, texture, identification, and so on.

Another activity that facilitates interhemispheric transfer is music therapy. In particular, musical instruments that require coordinated movements of the hands may be most useful in this regard. For example, playing the piano requires that musicians be able both to read treble and bass clefs and engage in bimanual coordination abilities simultaneously, rendering this an excellent therapeutic instrument for children with interhemispheric dysfunction. In a study of interhemispheric function across the life span of normal adults, Bellis and Wilber (2001) found that those subjects who played piano or a similar instrument for several years consistently demonstrated the greatest interhemispheric integrity in each age group. Although this finding may suggest a self-selection process in which individuals with good interhemispheric function excel at and enjoy playing such instruments, it may alternatively indicate that consistent playing of a musical instrument over time helps to strengthen those cross-modality callosal pathways through repeated stimulation.

Children with interhemispheric dysfunction may also benefit from activities involving singing, as this requires both linguistic output (a left-hemisphere function) and melodic expression (a right-hemisphere function). Similarly, listening to popular songs for purposes of answering content questions about the lyrics themselves also requires activity from both hemispheres of the brain. The recent resurgence of the popularity of music therapy suggests that these types of activities may be a fun manner in which to strengthen multimodality and interhemispheric skills in children.

Additional interhemispheric activities that can be implemented with children include video games requiring visual and auditory vigilance and bimanual coordination, dance lessons requiring bipedal coordination, drawing pictures from verbal directions (or having children describe the pictures as they draw them), and extracurricular sports. Although these activities may prove quite difficult for children with corpus callosum dysfunction, they are also inherently fun and interesting for most children as long as the emphasis is placed on enjoyment rather than on proficiency. Therefore, it has been my experience that children typically engage in interhemispheric exercises willingly and with enthusiasm. The selected interhemispheric exercises discussed in this section are listed in Table 9-5.

In conclusion, remediation activities should be chosen that are specific to children's deficit area(s) and levels of mastery. They may include techniques to facilitate auditory closure, binaural separation and/or integration abilities, auditory temporal patterning skills, discrimination of speech and nonspeech stimuli, temporal processing abilities, and interhemispheric integration. These intervention techniques can be incorporated into existing management programs for many children with CAPD, or can be performed on a one-on-one basis by a variety of professionals or at home, depending on the task demands. The most important factors in determining which type of activity should be implemented in any given case is the nature of the fundamental underlying deficit area(s) and the functional sequelae and interests of the children themselves.

Table 9-5
Summary of Selected Interhemispheric Exercises

- "Grab bag" verbal-to-motor transfers
- "Grab bag" motor-to-verbal transfers
- Music (e.g., piano, singing) lessons
- Listening to songs and answering questions about the lyrics
- Video games requiring auditory/visual integration and bimanual coordination
- Sports, games, or dance activities requiring bipedal and/or bimanual coordination

Computer-Assisted Therapy for CAPD

In recent years, we have witnessed a dramatic upsurge in the popularity of computer-assisted "therapy in a box" programs for remediating auditory, language, and related disorders. Moreover, public awareness of these programs has increased exponentially, mostly through anecdotal accounts of successes with them on web sites and Internet listservs and in the popular media. As a result, clinics currently are being inundated by requests for these programs from parents, teachers, and others. Although there are several computer-assisted auditory/language training programs on the market today, the two that have enjoyed the greatest popularity are Fast ForWord (Scientific Learning Corporation, 1999) and Earobics (Cognitive Concepts, 1998). A third, more recent, computer-assisted program that purports to address auditory discrimination and other listening skills, attention, and memory is SoundSmart (Braintrain, 2001).

Each of these programs approaches computer-assisted auditory and language training in slightly different manners. For example, Fast ForWord (and its upper extension, Step ForWord) focuses primarily on training perception of underlying temporal processing skills important for auditory discrimination. The program is based largely on the findings of Tallal et al. (1996) and Merzenich et al. (1996), suggesting that remediation of temporal processing deficits leads to greater auditory and language gains in children with specific language impairment. Disadvantages of the Fast ForWord program are that it is costly in terms of both time and money, requires data to be uploaded via the Internet to a central analysis site where progress is measured (thus making the clinician a technician), can only be implemented by a clinician certified by Scientific Learning Corporation, and does not allow for end-user clinical decision making and manipulation of task parameters.

Earobics, which is available in three age levels from 4 years through adult, also uses acoustically modified speech to train discrimination of minimally contrasting phoneme pairs. In addition, Earobics focuses on speech-to-print skills as well as a variety of other listening abilities, including auditory closure, attention, rhyming, and sequencing. Implementation of the Earobics programs does not require clinician certification, the program is available in both clinic and home versions, and it is less costly monetarily than Fast ForWord. In addition, Earobics allows for clinician-driven manipulation of stimulus presentation and response parameters, choice of which activities to include and in what order, and data interpretation. For example, instead of having all children begin at the easiest level and progress to more difficult tasks, Earobics allows clinicians to set activities at a beginning level of difficulty that is challenging for a given child. In addition, different games within the program can be set at different starting levels. I have also found it useful to require some children with auditory and language disorders to imitate the target stimuli verbally rather than using a mouse click response—a procedure that engages the perception/production loop and results in improved expressive skills as well.

Finally, SoundSmart is a relatively new computer-assisted program that focuses on auditory discrimination, attention, memory, and "self-control." At present, to my knowledge, there exist no data investigating the use of this product with children with CAPD; however, some of the activities included in this program appear promising.

Although each of these programs employs different auditory tasks and is reported to address different types of disorders, there are some significant similarities among them. They all consist of "games" that include visually engaging, child-oriented graphics. Each employs some type of algorithm that renders the listening task more difficult after correct responses and easier after incorrect responses. They all focus on a variety of fundamental auditory, language, and/or listening skills, with the greatest emphasis placed on speech-sound discrimination and phonological awareness. Finally, all of these programs offer an attractive alternative to intensive one-on-one clinician/child therapy and can be implemented in the home setting.

Clinicians should be aware, however, that the clinical efficacy of these programs has not been established to date. For example, although the developers of Fast ForWord have published reports regarding the effectiveness of their product, large-scale independent clinical trials have yet to be undertaken (Gillam et al., 2001b). A similar situation holds true for Earobics and SoundSmart. My own clinical experience has been that, although some children exhibit significant gains from intensive training using these programs, others do not. Unfortunately, it is not clear at present which children (or which types of auditory deficits) might benefit most from these programs.

One thing can be said for certain: no one program will ever be a "cure-all" for every case of CAPD. As such, the cost of each of these therapy programs, and those like them, should be weighed very carefully against the benefits one hopes to attain from them. The issue of who should undergo these training programs, as well as that of the minimum intensity and frequency needed to achieve maximum results, remains to be investigated. In the meantime, I recommend that clinicians carefully evaluate each activity within each program regarding the type(s) of auditory processes it taxes. Based on the nature of the auditory processing deficit that is present in a given child, programs (or games within programs) can be chosen that relate most directly to the child's deficit area(s). Thus, **these programs—like all aspects of CAPD intervention—should be deficit-specific, individualized, and never recommended in a blanket manner for all children with auditory processing disorders.** Finally, as discussed previously in this chapter, there is a possibility that any or all of these programs may be beneficial for some children with CAPD, regardless of the types of activities employed (Gillam et al., 2001a, b).

Lastly, I should mention that there are some other commercially available listening programs that have gained popularity in recent years and that focus primarily on auditory stimulation without the need for active participation on the part of the listeners. Some of these programs use music, tonal, or noise stimuli that have been altered in terms of frequency or intensity. Typically, the children's task is simply to listen to the stimuli for a set period of time daily. The creators of many of these programs make claims that they "normalize distortions in the audiometric configuration," "sculpt right-hemisphere frequency responses," or similar verbage. However, most of these claims are not consistent with the auditory neuroscience literature. Of even more concern is the fact that, following training with some of these programs, children may remain unable to use headphones even for leisure purposes and some reports of tinnitus and similar auditory complaints have been documented. Finally, data supporting the clinical utility of these programs for children with CAPD are either lacking or are extremely unconvincing at present (e.g., Yencer, 1998). The combination of lack of scientific bases, limited supportive efficacy data, and potential harm to listeners renders me unable to recommend these programs for children with CAPD.

In conclusion, computer-assisted auditory discrimination and related programs such as Fast ForWord, Earobics, and SoundSmart, among others, may hold promise for CAPD intervention. However, the efficacy, candidacy, and frequency/intensity of therapy parameters are areas of much needed study. Clinicians should research both the types of activities included in any computer-assisted auditory training program and the scientific bases for claims made by the program creators prior to recommending these activities for children with CAPD. Any listening program that does not appear to be solidly based in neuroscience, or that holds the potential for harm to the listener, should not be recommended for use.

Programming CAPD Intervention Based on Deficit Subprofiles

Chapter 7 presented the Bellis/Ferre model of CAPD in which three primary and two secondary subprofiles were delineated. Suggested environmental modifications and compensatory strategies were listed in Chapter 8, including what types of management strategies were indicated for the different subprofiles in the Bellis/Ferre model. Thus far in the current chapter, we have focused on deficit-specific remediation activities for specific processing areas. This section will summarize the information in these sequential chapters to illustrate how a comprehensive CAPD intervention program can be developed on the basis of functional deficit profiles.

Readers should again be cautioned that the **information contained in this section is not intended to be a step-by-step cookbook approach to CAPD management and remediation.** The relative appropriateness of each of the following suggestions will depend upon the behavioral auditory, language, learning, and communicative sequelae of each, individual child. Furthermore, not all children will fit neatly into one of the following subprofiles. Therefore, the nature of the primary auditory deficit area(s) and the secondary behavioral and functional difficulties should always take precedence in determining which management strategies to employ for children with CAPD.

PRIMARY CAPD SUBPROFILES
Intervention for Children with Auditory Decoding Deficit
- **Primary Deficit Area:** Auditory closure
- **Possible Secondary or Associated Deficit Areas:** Speech-sound discrimination, temporal processes
- **Environmental Modifications that *may* be appropriate:**
  - Acoustic modifications
  - Use of assistive listening device

- Preferential seating
- Frequent checks for comprehension
- Employment of multimodality cues
- Repetition
- Preteaching of new information/vocabulary
- Provision of a notetaker
- Gaining attention prior to speaking
- Generous use of positive reinforcement
- Avoidance of auditory fatigue
- **Compensatory Strategies that *may* be appropriate:**
  - Attribution training (if secondary motivational concerns are evident)
  - Whole-body listening techniques
  - Self-instruction, self-regulation, and problem solving (if analyzing, developing, and carrying out solutions are areas of concern)
  - Self-reflection and journaling
  - Mnemonic devices (if secondary "auditory memory" difficulties are present)
  - Recoding information into pictorial form
  - Setting steps to music or motion (if secondary "auditory memory" difficulties are present)
  - Formal and content schema induction (if not automatically employed)
- **Direct Remediation activities that *may* be appropriate:**
  - Auditory closure activities
  - Phoneme training and speech-to-print skills
  - Temporal processing training

Intervention for Children with Prosodic Deficit
- **Primary Deficit Area:** Auditory temporal patterning
- **Possible Secondary or Associated Deficit Areas:** Nonspeech discrimination
- **Environmental Modifications that *may* be appropriate:**
  - Acoustic modifications
  - Preferential seating
  - Frequent checks for comprehension
  - Employment of multimodality cues
  - Repetition or rephrasing (if prosodic cues are rendered more salient)
  - Preteaching new information/vocabulary
  - Provision of a notetaker
  - Gaining attention prior to speaking

- Generous use of positive reinforcement
- Placement with an "animated" teacher
- **Compensatory Strategies that *may* be appropriate:**
    - Attribution training (if secondary motivational concerns are evident)
    - Whole-body listening techniques (emphasizing attention to facial expression and body-language cues)
    - Self-instruction, self-regulation, and problem solving (if analyzing, developing, and carrying out solutions are areas of concern)
    - Self-reflection and journaling
    - Mnemonic devices (if secondary "auditory memory" difficulties are present)
    - Formal and content schema induction (particularly focusing on key words and social communication expectations)
- **Direct Remediation activities that *may* be appropriate:**
    - Prosody training and key word extraction
    - Basic temporal patterning training
    - Auditory discrimination using nonspeech stimuli (e.g., frequency, intensity, duration difference limens; tonal glides)
    - Speech-language intervention for pragmatics

Intervention for Children with Integration Deficit
- **Primary Deficit Area(s):** Binaural separation, binaural integration
- **Possible Secondary or Associated Deficit Area:** Sound source localization
- **Environmental modifications that *may* be appropriate:**
    - Acoustic modifications
    - Use of assistive listening device
    - Frequent checks for comprehension
    - Repetition
    - Preteaching new information/vocabulary
    - Provision of a notetaker
    - Gaining attention prior to speaking
    - Generous use of positive reinforcement
    - Avoidance of auditory fatigue
- **Compensatory Strategies that *may* be appropriate:**
    - Attribution training (if secondary motivational concerns are evident)
    - Self-instruction, self-regulation, and problem solving (if analyzing, developing, and carrying out solutions are areas of concern)

- Self-reflection and journaling
- Mnemonic devices (if secondary "auditory memory" difficulties are present)
- Formal and content schema induction (if not automatically employed)
- **Direct Remediation activities that *may* be appropriate:**
  - Interhemispheric exercises
  - Dichotic listening training
  - Speech-in-noise training
  - Localization training

SECONDARY CAPD SUBPROFILES
Intervention for Children with Associative Deficit
- **Primary Feature:** Difficulty applying rules of language to incoming messages
- **Environmental Modifications that *may* be appropriate:**
  - Acoustic modifications
  - Preferential seating
  - Frequent checks for comprehension
  - Employment of multimodality cues
  - Rephrasing using smaller linguistic units
  - Preteaching new information/vocabulary
  - Provision of a notetaker
  - Gaining attention prior to speaking
  - Generous use of positive reinforcement
- **Compensatory Strategies that *may* be appropriate:**
  - Attribution training (if secondary motivational concerns are evident)
  - Whole-body listening techniques
  - Self-instruction, self-regulation, and problem solving (if analyzing, developing, and carrying out solutions are areas of concern)
  - Self-reflection and journaling
  - Recoding information into pictorial form
  - Mnemonic devices (if secondary "auditory memory" difficulties are present)
  - Setting steps to music or motion (if secondary "auditory memory" difficulties are present)
  - Formal and content schema induction (particularly focusing on metalinguistic, including discourse cohesion, devices)
- **Direct Remediation activities that *may* be appropriate:**
  - Speech-language intervention focusing on receptive language skills

Intervention for Children with Output-Organization Deficit
- **Primary Feature:** Difficulty acting on/responding to auditory input
- **Environmental Modifications that** *may* **be appropriate:**
  - Acoustic modifications
  - Use of assistive listening device
  - Preferential seating
  - Frequent checks for comprehension
  - Employment of multimodality cues
  - Rephrasing using smaller linguistic units
  - Preteaching of new information/vocabulary
  - Provision of a notetaker
  - Gaining attention prior to speaking
  - Generous use of positive reinforcement
  - Avoidance of auditory fatigue
- **Compensatory Strategies that** *may* **be appropriate:**
  - Attribution training (if secondary motivational concerns are evident)
  - Whole-body listening techniques
  - Self-instruction, self-regulation, and problem solving (focusing on planning and implementing steps of a procedure or solution)
  - Self-reflection and journaling
  - Mnemonic devices (focusing on sequencing steps of a process)
  - Formal and content schema induction (if not automatically employed)
- **Direct Remediation activities that** *may* **be appropriate:**
  - Speech-in-noise training
  - Speech-language intervention focused on expressive language skills

Central Auditory Processing Disorders Management for Very Young Children

Much has been made in previous chapters of the need for children to be age 7 or 8 before diagnostic central auditory testing can be conducted. What, then, of very young children? Are we to wait until the disorder can be confirmed before beginning intervention for young children who are clearly exhibiting many of the behavioral signs and symptoms of CAPD?

Although it is true that comprehensive behavioral central auditory assessment cannot be undertaken in preschool-age children, the fact remains that early and aggressive intervention is imperative as soon as the presence of CAPD is suspected. Musiek and Chermak (1995, 1997) suggested that children suspected of having CAPD be involved in a program that focuses on auditory skills development. Several different activities may be used with children that maintain a high interest level while improving auditory perceptual skills.

The phoneme discrimination training activities discussed earlier in this chapter can be adapted for use with very young children in much the same manner in which auditory training activities are carried out with preschoolers with hearing impairment. Instead of associating the sound with the printed letter symbol, pictures may be used to illustrate the minimal contrast pairs (e.g., a picture of a tiger for /t/ and a dog for /d/). The remainder of the activity may be carried out as with older children, although the speech-to-print activities probably would not be necessary with preschoolers.

Musiek and Chermak (1995, 1997) suggested that reading aloud, a popular activity for young children, be conducted with specific goals in mind, namely, selective listening for designated target words identified prior to the story being read. In this manner, children must listen carefully to all aspects of the story in order to hear and identify the target words. To ensure comprehension of the story, readers should ask comprehension questions throughout and at the end of the story presentation. Games such as "Duck, Duck, Goose" and variations of "Musical Chairs" can also foster selective listening skills in very young children.

Likewise, additional remediation activities provided in this chapter may be adapted for very young children so that they may be conducted in the preschool classroom as a fun, group activity. Interhemispheric exercises such as grab bag activities offer an interesting diversion for any preschool child. Activities that require children to guess the emotion based on intonational characteristics may foster awareness of prosodic features of speech, and elementary verbal scavenger hunts and variations of "Simon Says" assist in the development of skills necessary for following verbal directions. Even temporal patterning activities can be developed that build on young children's inherent love of imitation and body movement.

Children who are suspected of having CAPD should be watched carefully in the classroom in order to identify areas of functional difficulty. As many preschool classrooms are experiential in nature, involving multimodality stimulation every step of the way, children should be monitored carefully for signs of confusion when more than one modality is introduced, a possible sign of Integration Deficit. Teachers or clinicians may discover that a child does much better when information is presented via one mode at a time, thus providing useful insight into the possible underlying deficit as well as into the child's primary learning mode.

In short, through the use of multidisciplinary information, as described in Chapter 4, a determination can be made whether a given child exhibits difficulties characteristic of CAPD. By looking at what children are able to do well, it is often possible to rule out one or more subtypes of CAPD and to narrow the list of possible contenders. Finally, those management and intervention techniques discussed in this and the previous chapters can be adapted to the children's language and functional skills levels. In this way, suspected CAPD can be treated through a "best-guess hypothesis" rather than a "shotgun" approach, with the clear understanding that *a CAPD has not yet been formally diagnosed and that confirmation of the deficit(s) should be undertaken when children are able to participate in the testing.* It is imperative that clinicians make this concept very clear to parents, teachers, and others so that no misunderstandings ensue and so that additional investigation into the other possible causes for children's difficulties continues.

There is one exception to this general rule. In Chapter 6, the topic of electrophysiologic assessment for CAPD was discussed. A diagnosis of CAPD may be enabled in very young children if auditory electrophysiologic measures are abnormal for age *and* children demonstrate functional behavioral sequelae suggestive of CAPD as opposed to a higher-order cognitive or related disorder. However, as discussed in previous chapters, I have found that abnormal auditory evoked potentials findings are of very little value in guiding the development of individualized, deficit-specific management and intervention programs. Instead, information regarding functional difficulties gleaned from the multidisciplinary team provides far greater insight into what types of strategies and activities might be appropriate for a given child.

Finally, it should be noted that these principles may also apply to others for whom behavioral testing cannot be completed due to the presence of hearing loss or another confounding variable. For example, looking for patterns across functional deficit areas may help to illuminate why a child with a hearing loss fares much poorer with oral/aural communication than would be expected, and also helps to guide (re)habilitative efforts. Similarly, I have used the screening, interpretation, and intervention principles discussed in this book for children with limited intellectual capacity, including Asperger's syndrome and high-functioning autism. These children cannot rightly be said to exhibit CAPD but, rather, demonstrate auditory difficulties arising from higher-order global processing deficits. However, many of these principles can help identify auditory areas of weakness and improve listening skills. It is critical, however, that parents and caregivers understand that, in doing this, we are not attributing a child's cognitive difficulties to underlying CAPD, nor are we implying that a misdiagnosis has been made.

In conclusion, although valid and reliable behavioral test procedures to diagnose CAPD in preschool-age children are not available at the current time, early intervention can and should be undertaken with children suspected of having CAPD. As with other auditory disorders, early intervention may help to dilute or avoid entirely later difficulties that will inevitably appear when a child exhibits CAPD.

Summary

Several remediation techniques for addressing specific auditory processing deficits have been delineated in this chapter. Some of these techniques are intended to maximize neuroplasticity and change the way the brain processes sound at the neurophysiologic level. Others represent compensatory skills designed to bridge the gap between fundamental bottom-up processes and higher-order spoken language comprehension in real-world environments. Intervention for CAPD should always include direct remediation and compensatory skills activities along with environmental modifications to maximize children's use of auditory information.

In addition, this chapter provided a general guide to the types of environmental modifications, compensatory strategies, and direct remediation activities appropriate for various subtypes of CAPD. However, readers are reminded that this was not intended to be a cookbook approach to CAPD intervention. Instead, it is critical that elements of the intervention program be chosen that are appropriate for each child. In addition, just as with all types of communication disorders treatment, the actual activities used to train specific auditory skills should be age-appropriate and targeted toward the language levels and interests of the children undergoing therapy.

Finally, strategies were suggested for developing management and intervention plans for very young children in whom a formal diagnosis of CAPD cannot be obtained. Through the use of these strategies, early intervention can begin as soon as a possible CAPD is suspected. However, it is important to make it very clear to parents and others that, unless direct physiologic findings of abnormal auditory pathway activity are present, the formal diagnosis of CAPD cannot be undertaken in children younger than age 7 or 8.

Readers should not assume that all means of treating CAPD have been covered in this chapter. New therapy techniques are appearing almost daily. Some of these are commercially available, and some of them are implemented by individual clinicians in their own clinics. Intervention for CAPD is really no different than intervention for any other type of communication disorder. It relies on clinicians' solid knowledge of science and theory, appropriate diagnosis, and—ultimately—the ability of clinicians to use their professional expertise and creativity to develop means of targeting deficit areas in an individualized manner.

On a final note, I have spoken with clinicians throughout the world who have developed and implemented novel techniques for treating auditory processing deficits but who, for various reasons, have chosen not to publish their achievements. I urge them to share their valuable information with the rest of the professional community. The activities presented in this chapter are those that have received attention in the literature, are currently popular, or that I have developed or implemented myself. They do not represent all of the possibilities, and many of them still await empirical validation of therapeutic efficacy. I feel that the greatest contribution to CAPD intervention ultimately will come from my clinical colleagues who are in the trenches every day. In the following chapters, we will explore the topics of service delivery, documenting treatment outcomes, and engaging clinicians in research endeavors. Only when information and data are shared freely among the scientific and clinical communities will the answers to many of the questions surrounding CAPD diagnosis and intervention finally be illuminated.

Review Questions

1. What three primary assumptions underlie the rationale for deficit-specific CAPD intervention?

2. Briefly discuss the following direct remediation techniques, including what type of CAPD the activity would be appropriate for use with:

> Auditory Closure Activities
> Binaural Separation/Integration Activities
> Temporal Patterning Activities

Auditory Discrimination and Temporal Processing
   Activities
Interhemispheric Exercises

3. Outline activities that may be undertaken with very young children suspected of CAPD.

4. Johnny is a 10-year-old male who is exhibiting significant difficulties in the classroom. His teachers report that he has difficulty following directions, appears confused much of the time, and exhibits difficulty in noisy situations. Upon central auditory assessment, Johnny exhibits a left-ear deficit on Dichotic Digits and a more pronounced left-ear suppression on Competing Sentences. In addition, his performance on the Frequency Patterns test indicates a bilateral depression when verbal report is required; however, the scores revert to within normal limits when Johnny is asked to hum his responses. His performance on Low-Pass Filtered Speech is within normal limits for his age.

   a. Is it likely that Johnny exhibits a CAPD and, if so, what underlying processes appear to be dysfunctional?
   b. What CAPD subprofile(s) does Johnny exhibit characteristics of?
   c. Design a management program based on Johnny's specific deficit(s), if any.

5. Mary is a 12-year-old female with difficulty understanding speech in noise. Although she is in the sixth grade, she reads at a second- to third-grade level, and her word attack skills are significantly depressed. Upon central testing, Mary exhibits poor performance bilaterally on the Dichotic Digits and Competing Sentences tests. Her scores for the Frequency Patterns test in the verbal report condition are well within the normal range; however, her performance on Low-Pass Filtered Speech is abnormally low bilaterally. When a Time-Compressed Speech test is administered, Mary scores just above the chance level for both ears.

   a. Is it likely that Mary exhibits a CAPD and, if so, what underlying processes are likely to be dysfunctional?
   b. What CAPD subprofile does Mary exhibit characteristics of?
   c. Design a management program for Mary.

6. Fred is a 9-year-old male who is enrolled in speech-language services for receptive language delay. He exhibits receptive language deficits in the areas of vocabulary, semantics, and syntax. His early academic history is unremarkable, but he began having difficulty in school upon beginning the fourth grade. Fred is looked upon as a social misfit by many of his peers and teachers. Central testing indicates bilateral deficits on Dichotic Digits and Competing Sentences; however, performance on all other tests is within normal limits.

   a. Is it likely that Fred exhibits a CAPD and, if so, what underlying processes are likely to be dysfunctional?
   b. What CAPD subprofile does Fred exhibit characteristics of?
   c. Design a management program for Fred.

7. Alex is a 14-year-old male who is reported to have a very difficult time making friends. Although he performs loosely within the normal range in all academic areas, he has relatively greater difficulty in geometry class. Alex does not qualify for special education services; however, he often has difficulty following complex directions in the classroom, exhibits very poor notetaking skills, and often reports that others are teasing or making fun of him. Speech and language testing is within the normal range; however, Alex is reported to speak in somewhat of a monotone. Central auditory testing reveals a left-ear deficit on dichotic speech tasks. His performance on Frequency and Duration Patterns tests is extremely poor in both the labeling and humming conditions. All other test results are within the normal range.

   a. Is it likely that Alex exhibits a CAPD and, if so, what underlying processes are likely to be dysfunctional?
   b. What CAPD subprofile does Alex exhibit characteristics of?
   c. Design a management program for Alex.

8. Lexy is a 9-year-old girl with reported difficulties following directions in the classroom and at home, especially if there is competing noise in the environment. However, when she knows what is expected of her, Lexy is able to follow through on tasks quite easily. She asks for repetitions fre-

quently, and sometimes appears not to be paying attention when spoken to. Her academic achievement is appropriate for her age, but her teachers have expressed concern about her "listening" skills. Lexy enjoys sports and piano lessons, but is not particularly talented in either area. On central auditory testing, Lexy exhibits a significant (slightly better than chance level) left-ear deficit on the Competing Sentences test. All other test results are within the normal range.

> **a.** Is it likely that Lexy exhibits a CAPD and, if so, what underlying processes are likely to be affected?
> **b.** What CAPD subprofile does Lexy exhibit characteristics of?
> **c.** Design a management program for Lexy.

9. Caleb is an 8-year-old boy who exhibits behavioral symptoms very similar to Lexy's. He is often accused of not paying attention in class and at home. On central auditory testing, Caleb exhibits a bilateral deficit on Dichotic Digits testing, a left-ear deficit on Competing Sentences testing, poor performance on Frequency and Duration Patterns in both the verbal and humming report conditions, and bilateral difficulty with Low-Pass Filtered Speech, especially for words near the end of the lists.

> **a.** Is it likely that Caleb exhibits a CAPD and, if so, what underlying processes are likely to be affected?
> **b.** What CAPD subprofile does Caleb exhibit characteristics of?
> **c.** Design a management program for Caleb.

CHAPTER

TEN

Considerations in Central Auditory Processing Service Delivery

C entral auditory processing disorders do not exist in a vacuum, and neither does the clinician involved in the assessment and management of such disorders. Instead, clinicians involved in the field of CAPD must interact with other professionals in the special education arena, medical personnel, administrators, parents, and additional key individuals in order to ensure the success of any CAP program.

This chapter provides recommendations for the development and implementation of CAPD service delivery programs. Included are methods of educating appropriate individuals as to the nature of CAPD and the justification for a comprehensive program to address CAPD, suggestions for report writing and other means of imparting screening, assessment, and management information to referral sources, the use of the Child Study process to detail management recommendations and foster appropriate follow-through on management suggestions, and the presentation of a model service delivery program that includes all levels of CAPD assessment and management, from screening to follow-through.

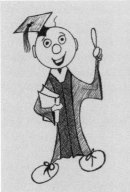

Learning Objectives

After studying this chapter, the reader should be able to:

1. Provide justification for the need for a comprehensive CAP service delivery program.
2. Identify methods of addressing questions and concerns most likely to be raised by colleagues, associated professionals, and parents.
3. Discuss methods of conveying salient information to referral sources and other appropriate parties.
4. Identify components necessary in any CAP service delivery program.

Education of Key Individuals

The first step in the success of any CAP service delivery program is the education of all individuals involved regarding the nature of CAPD, state-of-the-art methods of assessing and managing such disorders, and the justification underlying the necessary expenditures of time and money to ensure the quality of a comprehensive program.

It cannot be denied that there exists a general consensus regarding the need for means of addressing CAPD in the educational setting. Audiologists throughout the country are deluged by phone calls requesting information about CAPD. Special education professionals are hungry for recommendations regarding management of such disorders. Journal articles concerning CAPD proliferate in every professional arena, and CAP workshops and conferences are springing up in every region.

Therefore, it may surprise enthusiastic clinicians who charge to the forefront of their educational settings like knights in shining armor that many of the recommendations made regarding assessment and management of CAPD are met with resistance, reluctance, and perhaps even complete dismissal.

It appears that what is wanted is not just a method for addressing CAPD in the educational setting, but a method that is simple to implement, costs no additional money, and involves little additional time or training on the part of the individuals involved, yet will still yield the desired results. When confronted with the complexity of CAPD itself, combined with the need for training, equipment, and clinical time to implement a comprehensive, state-of-the-art CAP program, audiologists and other educational professionals may question whether the return is worth the cost. These individuals, already struggling with inflated caseloads and insufficient funding, may unconsciously search for ways to look the other way, while still expressing a desire for answers to the continuing problem of CAPD.

Citing the lack of consensus among special education professionals regarding best methods of assessment and management, these individuals may decide to wait until all the answers are in before taking action. Referring to screening tools already available and in use in many regions, they may determine that little additional information would be gained by the employment of assessment techniques such as those described in this book and, therefore, decide that the screening tools already in use are sufficient for diagnostic purposes. Emphasizing their own full schedules, combined with poor prospects for funding for additional personnel, they may decide that they simply don't have the necessary time or interest to engage in comprehensive CAP service delivery.

Flying in the face of the growing body of literature in the areas of neurophysiology, neuroplasticity, reliability and validity of assessment measures, management techniques, and the like, the search continues for the easy answer to the CAPD question.

It must be emphasized that there is no easy answer nor, in my opinion, is there likely to be one, for the sheer complexity of the central auditory system precludes a simplistic approach to the identification and treatment of disorders of that system. In addition, the heterogeneity of the CAPD population disallows the existence of one, easy, right way of addressing the needs of the population. And, as more and more is learned about auditory processing and its disorders, the entire topic of CAPD undoubtedly will become even more complex than it is currently.

However, it should be recognized that great strides have been made in the field of CAPD in recent years and, while recommendations for assessment and management will no doubt continue to change and evolve as more data are collected, sufficient information exists today to help us refine our identification and treatment approaches. Assessment procedures, such as those described in previous chapters, are available that have demonstrated validity in detecting disorders of the CANS. Likewise, there is increasing evidence that language, auditory, and educational management approaches, undertaken as early as possible, are likely to be of benefit to the child with CAPD.

Therefore, despite the complexity of the subject, **the only effective means of providing services to children with CAPD in the educational setting is through the development and implementation of a CAP service delivery program that incorporates current state-of-the-art screening, diagnostic, and therapeutic techniques while, at the same time, providing for continuing education so that modifications to the program may be made based on emerging data and recommendations for best practice.**

This is not an easy task. Clinicians entering the field of central auditory processing must be prepared to invest time and energy in the education of fellow audiologists, speech-language pathologists, psychologists, educators, administrators, and other associated individuals. In addition, all of these professionals are likely to bring to the table different questions and concerns related directly to their areas of expertise and involvement. Therefore, what follows is a discussion of common concerns likely to be raised by each of the disciplines involved in the implementation of a comprehensive CAP program and also suggestions for addressing those questions and concerns with an eye toward ensuring transdisciplinary cooperation and support.

Audiologists

Not surprisingly, the audiologist is the professional most likely to raise concerns regarding the components necessary in the implementation of a comprehensive CAP program, primarily because it is the audiologist to whom the task of leading the project will fall. Several concerns may be raised by audiologists; however, they will tend to fall into two general categories: lack of time and lack of training.

Audiologists in the educational setting have a formidable task. Often, they are responsible for their districts' hearing screening programs, including the provision of diagnostic audiological services to those children who fail the screening, as well as monitoring the audiological status of at-risk and hearing-impaired students. Staffings must be planned for and attended, and inservices must be given. Amplification and assistive listening devices used by the hearing-impaired, school-age population must be monitored and repaired.

And, to perform all of these duties, many school districts employ only one full-time, or even one part-time, audiologist.

There is no evading the fact that serving as the team leader for a CAP service delivery program is a time-consuming endeavor. When one takes into account the time investment necessary to guide the CAP screening team, review data collected during the screening process, engage in comprehensive assessment procedures, make recommendations for management, meet with teachers, parents, and other individuals to explain the recommendations made and ensure follow-through, and provide inservice training to all applicable persons, it can be seen that audiologists may need to spend up to several hours per child. This is a daunting prospect for even the most energetic and enthusiastic of audiologists.

Recent events in the federal government have virtually assured that educational funding will be cut drastically in the future, thus prohibiting the hiring of additional personnel. At the same time, more and more children are entering the school system every day. Thus, it is easy to see why many audiologists might approach the subject of CAP service delivery with a healthy degree of skepticism and trepidation.

Second, audiologists may balk at the amount of training necessary for the appropriate interpretation of central auditory assessment tools and development of management plans. As discussed in this book, it is not enough simply to become familiar with the various test tools that can be utilized. Instead, a thorough understanding of the underlying processes, including anatomical and neurophysiological bases, is necessary. The typical audiologist has received little education in this area.

A primary reason for this lack of education is that **few educational programs for audiologists deal with the subject of CAPD in sufficient detail to allow for independent clinical application.** In fact, I still occasionally encounter audiology graduate programs that devote one day or less to the subject of CAPD. When questioned, their program administrators reply with one of the widely held myths surrounding the subject: "We can't really test it, and we can't do anything about it if we diagnose it. Therefore, there's nothing to teach." As a result, graduates entering the field of educational audiology may carry similar misconceptions and lack of knowledge in the area and may be surprised and unprepared when they are asked to address CAPD on a more and more frequent basis.

A second factor contributing to the insufficient education of audiologists regarding CAPD is the **lack of consensus regarding best practices in CAP service delivery.** It is generally acknowledged that, in recent years, debate has raged as to how CAPD should be viewed, assessed, and managed. In general, it appears that the debate has cen-

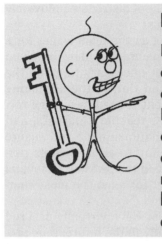

KEY CONCEPT

Familiarity with the administration of central auditory tests is not enough. In order to engage in comprehensive CAP service delivery, the clinician also must have the necessary background knowledge and competencies.

tered around finding the *one* best definition, the *one* best method of assessment, and the *one* best method of managing disorders of central auditory processing. During the 1994 CAPD consensus development conference in Albuquerque, New Mexico, it surprised some of us who attended as mere observers to hear the degree of emotional disagreement and debate. During the two-day program, leaders in the field of CAPD held faithfully to their own, particular viewpoints on the subject and, in many cases, refused to acknowledge the input of others.

Debate raged over such subjects as whether CAPD is fundamentally a language-based disorder, whether electrophysiological tests should be utilized to diagnose CAPD, and if management approaches should focus on auditory, phonemic decoding, or language-based skills. Interestingly, when approached from an objective viewpoint, it was apparent that very little actual disagreement was taking place. Instead, each of the participants seemed to be describing different manifestations of this heterogeneous beast called CAPD. Like the parable of the four blind men who, while each is feeling a different part of an elephant, disagree over what the animal actually is, leaders in the field of CAPD seemed to hold so closely to their own viewpoints that they failed to recognize that each was describing a different part of the same animal.

Since 1994, the situation has improved only negligibly, if at all. Despite the ever-increasing evidence that CAPD is a heterogeneous entity, we are still trying to define it, diagnose it, and manage it in one, simple manner. The more recent consensus conference convened at the Callier Center in Dallas in April 2000 led to recommendations that acknowledged the need for multimodality testing and mentioned the importance of considering higher-order factors (such as attention, language, and cognition) in diagnosing CAPD. However, it might be argued that the outcome of even this most recent effort at consensus was limited in scope. For the most part, members of the consensus committee were audiologists or hearing scientists. Additional attention was given to augmenting performance on behavioral tests of CAPD with physiologic measures, including electrophysiology and imaging techniques. But the need for also correlating performance on these assessment tools with standardized measures of language, cognition, and academic achievement was not adequately addressed. Although the lack of inclusion of professionals from a variety of disciplines may be thought of as an effort to focus on and arrive at a consensus regarding the auditory-specific nature of CAPD, it can also be perceived as reflecting an inaccurately narrow view of the disorder. After all, this is a disorder that is purported to affect learning, language, and communication and that must be differentiated from nonauditory cognitive, learning, attention, and related disorders. This is a difficult task at best when professionals involved in these other arenas are not included in the process of screening and diagnosis. Recommendations made for screening for CAPD were limited to the administration of a test or two and questionnaires addressing basic listening characteristics that can apply equally to individuals with many types of disorders, including attention deficit. As such, it is unclear how these recommendations will really decrease over-referrals for CAPD assessment. What the proceedings from this conference did serve to illuminate, however, is the desperate need for further research in virtually every area of CAPD screening, diagnosis, and management.

When one accepts the extreme heterogeneity of the CAPD population, one recognizes that, in some cases, the disorder may be more language-based than in others. While management appropriate for one child may focus more on language-related skills, management for another may be primarily auditory in nature. Thus, electrophysiological measures may add valuable information in many, but not all, cases of CAPD.

Although conclusive agreement has not yet been reached, when looked at objectively, it appears that some degree of consensus regarding CAPD assessment and management has, indeed, been reached, and involves the recognition and acceptance of the fact that **the CAPD population is a heterogeneous one and, therefore, assessment and management should reflect this heterogeneity.** To this end, and as discussed throughout this book, assessment of CAPD should include the collection of information regarding educational, speech-language, cognitive, and other appropriate aspects of the child, as well as the evaluation of a wide variety of auditory processes using assessment tools that have demonstrated validity in the detection of disorders of the CANS. Management should be as deficit-specific as possible and should be directed toward the individual child's presenting type of disorder. Rather than adopting one limited view of CAPD, clinicians would do well to recognize that, depending on the individual child, any of the views espoused may be the correct one in any given instance. Therefore, **clinicians should strive to keep an open mind and to avoid the adoption of one, limited view of CAPD.**

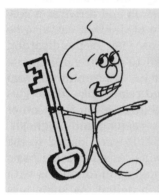

KEY CONCEPT

No one, easy, right answer to the CAPD question exists. Instead, the complexity of the "problem" reflects the complexity and heterogeneity of the disorder itself.

All of this having been said, audiologists would be correct in feeling that a great amount of education and training is involved in attaining the competencies necessary for CAP service delivery. This fact, combined with the lack of time to engage in training and service delivery activities, may result in reluctance on the part of many educational audiologists to become involved in the implementation of a CAP service delivery program, despite evidence of the need for such a program.

Educating Audiologists

To obtain the support of educational audiologists in the CAP service delivery program effort, it must first be acknowledged that the concerns they raise are reasonable and valid. The provision of CAP services is, indeed, time-consuming and requires specialized knowledge. On the other hand, the need for such services is undisputed. Therefore, efforts should be made to address the concerns of audiologists in a realistic manner.

The issue of lack of time is a difficult one to resolve. However, it should be noted that **it may not be necessary for every educational**

audiologist to engage in comprehensive CAP service delivery. Just as some physicians are better suited to certain specialties than are others, there may be some audiologists who, due to interest in the topic or other factors, may be more likely to become involved in the assessment and management of CAPD.

Later in this chapter, a model service delivery program will be presented that will provide for regional assessment centers to which all educational facilities in a given locale may refer for comprehensive central auditory assessment and recommendations for management. It may be possible, through interagency collaboration, for those audiologists who exhibit the desire and competence necessary to be primarily responsible for the delivery of comprehensive CAP services in a given location, thus eliminating the need for all audiologists to become involved in providing full-scale CAP services. In this manner, the responsibility for CAP service provision may be shared among several different educational agencies, and the waste of valuable time and resources that occurs with replication of services may be avoided.

Which brings us to the subject of training. It has been emphasized again and again throughout this book that **the provision of CAP services requires a working knowledge of the subject that can be obtained only through specialized education and training in the field.** Therefore, efforts to provide inservice and workshop education for audiologists should focus on the scientific and theoretical underpinnings of central auditory processing, as well as methods of practical application of scientific theory. In addition, it would behoove clinicians in the field to network with other professionals throughout the nation who, likewise, are involved in the provision of full-scale CAP services. Finally, we should encourage educational institutions to include in the graduate education of fledgling audiologists courses specifically designed to build the competencies necessary for the independent provision of comprehensive central auditory processing services.

The relatively recent advent of professional doctorate, or AuD, programs would seem to be an ideal venue for such additional training. However, it seems that, in many of these programs, the educational focus has moved away from a multidisciplinary view of auditory disorders and toward a more unitary model, heavily emphasizing issues such as hearing aids, third-party reimbursement, and audiology business practice. Although these are certainly important topics, they may not be the ones that are critical to audiologists entering the field of CAPD. Moreover, our recent self-imposed segregation from the field of speech-language pathology may enhance the autonomy of audiologists, but it also lessens the likelihood that audiologists investigating CAPD will obtain the education necessary to understand the language and related bases of this auditory disorder. Because the field of CAPD requires both knowledge of and collaboration with clinicians in fields such as speech-language pathology, neurocognitive sciences, psychology, and related areas, it would appear that even the emphasis on further education via the professional doctorate will contribute little, if any, toward these goals. Indeed, if the current trends hold true, audiologists may unfortunately find themselves even less prepared to interact with those in related fields and, as a direct result, less able to deal with the complexities of CAPD screening, assessment, and management.

In conclusion, as the professionals to whom the task of organizing a comprehensive CAP service delivery effort will fall, audiologists are likely to raise understandable concerns regarding time available for such activities, as well as the necessary specialized training. Therefore, through interagency collaboration and networking, efforts should be made to allow for sufficient clinical time and educational opportunities so that the audiologists involved may have the resources and support necessary for the provision of quality CAP services.

Speech-Language Pathologists

The speech-language pathologist is the professional who will probably be most involved in the implementation of management suggestions, particularly if recommendations involve direct therapeutic techniques that can best be handled in an individual therapy situation, or if the child in question exhibits a CAPD that requires more traditional language intervention. In addition, information from speech-language pathologists concerning individual children's speech and language capabilities is necessary for the CAP screening process. Therefore, speech-language pathologists, like audiologists, are apt to raise concerns that revolve around the time available for CAP-related activities.

Second, speech-language pathologists historically have been intimately involved in the central auditory assessment process. As discussed in Chapter 4, many of the speech-language tools on the market contain subtests that purport to assess auditory perceptual abilities. These professionals may require justification for the fact that these tools, which have until recently been utilized for diagnostic central auditory purposes, should actually be considered as screening tools only.

Educating Speech-Language Pathologists

Speech-language pathologists are key members of the CAP service delivery team. Therefore, it is necessary to obtain the cooperation and support from speech-language pathologists throughout the educational arena. In order to do this, speech-language pathologists must first be educated regarding the nature of CAPD and the validity and reliability of assessment tools. It must be shown that, while speech-language pathologists have much to offer in the CAP screening and management process, **assessment tools that have documented validity in the detection of disorders of the CANS must be utilized for the actual diagnosis and delineation of central auditory processing disorders.**

Second, and perhaps more important, the nature of CAPD management should be an issue in any educational program directed toward speech-language pathologists. Because they are the ones who will likely carry out many of the management suggestions made following comprehensive central auditory assessment, it is necessary that speech-language pathologists attain a working knowledge of categories of CAPD, types of underlying processes that may be dysfunctional, purposes and goals of each management technique described, and methods of implementing management recommendations. In addition, the contribution of auditory processing to speech perception, speech production, language, and learning should be addressed in any educational program for speech-language pathologists.

Finally, in cases of children who may already be on a speech-language pathologist's caseload, suggestions for infusing CAP therapeutic techniques into existing therapy plans will be quite helpful, as will suggestions for home-based and resource-based therapy. In this way, the additional time investment on the part of speech-language pathologists for CAPD management may be kept to a minimum.

Educators

Classroom teachers have the responsibility of addressing the educational needs of all the students in their classrooms, and may be responsible for twenty-five to thirty-five students in addition to the one child who exhibits CAPD. Although these educators may be extremely motivated to do whatever is necessary to help the child in need, it cannot be denied that little additional time is available for implementation of direct management suggestions in the classroom. Conversely, educators may be unaware of the nature of CAPD and the unique needs such a child demonstrates and, instead, feel that the child in question is just "not trying hard enough" or "not paying attention."

Special education or resource teachers may be more aware of the difficulties exhibited by a given child; however, they may be unfamiliar with educationally based methods of management appropriate for use with various types of CAPD.

Educating Educators

The key focus of educating educators should be on the educational impact of CAPD and methods of classroom-based management. Educators are much less likely to be interested in the diagnostic process than in compensatory strategies, environmental modifications, and other educationally based methods of CAPD management. Also, educators should receive information regarding the common indicators of CAPD for CAP screening purposes.

Therefore, activities directed toward education of educators should center around developing an understanding of the characteristics of CAPD in general, the nature of a given child's CAPD, and the academic impact of such a disorder, as well as the rationale behind each management suggestion made. In addition, regular education classroom teachers will benefit from guidance in how to implement classroom-based suggestions with the least amount of additional time investment.

Resource teachers may be in the position of implementing remediation techniques. For example, children who exhibit Auditory Decoding Deficit and are receiving remedial reading services may benefit greatly from the addition of phonemic decoding activities, including speech-to-print training, which can be added to the reading-based therapy program already in place.

Finally, educators should be familiarized with the various compensatory strategies that the child is being trained to use in the therapy situation so that the appropriate generalization and use of such strategies in the classroom can be monitored.

Educational Psychologists

Like speech-language pathologists, educational psychologists have in their armament various test tools that have traditionally been utilized for diagnosis of CAPD. Indeed, in my experience, many of the children who come to school with a "CAPD label" often have been "diagnosed" by someone in the profession of psychology. Therefore, it should be recognized that a degree of territoriality may exist, and suggestions made regarding the appropriate methods of assessing CAPD may be met with some skepticism and distrust.

On the other hand, many children with CAPD may be under the care of a psychologist for associated symptoms of frustration and depression that may occur with continual academic and communicative struggles. Therefore, psychologists are important members of the CAP team in that they may be in the unique position to provide valuable information regarding the social-emotional impact of the disorder, as well as cognitive and academic functioning and scatter of skills.

Educating Psychologists

Through inservice training or other methods, all attempts should be made to educate the psychological profession regarding the neurophysiological bases of CAPD and the appropriate, valid measures of diagnosing the disorder. Once an understanding of the auditory nature of CAPD is fostered, psychologists become much more likely to serve willingly as key members of the CAP service delivery team.

In addition, psychologists should become familiar with the CAP screening process and their contribution to CAP screening. The need for accurate measures of cognitive ability and other psychoeducational skills should be addressed. Finally, the potential impact of CAPD on a child's overall social and emotional well-being should not be overlooked, as psychologists may be called upon to provide individual or family counseling services to those children in need of additional aid.

Special Education Administrators

Administrators are responsible for providing the full range of special education services for all qualified children from a pool of ever-dwindling resources. As such, **they are less likely to be interested in the theoretical underpinnings of auditory processing and its disorders and much more concerned with how CAP services can be provided with the least amount of drain upon current personnel and funding sources.**

A principal concern for administrators is the need for such a service delivery program. Administrators are likely to have questions regarding the numbers of children affected in their schools or districts, the purpose of each member's involvement in the program, and the time and equipment neecessary for implementing a comprehensive CAP program. If a regional assessment center approach is proposed, such as the one described later in this chapter, administrators may have additional questions as to who will provide the direct diagnostic services for such a center, who will pay for assessment services, and how current caseloads will be affected by the additional duties required of those directly involved in the CAP endeavor.

Educating Administrators

The key to obtaining administrative support for a CAP service delivery program is to foster an understanding of the rationale for comprehensive CAP services. Clinicians should be prepared to address the estimated prevalence of CAPD, providing specific examples of children affected in a given school or district whenever possible; the academic, communicative, and emotional impact of such disorders; and current, state-of-the-art recommendations for service delivery. In addition, clinicians should collect data regarding the number of CAP-related requests for information and assistance received in a given time period from professionals throughout the district or region. In this way, clinicians can help to foster an understanding of the need for CAP services, as well as the rationale behind the comprehensive program being proposed.

Regarding resources, although all attempts should be made to spread the responsibility for CAP service delivery among all involved professionals, it must be accepted that additional time or funding may be required for the implementation of such a program. If the presenting difficulties of a given child are deemed by the educational professionals working with the child to require further investigation, it will ultimately fall to the educational system to provide the funding for such additional services. Therefore, along with administrators, clinicians should be prepared to develop plans for defining minimum referral criteria for CAP services and identifying methods of acquiring or allocating funds and personnel for CAP service delivery endeavors.

Education of Other Appropriate Individuals

Medical professionals, private practice audiologists and psychologists, parents, and other individuals are appropriate targets for inservice and other educational activities concerning auditory processing disorders in the educational setting.

It is not uncommon to find professionals in the private practice setting becoming more and more involved with CAP service delivery. From neurologists and other medical professionals to audiologists, speech-language pathologists, and psychologists, interest in CAPD and its clinical manifestations is blossoming nationwide. Of primary concern to clinicians in the educational setting is the education of such professionals regarding appropriate methods of assessment and the educational impact of such disorders.

Due to lack of familiarity with the educational setting in general, **private practitioners may be more likely to approach CAPD from a limited viewpoint, failing to take into account academic, cognitive, and communicative sequelae. As a result, the diagnostic and interpretive process may be limited in scope to only those skills that are auditory-based. Suggestions for management may fail to address the individualized academic and classroom-based needs of the child or, conversely, may address those needs in such a manner as to be impractical or inappropriate for the given child's educational setting.**

In addition, as federal funding for special education services undergoes further changes in the coming years, it is likely that many specialized services may be contracted out to private practitioners. Therefore, the education of those in the private practice milieu is of utmost importance.

The need for these individuals to work closely with educational professionals through inservice education and networking must be emphasized. Private practitioners should be encouraged to consult with and involve the child's educators in all aspects of assessment and management. The whole-child approach to diagnosis and management of CAPD should be advocated strongly, and open lines of communication between private practitioners and educational professionals should be made available at every step along the way. Through these efforts, the private practitioner becomes a member of the greater CAP team, and the likelihood of follow-through and success of management endeavors is greatly increased.

A final, critical component of the CAP team is the parents. Without understanding and support from the home environment, no CAP service delivery program can attain its full potential.

Parents of children with CAPD are likely to be in need of a great deal of information regarding the nature of the disorder, management suggestions, and prognosis for success. Even greater is the need for general, emotional support from clinicians and professionals in the educational arena. As discussed in Chapter 7, sufficient time should be made available during the diagnostic process to sit with the parents and explain the implications of assessment findings. Certain therapeutic techniques, such as interhemispheric exercises, may be particularly well suited for implementation in the home, and the rationale behind and methods of carrying out such activities should be delineated clearly. Parent support groups may be established to provide parents with emotional support and new information. The more the parents understand about their child's presenting disorder, the more likely appropriate follow-through will occur. Therefore, education of parents and other family members is of utmost importance for the success of any CAP service delivery program.

Information regarding CAPD and its treatment has become more readily available to parents in recent years through increased public awareness. Internet-based support groups, web sites, and similar sources have been invaluable to many parents of children with this puzzling disorder. However, the accuracy and completeness of the "facts" available from these sources vary greatly from site to site and, although valuable information may now be available to parents searching for answers, common misconceptions and outright inaccuracies are often perpetuated as well. Due to the presence of anecdotal stories of treatment techniques that "cure" children with CAPD, children with autism or mental retardation who were found to have CAPD instead, and similar dramatic stories, we are currently witnessing a "CAPD bandwagon phenomenon" that was, until recently, unimaginable. Clinics and schools are filled with parents demanding the one specific treatment that will ameliorate the disorder. Many parents are convinced that their children are suffering from CAPD even if no diagnosis has been obtained. Conversely, other parents may believe that a diagnosis of CAPD *has* been obtained through a family physician, psychologist, or educator simply because the possibility has been raised. Some may even question the need for careful diagnostics, especially if their children appear to exhibit the behavioral symptoms described in lists of key indicators for CAPD, and may be unaware that those same symptoms are quite typical of a host of other disorders as well. Mediations and due process hearings are increasing because many parents are unaware of the special education laws and how they pertain (or, rather, *don't* pertain) to CAPD and have been told that their children are entitled to intensive interventions through the school system. Finally, some parents of children with autism, mental retardation, attention deficit/hyperactivity disorder (AD/HD), and similar conditions are now discounting those (often accurate) diagnoses and attributing all of their children's difficulties to CAPD instead. In the court of public opinion, CAPD has become the preferred disorder *du jour*, and careful, accurate education of parents regarding the nature of CAPD and its diagnosis and treatment is desperately needed to correct these misconceptions.

To conclude, education of key individuals is a primary step in the development of any CAP service delivery program. However, it must be recognized that individuals involved in CAP service delivery likely will have different educational needs depending on their specific disciplines and degree of involvement. This section has attempted to identify some of the questions and concerns most likely to be raised by each member of the CAP team, and to suggest CAP-related topics most applicable for each discipline. Therefore, rather than approaching CAP education from a generic perspective, it is recommended that clinicians entering into the development and implementation of CAP service delivery programs make every attempt to establish methods of addressing the concerns of each team member. The information presented in this section is summarized in Table 10-1.

Table 10-1
Summary of Educational Needs of Key Individuals

Team Member	Education Should Focus on
Audiologist	Training and knowledge base necessary for comprehensive CAP service delivery, theoretical underpinnings and methods of practical application of scientific theory, time management
Speech-Language Pathologist	Appropriate methods of diagnosing CAPD, CAPD management
Educator	Educational impact of CAPD, classroom management suggestions
Educational Psychologist	Neurophysiological bases of CAPD, appropriate methods of diagnosing CAPD, need for accurate measures of cognitive and psychoeducational abilities, emotional impact of CAPD
Administrator	Prevalence of CAPD, rationale for comprehensive CAPD services, current recommendations for service delivery, funding issues
Other Professionals	The nature and impact of CAPD, appropriate methods of diagnosing CAPD, and the need for private practitioners to work closely with educational professionals
Parents	The nature of CAPD, diagnosis methods, management suggestions, and prognosis for success

Methods of Imparting Diagnostic Information

No matter how well organized and state-of-the-art any CAP service delivery program is, all efforts will be wasted unless the results of screening and diagnostic assessment and recommendations for management are reported in a clear, understandable way to the referring party, parents, and other appropriate individuals. Therefore, this section will focus on ways of imparting information through report-writing, handouts, and use of the Child Study process.

Writing Reports

When writing a report, it is important to make sure that the writing style is clear, that all salient points are covered, and that any potentially unfamiliar information or terminology is explained carefully. This is certainly the case with central auditory processing diagnostic reports, in which it may be assumed that the reader is unfamiliar with many of the tests utilized and the concepts presented therein.

This section describes the major components that should be included in the CAP diagnostic report: a discussion of relevant background information, results of audiological evaluation, description and report of central auditory evaluation results, impression of results, and recommendations for management (Table 10-2). It should be noted that it is not my intent to suggest that this is the only manner in which diagnostic reports may be written. The suggestions offered here are intended merely as suggestions so that issues of importance are covered adequately in the report-writing process.

Background Information

The background information section of the CAP report should include relevant information collected during the screening and parent interview process related to primary referring concern; results of academic, cognitive, communicative, and other testing; medical and family history; and areas of difficulty in listening situations reported by the child or parents. Emphasis should be placed on inclusion of those issues that led to the referral for comprehensive central auditory assessment; however, if a screening issue is "negative," that fact should be mentioned briefly (e.g., "Otologic history appears unremarkable" or "There does not appear to be a family history of learning problems") so that readers understand that the issue was investigated.

Any observations made regarding the child's educational environ-

Table 10-2

Components of the CAP Diagnostic Report

- Background Information
  - primary referring concern
  - results of academic, communicative, and other testing
  - medical and family history
  - areas of auditory difficulty
  - observations regarding the child's educational environment
- Results of Audiological Evaluation
- Central Auditory Assessment Results
  - description of test tools used
  - description of child's demeanor, attention, and behavior during testing
  - results of each test of central auditory processing
- Impressions
  - description of underlying process(es) indicated as dysfunctional by test results
  - description of CAPD subprofile suggested by test results
  - relationship of central auditory findings to information presented in background information section of report
- Recommendations
  - detailed description of any management suggestions made
  - recommendations for further testing, reevaluation, or medical follow-up, as needed

ment are also important. It has been my experience that, by including presenting symptomatology and other salient background information in the final diagnostic report, pieces of the puzzle that were not otherwise apparent often seem to fall into place. In addition, by carefully leading readers through the history and presenting complaints of the child in question, findings on central auditory assessment and, particularly, recommendations for management often tend to make more sense, thus helping to ensure appropriate cooperation and follow-through.

Results of Audiological Evaluation

If not mentioned during the background information section of the report, the results of any audiological testing performed should be delineated next. In this way, readers are assured that the peripheral auditory system has been evaluated, and that the presence of peripheral hearing loss as a primary cause of the reported symptoms can be ruled out.

Central Auditory Assessment Results

I recommend that this section begin with a brief description of each test utilized in the assessment process, including the task required from each test as well as the process or processes investigated. The primary reason for this is that many individuals are unfamiliar with tests of central auditory processing, and will require information regarding testing methodology. In addition, other clinicians who themselves are engaging in central auditory assessment will want to know the final results of testing and the methods through which those results were obtained. Therefore, the test protocol should be explained briefly, but with sufficient detail to foster an understanding of the methods through which the diagnostic impressions were derived.

Following the discussion of test protocol, the child's general demeanor, attention, and other behavioral factors during testing should be addressed, as well as the possible impact, if any, on reliability of the results. For example, if the child in question demonstrated inappropriate behavior during testing, or was easily distracted despite the carefully controlled environment, this finding should be mentioned, as should the fact that findings on test results may be confounded due to the observed behaviors. Conversely, if the child attended and cooperated well throughout the test session, such should be noted.

Finally, results of each test of central auditory processing should be reported. Rather than merely listing percentages or raw scores obtained, I recommend that each score be reported in terms of how it compares to normative values for the given age range, as raw score values rarely convey diagnostic significance when utilized alone. Significant differences between ears, or ear effects, should be noted whenever obtained. The purpose of this section of the report is not to interpret the test results, but to present them in a coherent fashion.

Impressions

In this section of the report, the conclusions drawn from the assessment findings are delineated. All attempts should be made to describe results in terms of the underlying process(es) found to be dysfunctional, and the likely behavioral, communicative, and academic impact of such dysfunction. Relating the findings to information presented in the background information section of the report is useful in helping readers to understand the possible contribution of the given CAPD to the individual child's presenting history and complaints. If possible, the use of CAPD subprofiling, including a brief description of the appropriate profile(s), may also be useful in fostering reader understanding of the impact of the child's CAPD.

Recommendations

If the presenting history, test results, and impressions have been presented with sufficient detail and clarity, the recommendations made should appear to follow logically to the reader. In addition, it is helpful to separate recommendations for management into those that will occur in the classroom and those that will be addressed in a therapy situation or at home.

In some cases, no therapeutic recommendations will be made, either because the assessment results do not suggest a need for therapy, or because the child is already receiving adequate services, as is frequently the case in language-based auditory processing disorders. In these situations, it is best to discuss *why* additional therapy suggestions are not being made, as well as the services currently in place that appear to be addressing the child's CAPD appropriately. Thus, readers understand that intervention is, in fact, needed; however, the current program appears, at the present time, to be addressing the needs adequately. On the other hand, if the need for auditory processing intervention is not indicated by the results of central auditory evaluation, this should be discussed as well.

Finally, it should be remembered that the intervention strategies discussed in Chapters 8 and 9 may not be familiar to many educational professionals. For this reason, recommendations for management should be described as clearly as possible. Remediation techniques should be supported with rationale, and examples should be given. In the next section, I will discuss the use of handouts to explain in detail

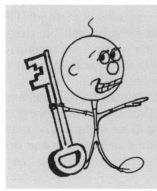

KEY CONCEPT

If no recommendations for management are made, the report should specify the reasons why additional intervention is not indicated.

the intervention methods that may be recommended. Handouts are an excellent way to guide readers through management approaches, while reducing the report-writing and postevaluation counseling time investment on the part of the clinician providing comprehensive central auditory assessment services.

In conclusion, the diagnostic report is a key method of conveying information gleaned during the screening and assessment process. However, it is imperative that information contained in the report be written as clearly as possible, with sufficient detail so that readers are able to understand the methodology used and the implications of the findings. When background history and screening information, test protocol, assessment results, and impressions of findings are explained in detail, recommendations for management will seem part of a logical progression, and the likelihood of appropriate follow-through will be enhanced.

Handouts

Handouts and other preprinted material can be invaluable resources for busy clinicians. In my clinic, each of the management techniques discussed in Chapters 8 and 9 is described in some detail, with step-by-step directions and examples of stimulus items. When a recommendation is made for a given type of remediation activity in the diagnostic report, the handout corresponding to the recommendation is attached. This practice saves valuable time and helps to ensure that remediation activities are conducted in a proper manner.

In addition, clinicians engaging in comprehensive CAP service delivery are likely to receive numerous requests for general information related to central auditory processing and its disorders. I have found it helpful to develop a general information packet that includes many of the key concepts presented in this book, from common indicators and definitions of CAPD to appropriate assessment methods. Of particular emphasis in my packet is the need for valid, reliable diagnostic procedures, as well as the heterogeneity of the CAPD population, which makes the presentation of general recommendations appropriate for every child with CAPD impossible.

To conclude, the use of preprinted handouts can be an excellent time-saving device for clinicians providing CAP services. However, caution should be exercised when developing these materials so that readers clearly understand that the handouts are merely aids and do not take the place of valid diagnostic assessment and individualized management.

The Child Study Process

All special education programs have in place methods of bringing a variety of service providers together to discuss the educational concerns and needs of a particular child. This is done either before an Individual Educational Plan (IEP) staffing takes place, or at any time during the child's educational career when it is felt that additional concerns need to be addressed or the child's educational plan needs to be changed. These meetings usually involve the educators and service providers working with a given child, as well as the parents and, in some instances, the children themselves. The name by which these meetings are called varies from region to region but I will call them *Child Studies.*

The Child Study process is an appropriate vehicle for disseminating information regarding auditory processing. It may be used before diagnostic assessment to discuss and delineate auditory-related concerns, as well as after central auditory evaluation to convey findings and recommendations for management. Through the use of the Child Study process, time is saved by addressing all appropriate individuals simultaneously, and questions can be answered promptly and within earshot of all involved. Finally, understanding of the disorder and management recommendations is fostered more easily when all persons involved in the education of the child are brought together.

We recommend that clinicians providing comprehensive CAP services set aside time to attend such meetings. In this manner, everyone involved with the child can approach the issue from the same perspective, questions and misunderstandings can be clarified from the outset, and valuable time can be saved that might otherwise have been spent on individualized consultation with each service provider involved.

This section has discussed methods of imparting salient information to involved professionals and parents. Suggestions for clear, concise report-writing, the use of handouts and other preprinted material, and the Child Study process as a means of meeting face-to-face with service providers were included. Clinicians should make use of these and other devices that will allow for better dissemination of information, while saving valuable time for everyone involved.

Comprehensive Central Auditory Processing Service Delivery

Throughout this text, I have discussed various aspects of central auditory processing, from neuroanatomy and neurophysiology to screening methods, assessment tools, and approaches to CAPD management. Because of the complexity of the subject, any service program designed to address central auditory processing will, likewise, be complex. This section will discuss those components necessary for developing and implementing a comprehensive CAP service delivery program. Also included will be the presentation of a model service delivery program which, through the use of regional assessment centers, may help to save time and money investment for each individual school or district, while still providing for quality service delivery.

Components of a Comprehensive CAP Service Delivery Program

Several components must be in place for a CAP service delivery program to be successful. These components are outlined in Table 10-3, and are reviewed in this section. Methods of funding a program such as that described in this book will differ depending upon regional characteristics. Therefore, beyond the general suggestions that have been made herein, funding will not be addressed. Clinicians involved in the development and implementation of CAP services should discuss funding-related issues with their respective administrators.

Training and Education

The first step necessary for the development and implementation of any CAP service delivery program is training and education of involved professionals. The level of training will vary depending on the degree of involvement. As discussed earlier in this chapter, the educational needs of educators and associated professionals will be different from those of primary clinicians providing comprehensive CAP services.

Table 10-3
Necessary Components of Any Comprehensive CAP Service Delivery Program

Training and education of key individuals

Screening procedures

Resources for carrying out comprehensive central auditory assessment

Resources for implementing management suggestions

Methods of data collection and research to document program efficacy

The CAP team leader, by necessity the audiologist, will need to receive training in all aspects of central auditory processing. Education in the scientific bases of CAP, screening and assessment methods, interpretation of central auditory assessment results, and management approaches is essential for any clinician entering this complex field. **It is my opinion that it is more harmful to provide these services with poor or inadequate training in all aspects of CAP than it would be not to provide any CAP services at all.** The need for appropriate training of any individual entering the greater CAP arena cannot be overemphasized. Clinicians desiring to provide comprehensive CAP services should seek out sources of the training needed, using the suggestions provided earlier in this chapter.

In addition to the need for training for audiologists providing the bulk of the services, educational inservice opportunities must be provided for all professionals involved in the CAP effort. In many cases, the CAP team leader will provide such inservice training. The educational needs of each of the disciplines involved were presented in some detail earlier in this chapter.

Finally, the need for keeping up with new trends and information in the field of CAP cannot be overlooked. Therefore, in addition to initial training and inservice education, a system of continuing education must be in place for professionals involved in any CAP service delivery program.

Screening

The topic of CAP screening was dealt with in detail in Chapter 4. Therefore, I will not reiterate here what has already been covered. Readers should be aware, however, that a screening program for CAPD is an integral part of any comprehensive CAP service delivery program. It should also be remembered that the screening program should be based on a multidisciplinary team approach, allow for appropriate referral for comprehensive assessment when indicated, and include methods of data collection for monitoring program efficacy.

Comprehensive Central Auditory Assessment

The next integral component is the CAP diagnostic program itself. Once a child has been identified through the screening process as needing further central auditory assessment, there must be in place a means of performing diagnostic testing. This component includes the actual assessment procedures and methods of reporting the results to the referring party, as well as making recommendations for management.

The comprehensive assessment portion of the CAP service delivery program need not be available at the school, or even the district, level. Instead, a school or district may choose to refer to a regional assessment center for such services. **What is critical is that comprehensive CAP assessment services are available in a given region and that access to such services is ensured as part of the overall CAP program.**

Management

A critical component of any CAP service delivery program is the implementation of management suggestions. Methods of providing therapeutic intervention must be in place for children who are in need of such services, as well as classroom-based modifications and other management strategies. The decision regarding who should oversee the management effort or be primarily responsible for implementing therapy suggestions (e.g., speech-language pathologist, audiologist, resource teacher) will depend on the personnel constraints of the given school or district as well as the intervention needs of the individual child.

Regardless of which professional is primarily responsible for implementing management suggestions, it is imperative that the lines of communication among diagnosticians, educators, therapists, and others involved in the CAP effort be kept open for ongoing monitoring of treatment efficacy.

Data Collection and Research

In addition to the provision of clinical services, it is important that the CAP service delivery program also be equipped for collecting data and generating research. At the very least, clinicians providing diagnostic services must be knowledgeable regarding the collection of normative data for each test tool in use. Data collection related to screening program efficacy is also necessary, as mentioned previously.

Although these data collection activities are generally considered to be integral parts of the CAP service delivery program, I also recommend that clinicians become familiar with scientific methodology and, as practitioners, take on the responsibility of contributing to the growing body of CAPD literature. The need for further research has been mentioned frequently throughout this book, particularly in the areas of treatment efficacy and assessment methodology. **No one is better suited for generating treatment-related data than those practitioners**

engaged on a regular basis in providing CAP management services, and it is my opinion that a large portion of the much-needed data regarding treatment efficacy ultimately will come from these same practitioners.

Moreoever, given today's focus on outcome measures in all aspects of health care delivery, the collection and analysis of data has become integral to our professions. Outcome measures focus on the impact of care or intervention. Outcomes of a screening program, for example, may include the number of children screened, the number who failed the screening, and the number of those who turned out to, indeed, exhibit the disorder in question. In this way, the efficacy of the screening program may be demonstrated objectively. Data regarding entrance and dismissal criteria for therapy, expected rate of progress, optimal frequency and intensity of therapy sessions, and relative efficacy of different therapy approaches are necessary for planning and justifying intervention services. Outcome measures from virtually all areas of audiology and speech-language pathology are important both for the enhancement of knowledge in the field and to influence third-party reimbursement companies, legislators, and others as to the value and cost-effectiveness of our services. They also help to guide clinicians in developing programs, planning diagnostic and intervention services, prioritizing clients within their caseloads, and obtaining third-party reimbursement.

The documentation of outcomes is mandated by federal law under the Individuals with Disabilities Education Act (IDEA) for children receiving special education services. Collection of data relating to treatment efficacy and related issues is also considered an important responsibility of audiologists and speech-language pathologists under the ASHA Code of Ethics. As such, clinicians must engage in data collection activities as part of their regular professional duties, and have an ethical obligation to demonstrate the effectiveness of their services and to share the information they obtain with others in the field.

Therefore, I encourage clinicians engaged in CAP service delivery to commit themselves to the journey from practice back to science, and to engage in research-related activities that will further our knowledge of this complex field. General principles of scientific methodology and data collection will be discussed in the final chapter of this book.

In conclusion, the necessary components of the CAP service delivery program consist of education and training, screening, comprehensive diagnostic assessment, management, and data collection for the purposes of development of normative values, program monitoring, and future research needs.

A Regional Assessment Center Model
Service Delivery Program

Over the past several years, I have served as a consultant to several regions and states throughout my own country and to others who are struggling with the need to implement some type of CAPD service delivery program yet are challenged either financially, geographically, or both. For the most part, each of these regions has an inadequate number of trained clinicians to meet the increasing demands, limited funding to support clinical programs in CAPD, and large areas that are covered by a single educational unit. For areas such as these—as well as smaller, more populated, regions—a collaborative regional assessment center model for CAPD service delivery such as that outlined in Figure 10-1 has proven to be the most economical and efficient way of meeting the demand for quality CAPD screening, assessment, and management services.

In this type of program, regional assessment centers, headed by trained audiologists, are established. Audiologists at the regional assessment center carry the responsibility for heading screening efforts and reviewing screening data, providing diagnostic evaluations, and making recommendations for management for all of the schools or districts in their regions. Depending on population and geographical distance, each assessment center may be responsible for one or more school districts.

CAP screening is carried out at the school or district level. Educational personnel are provided with inservice training in order to delineate screening activities and other salient information necessary for screening and follow-through. Occasionally, the screening may, itself, be contracted out, particularly in difficult-to-interpret cases. Because this screening procedure consists primarily of a paper review, as discussed in Chapter 4, it can be done by anyone trained in pulling the pieces of the academic, cognitive, speech/language, and auditory puzzle together, even if that professional is located in another state (or, indeed, in another country). Although it is always more desirable to have members of the educational team working with the child make the decision whether to refer for central auditory assessment, this is not always possible and additional expert input may be sought. In these cases, it is common for the screening party to charge a fee for the record review. When the screening party is not located at the regional assessment center for the educational unit(s), the fee for the screening is usually deducted from the cost of the diagnostic eval-

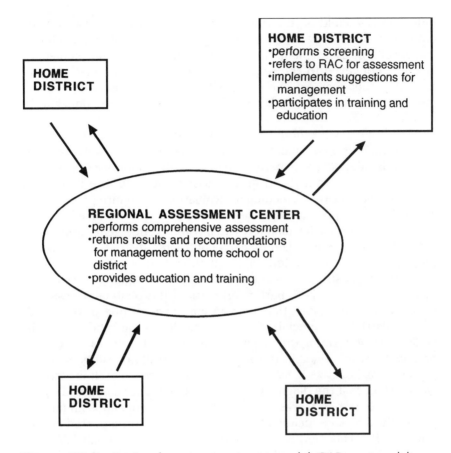

Figure 10-1. Regional assessment center model CAP service delivery program.

uation as part of a contractual agreement. On the other hand, when the screening is carried out by the educational team or by the designated regional assessment center, a fee is usually charged only if referral for a full diagnostic evaluation is *not* recommended. When referral for a full assessment is undertaken, the records review is then considered part of the diagnostic process, and is absorbed in the fee for the diagnostic assessment. In any case, results of the screening and recommendations based on records review should be communicated in writing, as discussed in Chapter 4.

When screening data suggest that further diagnostic evaluation is indicated, the child is referred to the regional assessment center for comprehensive central auditory testing. Upon completion of such testing, results of assessment and recommendations for management (if any) are conveyed to the referring school through the methods discussed in this chapter. The responsibility for implementing management suggestions is then taken up by the appropriate personnel at the school level.

The issue of who shoulders the financial burden for district-initiated screening or assessment procedures, as well as for salary-related costs if the audiologist is performing the central auditory diagnostics, differs from program to program. Most frequently, the district or school requesting the screening or evaluation procedure pays for that service, and the program may also be additionally subsidized in a collaborative, interdistrict manner. Often, the revenue generated, along with additional monies paid by each contracted district, is pooled for the purpose of hiring additional audiology staff so that the central auditory diagnostician has release time for the regional assessment center activities. This is particularly true if the regional assessment center (and the diagnostician) is an employee of one of the area's school districts or special education unit. If, on the other hand, the audiologist performing the diagnostic and related services is a clinical or private practitioner in the area, most districts or schools simply pay on a case-by-case basis via a contractual agreement. It is extremely important that the diagnostic audiologist, whether employed by the area schools or not, works closely with each school and is an integral part of the special education team for children with suspected or confirmed CAPD. This method is a useful way of ensuring quality CAP services for all children in a given region while, at the sime time, lessening the time investment requirements on many of the professionals involved. An additional advantage to the program is that only those audiologists with the interest and energy to devote to training in the area of auditory processing need commit to the provision of comprehensive CAP services. **Those audiologists without the time, interest, or other means to invest in such pursuits are provided with the option of referring out for those CAP services for which they are not trained.**

The program described here represents just one example of how a CAP service delivery program can be established to address the needs of the given population. What is most important is an understanding of the necessary components of any CAP service delivery program. Once that understanding is attained, we urge the clinician to be creative and to take advantage of all available resources when developing ways of implementing CAP services.

Summary

This chapter has discussed a variety of considerations in CAP service delivery, including the need for education for all individuals involved, methods of conveying salient information to appropriate persons, and components necessary for inclusion in any CAP service delivery program.

The development and implementation of a CAP service delivery is a complex, time-consuming endeavor requiring input and cooperation from a variety of professionals and other individuals. However, it must be emphasized that each of the components described in this chapter, from education and training to screening, assessment, and management, must be included for any program to demonstrate effectiveness and overall success. A CAP service delivery program that employs poorly trained individuals, is poorly planned, poorly executed, and lacks one or more of the necessary components discussed in this chapter is no better, and may actually be worse, than no CAP service delivery program at all.

Finally, clinicians must remain aware at all times of the ever-changing nature of central auditory assessment and management and make every effort to adapt and incorporate such changes into their comprehensive CAP service delivery programs.

Review Questions

1. What purpose(s) does education of individuals involved in the delivery of CAP services serve?

2. Identify key topics important in the education of the following persons:

Audiologists	Speech-Language Pathologists
Educators	Psychologists
Parents	Private Practitioners

3. What components should be included in a central auditory diagnostic report?

4. How should the lack of significant findings upon diagnostic testing be addressed in the written CAP report?

5. How can the use of handouts aid the clinician in imparting CAP-related information?

6. What is a child study and how can it be used in the dissemination of CAP-related information?

7. What are the primary components of any CAP service delivery program?

8. Why is knowledge of data collection and scientific methodology important in CAP service delivery?

9. List the primary purposes of outcome measures, and briefly discuss why clinicians in speech-language pathology and audiology should be involved in the collection of outcomes data.

10. For your own setting, identify obstacles that are most likely to surface in the development and implementation of a comprehensive CAP service delivery program, and design a plan for addressing each of these obstacles.

CHAPTER

ELEVEN

Back to Science

Note to readers: There was some question following the publication of the first edition of this text concerning the applicability of a chapter on basic research methods in a book on CAPD. Despite several years having passed, however, I find that clinically applied research in the area of CAPD remains just as desperately needed now as it was in the mid-1990s when the first edition of this book was published. Moreover, with the advent of the professional doctorate in audiology (AuD), the dichotomy between clinician and researcher has widened even farther. Presently, there is a good deal of controversy surrounding the need for clinical preparation (AuD) programs to provide training in or require students to complete basic research projects. Many contend that research is a fundamental component of what clinicians do on a daily basis and that some training in research methods is critical so that clinicians can become better consumers (and producers) of literature in the field. This is a view I adhere strongly to and that is emphasized in this chapter. Others, however, feel that research methodology is a topic best left to academicians and PhD programs and that it has no place in the clinical arena. As an audiologist who has worked clinicially in the field for more than sixteen years and who is now also an academician, having earned my PhD since the publication of the first edition of this text, I continue to feel that the most needed areas of research in CAPD—those of treatment efficacy and of defining categories of the disorder—require the involvement of clinicians who are working with large numbers of these children on a daily basis. To truly bridge the gap between science and practice, we must involve practitioners in the collection and dissemination of science. Therefore, this chapter is included in this revised edition because the issues it raises continue to be as—if not more—important than they were before.

T he preceding chapters of this book have focused on the practical application of scientific theory regarding central auditory processing. The purpose of this chapter is to provide readers with a brief introduction to scientific methodology in the hopes of generating interest in the fascinating journey from practice back to science. In addition, this chapter will assist readers in developing an understanding and appreciation of the need for research-based activities on the part of clinicians engaged in central auditory processing service delivery. This chapter discusses the need for clinicians to perform as scientists in their daily settings; fundamentals of the scientific method, including terminology and basic concepts of research design; a brief overview of commonly used statistical formulas; and areas of need for further study within the field of central auditory processing and its disorders.

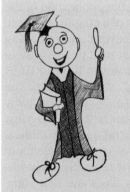

Learning Objectives

After studying this chapter, the reader should be able to:

1. Discuss the justification underlying the need for clinicians to engage in research-based activities in their daily settings.
2. Identify and discuss key concepts related to scientific methodology.
3. Define common terms related to research design.
4. Identify the purpose of several commonly used statistical procedures.
5. Delineate several areas of need for future research in central auditory processing.

Why Should Clinicians Engage in Research?

Although the word *research* strikes fear in the hearts of many audiologists and speech-language pathologists in the trenches, **it should be recognized that what many of us do on a daily basis is essentially scientific study.** For example, when a patient enters the clinic for a standard audiological examination, the audiologist must first identify a clear objective of the clinical session (e.g., to identify whether a hearing loss is present and, if so, what type and to what degree). Then, data collection activities must be performed in order to gather information that will, hopefully, meet the objective (e.g., obtaining pure-tone air- and bone-conduction thresholds, word recognition scores, immittance measures), while simultaneously assessing the reliability of the data being collected (e.g., determining the degree of agreement between pure-tone average and speech recognition threshold, using a bracketing approach, and varying the rhythm of stimulus presentation to control for false responses). Finally, the data collected must be interpreted in light of what is known about auditory function in order to address the initial objective.

Likewise, (re)habilitative activities must follow the general principles of scientific research. The initial problem must be identified, baseline data collected, and a hypothesis must be formed regarding the effective treatment of the problem. Then, rehabilitative activities must be undertaken over a period of time, with repeated data collection occurring at regular intervals. Finally, the data must be interpreted in order to determine whether treatment has been effective, as well as to identify future directions for intervention.

In short, what each of us does every day in our respective settings is nothing short of scientific research. As Silverman (1977, p. 15) stated, **"There should be no difference, therefore, in the way you would go about answering clinically relevant questions or testing clinically relevant hypotheses for clinical and research purposes."**

Nevertheless, it appears that a general dichotomy exists between those engaged in clinical practice and those engaged in scientific research (Goldstein, 1972; Hamre, 1972; Jerger 1963). In other words, clinicians, although they are of necessity consumers of research, rarely engage in research-related activities for mass dissemination, whereas scientists spend their careers performing research-related activities for use by clinicians in the practical setting. This separation of the researcher from the clinician fails to acknowledge the interdependency of the two activities and results in a paucity of clinically relevant research for use in daily practice. Some even suggest that this lack of clinical research could ultimately lead to the downfall of the future of our profession unless we are able to turn things around soon.

Silverman (1977) listed several benefits that a clinician may realize from functioning in the dual role of practitioner and scientist, including an increase in job satisfaction and stimulation; improvement in one's effectiveness as a clinician; and the provision of much-needed data regarding clinical diagnostic and treatment methods (Table 11-1). For example, because the daily clinical activities required of audiologists and speech-language pathologists are so closely tied to research methodology, engaging in research activities would serve to improve clinical skills by helping to develop a more scientific approach to clinical decision making. Instead of asking whether a particular treatment approach has been effective, for instance, clinicians would learn to phrase clinical questions in a manner such that answers can be more specific and measurable (e.g., did therapy result in certain desired behaviors?). In addition, familiarity with the scientific method would aid clinicians in the collection of normative data for nonstandardized and new diagnostic procedures, as well as in the development of new diagnostic and treatment procedures.

Data generated by clinicians also can help to provide much-needed answers to questions that are difficult to address outside the clinical venue. Take, for example, an issue mentioned repeatedly throughout this text, that of CAP treatment efficacy. Who better to engage in research and generate data regarding CAP treatment efficacy than those clinicians actively engaged in such pursuits in their daily practice? **Because of the nature of treatment efficacy research, which must be gathered over a period of time and is best generalized when obtained from situations most resembling the "real-life" treatment environment, clinicians may be in the best position to generate such data.** Additionally, clinicians may not only have access to the patients, opportunity, and setting that are needed for research of this type, but they also may have better ideas of what questions are clinically relevant than would scientists not actively engaged in clinical practice.

Clinicians may be hesitant to engage in clinical research because of

Table 11-1

Ways in Which Engaging in Research Can Be of Benefit to Clinicians

Engaging in research activities can
- Increase job satisfaction and stimulation, and reduce boredom
- Improve clinical skills by developing a scientific approach to clinical decision making
- Provide answers to clinic-related research questions regarding diagnostic methods and treatment efficacy

the feeling that such activities require more time than is available. However, as stated previously, the types of activities required of clinical researchers are the same as those required for daily clinical practice. Naturally, although some additional time and support would be required for the analysis and presentation of data, clinicians should realize that the sources of such data may well lie within their current caseloads. **By incorporating the scientific method into daily practice, all activities performed in the daily routine can be used for data collection purposes, and clinicians would be in a better position to judge the efficiency and effectiveness of their clinical activities.**

In conclusion, by engaging in research-based activities, clinicians can not only help to improve their own efficiency as service providers, but also can help to answer important research questions that may best be addressed by those who are in the clinical setting. For these reasons, I encourage clinicians entering the CAP arena to become familiar with scientific methodology and to perform their own CAP-related duties with an eye toward generating data that will help to clarify those areas that remain largely untested and untried, but critical to the overall big picture of CAPD assessment and management.

Fundamentals of the Scientific Method

When we set out to incorporate the scientific method into daily clinical practice, we must become familiar with certain concepts and terms implicit in research methodology. This section will focus on critical elements of the scientific method and will introduce selected terminology, concepts, and types of research designs. These concepts should not be new to experienced clinicians; however, a review may help to remove some of the rust if they have not been used for a while.

Terminology

When discussing research, various terms are used to describe a variety of facets of the scientific method. Many of these terms are frequently encountered when reading journal articles or materials such as this book, and the reader may be somewhat familiar with their meanings. The purpose of this section is to clarify some of the more commonly used terms in research.

Data

The term *data* refers to those attributes or events that are observed (or collected) during research activities. Data may be quantitative, or numerical (e.g., scores on a test, ages, percentile ranks, response time) or they may be qualitative, or descriptive (e.g., race, hair color, attention). What is critical when considering what data to collect during a research activity is that the attributes be measurable in some way, and that a clear plan for assigning values or coding the data is established prior to data collection.

To illustrate, if investigators wish to look at attention during testing as an attribute critical to a study, they must make sure that *attention* is defined in such a way as to be measurable. It may be decided that the percent of time spent on task will be an indicator of *attention*. On the other hand, *attention* may be assigned a value on a continuum from good to poor. In any case, the attribute or event being observed must be defined in a manner that allows it to be measured and coded as data.

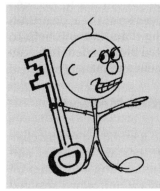

KEY CONCEPT

The attribute or event under study must be defined in such a way as to be measurable and able to be coded as data.

Variables

A variable is an outcome that can take on more than one value. For example, response time is a variable that can take on several numerical values. Likewise, race is a variable that can take on values such as Caucasian, African-American, Hispanic, and Asian.

To take our discussion of variables one step further, a *dependent variable* is one that measures the outcome of a research study. Conversely, an *independent variable* is a condition that is controlled by the researcher in order to test its effect on the outcome. For example, if one is studying the effect of age on performance on a test of central auditory processing, then age would be the independent variable, and the actual scored performance on the test would be the dependent variable.

When engaging in research activities, one must be aware of and control for additional confounding variables that may affect the ultimate outcome of the study. For example, in the above illustration, while age certainly has an effect upon central auditory test performance, so might variables such as cognitive capacity, history of otitis or other otologic or neurologic disorders, family history of learning disabilities, and so on. Therefore, in this example, one would want to choose a sample of children who exhibit normal cognitive capacity and have no significant medical or family history in order to isolate, as much as possible, the effect of age alone on the test being studied.

Sample

Because it would be virtually impossible to include every person in the world in a given research study, we must select a sample that is as representative of the population being studied as possible. The more representative the chosen sample is of the target population, the more likely it will be that the findings of the study can be *generalized*, or applied, to the population as a whole. This process of inferring the results from a sample to a population is the basis for the *inferential method* upon which many of the studies discussed in this book are based.

To provide a simplified illustration, if clinicians are collecting data for the purpose of developing clinic-specific normative values for a selected test of central auditory processing, they will want to make sure that the sample that is chosen is representative of the population as a whole. In order to do this, clinicians will want to select children from different classrooms in a given school or region while simultaneously controlling for independent variables that may have a detrimental effect on test performance. In other words, all children within the desired age ranges who exhibit normal cognitive capacity and negative medical and family history should have equal chances of being selected for the normative study. Readers should be aware that those variables mentioned above may not be the only ones that might be considered when choosing a representative sample from a given population, but, rather, are intended here for illustrative purposes only.

A final consideration when discussing samples is that of sample size. As a general rule of thumb, the larger the sample size, the smaller the chance for error. However, due to constraints upon time and resources, it will usually be desirable to limit the sample size to a workable number that will still yield the desired results and minimize the chance for error. I recommend that, in multisubject studies designed for the purpose of developing representative data for a population (e.g., development of normative values for specific age groups), the sample size (N) be at least fifteen to thirty within each group. As the study becomes more complex in terms of number of independent and dependent variables, as well as estimated variability within the population, then the size of the sample might need to be increased in order to minimize error. Likewise, if the target population is quite homogeneous, and the desired outcome is likely to demonstrate very little variability, then the sample size may be smaller and still yield reliable results that can be generalized to the target population as a whole.

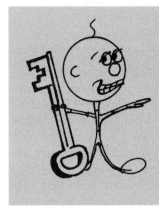

KEY CONCEPT
The number of subjects needed for results of a given study to be reliable will depend upon the complexity and number of variables and the homogeneity of the population under scrutiny.

Variability

Variability refers to the degree of spread that characterizes a group of scores within a sample or a population. In other words, scores that are closer together demonstrate a lesser degree of variability than do those that are farther apart. Measures of variability are those statistical procedures that determine the degree of heterogeneity of a selected characteristic of a sample. Specific measures of variability will be discussed in the section on statistical analysis.

Significance

Statistically speaking, *significance* refers to a finding that two experimental groups are different. The degree of significance is expressed in terms of *probability* (p). For example, $p < 0.05$ can be interpreted to mean that there is less than a 5% chance that the differences observed in an experiment were due to chance or error or, conversely, that there is a 95% chance that the differences observed were real and not merely an artifact. Tests of significance are utilized in research in order to determine the level of confidence that can be placed in the findings. The two most commonly used confidence levels in clinical research are 0.05 and 0.01.

The concept of *statistical significance* should be distinguished from that of *clinical significance*. Suppose, for example, that the performance of a very large number of boys on a test of central auditory processing was compared to the performance of the same number of girls, and the results indicated that the girls performed 1% better on the test than did the boys. Even if a statistical test of significance indicated that the probability of the finding was less than 0.01, indicating that the finding was statistically significant, a difference in performance of a mere 1% on a central auditory test is likely to be so negligible as to be clinically insignificant. **Therefore, it should not be assumed that results of a study are clinically relevant simply because the findings are statistically significant.** The reverse may also be true in some cases. That is, it is possible for a patient to perceive a subjective difference in quality between two hearing aids or treatment conditions even if statistical measures indicate no significant difference between them. Therefore, the degree to which the findings can be utilized in the real-life, clinical setting will determine the degree of clinical significance a given study exhibits. Some common tests of statistical significance will be discussed later in this chapter.

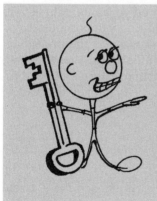

KEY CONCEPT

Statistical significance does not necessarily imply clinical significance. In order for findings of a study to be clinically significant, they must be applicable to the clinical setting.

Correlation

A correlation is a relationship between two or more variables. For example, the finding that the right-ear advantage (REA) decreases with increasing age indicates that the two variables—REA and age—have something in common, or are correlated. The higher the degree of relatedness among two or more variables, the higher the correlation is said to be.

Statistical tests for correlation can indicate whether the variables are *negatively* or *positively correlated*. A negative correlation is one in which an inverse relationship exists, or the value of one variable increases as the other decreases. The example provided above, in which the REA decreases with increasing age, would be an example of a negative correlation.

Conversely, two variables are said to be positively correlated when they change in the same direction. For example, the percentage of total correct responses on the Frequency Patterns Test increases with increasing age. This would be an example of a positive correlation.

Correlations are expressed in values referred to as *correlation coefficients*. Correlation coefficients range in value from -1.00 to +1.00. The size of the number is an indicator of the strength of the correlation, regardless of whether the number is negative or positive. **Therefore, a correlation coefficient of -0.78 indicates a stronger relationship between variables than does a correlation coefficient of +0.50.** Likewise, a correlation coefficient of -0.90 indicates that two variables are strongly negatively correlated, whereas a correlation coefficient of +0.90 indicates that two or more variables are strongly positively correlated.

This section has introduced some of the more common terms used in research and is by no means intended to be an exhaustive overview of research-related terminology. Additional important terms, such as reliability and validity, have been discussed in the preceding chapters. It is hoped that, by becoming familiar with these terms, readers will be better able to understand technical terms utilized in the literature, as well as begin to gain the knowledge fundamentals for engaging in research activities, themselves.

Types of Research

Research can take on many forms, and the form chosen for a given study will depend upon the question being asked. **Scientific research serves a variety of functions, including identifying the causative factors that lead to a given event, describing characteristics of a population or phenomenon, determining the nature of events that have occurred in the past, and identifying the relationship between two or more variables.** A discussion of the types of research designs that perform these functions, as well as considerations for engaging in each type, follows.

Experimental Research

The primary goal of *experimental research* is to determine the effect of a given variable on the outcome variable. In order to do this, subjects are assigned by the investigator to different groups, with each group receiving a different possible treatment in order to assess the differential effects of the treatment on the outcome. For example, if one wishes to compare the effect of daily phoneme training on performance on Low-Pass Filtered Speech Tasks to the effect of no training whatsoever over the same time period, one would assign matched subjects to the two groups. Group One, no therapy, would be considered the *control group*, while Group Two, the group receiving daily therapy, would be considered the *experimental group*. Baseline data, in the form of Low-Pass Filtered Speech scores, could be obtained from both groups before the experiment, with repeated data collection at various times throughout the allotted time period. The improvement in scores, if any, that occurs in Group One could be compared to those obtained from Group Two using selected tests of significance, which will be discussed later in this chapter.

Advantages to the experimental method include a high level of control over subject variables, group assignments, and treatment variables. However, it may not always be possible or ethical to assign subjects to groups and manipulate the treatment each group receives in order to determine relative effects. For example, if one wishes to study the effect of early otitis media on central auditory processing abilities, it would not be possible or ethical to assign children to two experimental groups, and then induce otitis in the members of one of the groups in order to assess its effect on auditory skills. In these situations, rather than conducting a true experimental research study, the investigator would need to utilize the type of research known as *causative-comparative research* (Salkind, 1991).

In causative-comparative research, the investigator has no control over the assignment of subjects to a particular group. Instead, subjects are assigned to groups based upon some characteristic that they bring to the investigation (e.g., history of early chronic otitis media). Although other factors, such as socioeconomic status, cognitive functioning, age, and academic achievement, can be controlled for, the actual variable of interest—history of otitis—is already established and cannot be manipulated by the investigator. Data collection would then occur "after the fact," and tests for significant differences between groups would be conducted as in experimental research.

Much of the research completed in the area of central auditory processing is of the causative-comparative type of research design. Studies of lesion effects on various tests of central auditory function, for example, would be an example of this type. Conversely, much of the research that occurs in the area of treatment efficacy is likely to fall into the experimental research design category, because the treatment variable can be manipulated during the investigation process in order to determine cause and effect.

Descriptive Research

The goal of *descriptive research* is to describe the characteristics of a selected phenomenon (Salkind, 1991). For example, the collection of data for purposes of establishing normative values on tests of central auditory function could be considered descriptive research. In this type of study, the investigator is merely collecting information (in the form of performance on selected tests) from a group of subjects, and then describing the characteristics of the group's performance, without comparing the results to the findings from another group. Statistical formulas used in descriptive research design, including the mean and standard deviation, will be discussed later in this chapter.

Correlational Research

Correlational research helps to determine if and how two or more variables are related to one another, without implying cause and effect. In addition, correlational research is useful in making predictions based

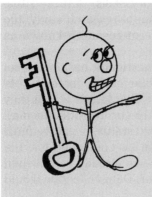

KEY CONCEPT

A significant correlation between two or more variables indicates that the variables are related; however, cause and effect cannot be inferred from the results of correlational analysis.

upon relationships among variables. For example, a study may be undertaken to determine the relationship between articulatory disorders (as measured by performance on a standardized test of articulation) and auditory closure deficits (as measured by performance on a monaural low-redundancy speech task). Results may show that, indeed, articulation disorders and auditory closure deficits are positively correlated. However, it should not be assumed that one factor (e.g., a deficit in auditory closure) causes the other (e.g., articulation disorder). Instead, **this information can be used only to document an association between the two variables and not to determine cause and effect.**

Historical Research

Historical research is primarily concerned with describing the nature of events that have occurred in the past for the purpose of examining trends in data. To perform historical research, the investigator can use historical documents, journal articles, and personal interviews, among other tools, in order to perform data collection activities. For example, an investigator may wish to determine the effectiveness of a screening program for CAPD that has been in place over the past year. The investigator might review the records of the past year to determine the number of children who, after having "failed" the screening and been referred on for comprehensive central auditory assessment, actually exhibited a central auditory processing disorder. The information obtained might be used to modify the screening protocol so that the number of inappropriate referrals is decreased, or it might serve to confirm that the majority of children referred did, indeed, exhibit a CAPD.

The types of research discussed in this section are summarized in Table 11-2.

Final Considerations Regarding the Scientific Method

To summarize, the scientific method is a system of asking and answering questions. The question itself will determine the ultimate form the research design takes. By undertaking studies in which variables are carefully controlled and questions are asked in ways that allow for measurable data to be collected and analyzed, information regarding cause and effect, relationships among variables, characteristics of a phenomenon, and past trends can be obtained.

Table 11-2
Overview of Types of Research

Type	Description
Experimental	Goal: to determine the effect of a given variable on the outcome variable. Clinician has control over the treatment variable and the assignment of subjects to groups.
Causal-Comparative	Goal: same as experimental; however, clinician has no control over the treatment variable and the assignment of subjects to groups.
Descriptive	Goal: to describe the characteristics of a selected phenomenon.
Correlational	Goal: to determine if and how two or more variables are related. Cause and effect cannot be inferred from the results of correlational research.
Historical	Goal: to describe the nature of events that have occurred in the past for the purpose of examining trends in data.

It should be emphasized, however, that answers obtained through the use of the scientific method should be considered tentative, and the reliability of findings depends upon such factors as control of extraneous variables, how representative the chosen sample is of the target population, and the methods chosen to investigate the topic. Even in cases of exceptional research design and variable control, results of any research study should be regarded as subject to change if new information becomes available that suggests the necessity of such a change. **Investigators should avoid at all times the tendency to consider the results of any study or series of studies as absolute fact and should be willing to modify their own hypotheses if subsequent evidence should cast doubt upon them.** Finally, rather than expecting an unequivocal answer to research questions, investigators should realize that the ultimate result of scientific inquiry is the generation of new questions and new directions for further research.

Basic Statistical Procedures

After data are collected, they must be organized and analyzed. It is the topic of statistical analysis, and the unavoidable mathematical formulas that go along with statistics, that turn many would-be scientists away from the fascinating realm of research. However, armed with a little understanding and a calculator or computer, many of the most commonly used statistical procedures can be performed with very little effort.

This section will describe several common statistical procedures used to analyze data for the purpose of answering research questions. It should be noted that a variety of computer programs exist that will perform the statistical procedures discussed here with a mere click of the mouse. Formulas will be provided for the first two categories of statistical procedures, measures of central tendency and measures of variability, as these procedures are likely to be used frequently in clinical practice and can be performed with very little effort by clinicians. Other statistical procedures that will be discussed in this section include tests of significance and measures of association.

Measures of Central Tendency

Measures of central tendency are designed to indicate the individual value that is in some way representative of the group of scores or values obtained. There are three measures of central tendency:

(a) the *mean*, which is the sum of the scores divided by the total number of scores. The mean is commonly referred to as the average, and can be computed using the following formula:

$$\overline{X} = \frac{\Sigma X}{n}$$

where $\overline{X}$ = mean
Σ = sum
X = individual score
n = number of scores in the sample

(b) the *median*, which is the score in a distribution above which half of the scores lie. In other words, the median represents the midpoint in a group of scores. The median can be computed simply by ordering the scores from lowest to highest value, counting the number of scores, and choosing that score which occurs at the midpoint or, in the case of an even number of scores, the average of the two middle scores. For example, for the following scores, the median value would be 14 since 3 of the scores occur below 14 and 3 occur above 14.

$$3 \quad 10 \quad 12 \quad \textcircled{14} \quad 16 \quad 25 \quad 90$$

(c) the *mode*, which is the score that occurs most frequently in a distribution. In order to compute the mode, simply look at the values and determine which score occurs more often than the others. For example, for the following distribution, the mode would be 10 since it occurs three times.

$$3 \quad 8 \quad \boxed{10} \quad 11 \quad 5 \quad \boxed{10} \quad 4 \quad 5 \quad \boxed{10} \quad 9 \quad 6$$

For purposes of descriptive statistics, it is the median, or average, that will likely be the most common measure of central tendency used.

Measures of Variability

As previously mentioned in this chapter, variability refers to the spread or dispersion of scores in a sample. It can also be thought of as the degree to which the scores differ from a measure of central tendency, usually the mean. The two most commonly used measures of variability for our purposes are the range and the standard deviation.

The *range* is simply the difference between the highest and lowest scores in the distribution. Therefore, in the following example, the range would be 10 – 4, or 6.

$$4 \quad 5 \quad 7 \quad 9 \quad 10$$

The *standard deviation* represents the average amount that each individual score differs from the mean. The larger the standard deviation, the more variability exists in the sample. The standard deviation can be computed using the following formula:

$$SD = \sqrt{\frac{\Sigma(X - \bar{X})}{n - 1}}$$

where SD = standard deviation
Σ = sum
$\bar{X}$ = mean
X = individual score
n = number of scores in the sample

The standard deviation is particularly important in the development of normative values. **For most tests of central auditory processing, performance is considered to be within normal limits if it falls within 1 to 2 standard deviations of the mean.** The decision regarding which value to use is based on the overall variability of the sample. If the choice of 1 standard deviation for the determination of "normal

Table 11-3
Procedure for Establishing Clinic-Specific Normative Values for a Test

Step One
  Choose appropriate subjects, making sure to match for age and controlling for confounding variables. Number of subjects should be no less than thirty.
Step Two
  Administer test, making sure to keep test conditions uniform across subjects.
Step Three
  Score test using the appropriate scoring methods for the given assessment tool.
Step Four
  Calculate mean and standard deviation of scores from the sample.
Step Five
  Determine normal cutoff value. For example, if 2 standard deviations below the mean is determined to be the appropriate cutoff value, use the following formula:
  $$\text{Cutoff} = \text{Mean} - (\text{Standard Deviation} \times 2)$$

cutoff" means that several of the scores obtained from the normative sample would "fail" the test, then it would be more prudent to use 2 standard deviations for interpretive purposes. On the other hand, if the scores in the sample for a given test are very close together, 1 standard deviation may be sufficient for determining the normal cutoff.

The procedure for establishing normative values for a given test of central auditory processing is outlined in Table 11-3, and involves choosing an appropriate sample (controlling for age and other variables as discussed previously in this chapter), administering the test and obtaining individual scores, computing the standard deviation, and determining the minimum value necessary for performance on the test to be considered "within normal limits."

Tests of Significance

The concept of significance was discussed earlier in this chapter, and involves determining the probability of whether a given finding can be attributed to chance. There are numerous tests of significance that can be used; however, the most common are the *t* test and analysis of variance.

The *t* test is designed to determine whether scores for two groups are significantly different. For example, in the example previously provided in this chapter in which the effect of phoneme training on Low-Pass Filtered Speech performance was being compared to the effect of no training on the same task, the scores obtained from Group A (therapy) could be compared to Group B (no therapy), and the probability of the presence of a significant difference between the groups could be determined using a *t* test for statistical significance.

Analysis of variance (ANOVA) (or *F* test) is similar to the t test, except that it is designed for use with more than two groups. The use of ANOVA in statistical analysis can determine whether significant differences exist overall in the means of three or more different groups.

Suppose that an investigation were designed to investigate the effects of three different types of therapeutic activities for a given disorder. In this example, there would be three experimental groups, one for each type of therapy. To determine if a difference exists among post-therapy scores obtained from the three groups, ANOVA could be utilized. A word of caution is warranted here: a finding of significance on analysis of variance indicates only that a significant difference exists *somewhere* in the groups, but does not suggest that all three groups are significantly different from each other. In order to determine relative differences, the data must be more closely scrutinized using additional analysis procedures.

Again, it should be emphasized that the two tests of significance discussed herein are offered merely as representative samples. A variety of significance tests can be used to analyze limitless combinations of data.

Measures of Association

Measures of association are intended to determine relationships, or correlation, among variables. As discussed previously, measures of association result in a correlation coefficient, or an indicator of the strength and direction of a relationship between two variables. Probably the most commonly utilized index of association, or correlation, in the field of communication disorders is the Pearson product-moment correlation coefficient (Pearson *r*), which is an indicator of relationship between two continuous variables. For example, in order to determine the relationship between a sample's performance on a test of auditory closure and a test of articulation, the Pearson r may be the statistical procedure of choice.

This section has provided readers with methods of computing measures of central tendency and variability, and has briefly reviewed tests of significance and measures of association in an attempt to dispel some of the mystery and confusion that surround the entire topic

Table 11-4

Overview of Basic Statistical Procedures

Procedure	Description
Measures of Central Tendency	Designed to indicate a value that is, in some way, representative of a group of scores. Includes the mean (average), median (the score above which half of the scores lie), and the mode (the score that occurs most frequently).
Measures of Variability	Indicates spread or dispersion of scores in a sample. Includes the range (difference between highest and lowest scores), and the standard deviation (the average amount that each score differs from the mean).
Tests of Significance	Determines the probability of whether a given finding was due to chance. Includes the t test (determines whether scores for two groups are significantly different) and ANOVA (designed for use with more than two groups).
Measures of Association	Indicates relationships or correlation among variables.

of statistical analysis. For further information regarding specific tests of significance and association, as well as the myriad of other statistical procedures that can be utilized for data analysis, readers are referred to their area bookstores or public libraries, where large numbers of statistical manuals can be found. The information presented in this section is summarized in Table 11-4.

Meeting the Research Challenge

The arena of CAPD holds unlimited opportunities for clinicians wishing to contribute to the general bank of knowledge by engaging in research activities. Further study is needed in virtually all CAP-related areas, from identification to management and everything in between, and many of these topics lend themselves particularly well to studies conducted in the clinical setting. In this text, I have mentioned the need for research in treatment efficacy, an area plagued by a paucity of empirical data. Perhaps no other topic in the field of CAPD is in greater need of clinician involvement in research design and data collection than the study of the efficacy of methods of CAPD management and treatment.

Treatment efficacy is not the only research area in which clinician involvement could contribute significantly to the understanding of CAPD. In Chapter 7, I discussed several subprofiles of CAPD. Although there are some data to support the use of these, or similar, subprofiles—data that have been collected in collaboration with clinicians throughout the world and that have led to the revision and clarification of these subprofiles since the publication of the first edition of this text—this approach to CAPD categorization remains largely theoretical at the present time. What is needed are large-scale correlational or factorial studies in which results of performance on tests of central auditory processing are considered along with measures of cognition, academic achievement, language, and social/emotional function. Further, the neurophysiologic representation of speech and nonspeech stimuli should also be studied in these same children through the use of electrophysiologic measures. Clinicians have access to the large numbers of children and the types of multidisciplinary data required for such a large-scale collaborative effort. Therefore, clinician involvement is critical for ultimately defining CAPD and for determining the real-world implications of basic science findings in the field.

Causative factors contributing to the development of CAPD in children is another area of need for further study. When a child is diagnosed as exhibiting CAPD, the next question is invariably, "Why?" The possible contribution of various pre- and postnatal conditions, maternal or paternal drug or alcohol use, and a variety of other factors that contribute to the incidence of CAPD in children needs to be examined closely.

And, speaking of incidence, it was mentioned in Chapter 4 that the actual incidence of CAPD in the school-age population is currently unknown. Studies need to be undertaken to determine the incidence of CAPD in the regular educational population as well as in the learning-disabled population, studies that will require large numbers of children available only to those investigators with access to the schools.

Regarding assessment, further research needs to be conducted into the development of assessment tools for very young children, and valid, reliable screening procedures for all ages. Predictors of future CAPD problems in the very young child need to be identified, and methods of assessment for the hearing-impaired and other hard-to-test populations need to be investigated and developed.

Further research needs to be done in the area of CAP assessment as well. Performance on central auditory tests needs to be compared to performance on similar tests within other modalities in order to determine the modality-specificity of the tests currently in use (Cacace & McFarland, 1998; McFarland & Cacace, 1995). Reliability of several of the test tools discussed in this book needs to be investigated more fully in the school-age population, as do relationships among these test tools and both the underlying neurophysiologic representations of acoustic stimuli and higher-order function on tests of cognition, academic achievement, language, social/emotional function, and related sequelae. New tests also need to be developed that will help us define the auditory capabilities of children with CAPD more accurately.

These are only a few of the CAP-related areas in which further research is indicated, and in which clinicians in the educational setting can and should become involved. For, when considering assessment and management of CAPD in the educational setting, it is the clinicians in that very setting who ultimately must generate the data that remain so badly needed within the area of central auditory processing and its disorders.

Summary

This chapter has provided readers with a brief introduction to various facets of scientific research, including terminology, types of research designs, and basic statistical procedures. In addition, the need for clinician involvement in CAP-related research was emphasized. It is my strongly held view that, unless and until clinicians within the educational setting become involved in asking and answering questions related to CAPD, the area of CAPD in children will remain as much a mystery as it is today.

This chapter, while barely touching upon the research-related topics selected for inclusion, should at least serve the function of whetting the appetites of clinicians in the educational setting for confronting the challenges of the unknown and embarking on the journey toward knowledge. In this great, uncharted frontier of CAPD, it is the clinicians who quest for enlightenment and pattern their activities accordingly who have the opportunity to map the territory and light the way for the rest of us.

Review Questions

1. What are some benefits that clinicians may enjoy by functioning in the dual role of scientists and practitioners?

2. How does the scientific method apply to everyday clinical activities?

3. Define the following terms:

   data   variable
   independent variable   dependent variable
   sample   inferential method
   variability   significance
   correlation

4. Regarding samples, what factor(s) helps to determine the degree to which the results of a study can be generalized to the population as a whole?

5. Contrast the concept of statistical significance with that of clinical significance.

6. What is the fundamental difference between negative and positive correlations?

7. List and define the four types of research discussed in this chapter.

8. How do experimental and causative-comparative research differ?

9. Using the following fictitious scores, compute the mean of the sample:

95	74	83	85	89	99
68	93	92	88	82	87
99	86	88	99	65	77
76	74	89	75	99	92
94	95	89	90	90	92

10. What is the median of the above sample? What is the mode?

11. What is the purpose of tests of significance?

12. How do t tests and ANOVA (F tests) differ from one another?

13. What is the primary purpose of measures of association or correlation?

APPENDIX

Answers to Review Questions

Chapter One

1. *sagittal:* A cut dividing the brain into right and left sides.
   coronal: A cut dividing the brain into front and back sections.
   horizontal: A cut dividing the brain into upper and lower portions.
   transverse: A cut that is diagonal to the horizontal plane.
   anterior: Toward the front.
   posterior: Toward the back.
   rostral: Toward the head and away from the tail.
   caudal: Toward the tail and away from the head.
   lateral/distal: Away from the midline.
   medial/proximal: Toward the midline.
   dorsal: Toward the back.
   ventral: Toward the belly.
2. **a.** *central sulcus:* The fissure or valley that separates the frontal and parietal lobes.
   b. *frontal lobe:* This lobe lies posterior to the central sulcus and anterior to the occipital lobe. The primary motor cortex is located along the posterior portion of the frontal lobe.

c. *lateral (Sylvian) fissure:* This sulcus marks the superior boundary of the temporal lobe.

d. *occipital lobe:* The occipital lobe makes up the posterior-most portion of each cerebral hemisphere. The primary and secondary visual cortices are located here.

e. *temporal lobe:* This lobe is located inferior to the frontal and parietal lobes and anterior to the occipital lobe. It contains the primary auditory cortex, portions of the auditory association areas, and portions of the language association areas.

f. *parietal lobe:* This lobe lies posterior to the central sulcus and anterior to the occipital lobe. Its primary functions include perception of somatic sensation and integration for multimodality information.

g. *longitudinal fissure:* This is the sulcus or valley that separates the right and left hemispheres.

3. *limbic system:* The limbic system is responsible for providing emotional drive for various functions necessary for survival.
   ventricles: These cavities within the brain function in the production and circulation of cerebrospinal fluid.
   meninges: The meninges are three fibrous tissue layers that form a protective covering for the brain and central nervous system.

4. a. putamen
   b. external capsule
   c. caudate
   d. internal capsule
   e. claustrum
   f. globus padillus

5. Excitatory transmitters lower a postsynaptic neuron's membrane potential, allowing the cell to fire and transmit an impulse. Conversely, inhibitory neurotransmitters elevate the membrane potential of a neuron and make it less likely to fire.

6. The three main divisions of the brainstem are the midbrain, pons, and medulla oblongata.

7. Primary characteristics of acoustic signal encoding in the auditory nerve include sharp frequency tuning, representation of periodicities via phase-locking, tonotopic organization, adaptation, and suppression for relay to higher CANS structures. Thus, the auditory nerve serves to break down incoming signals from the cochlea into their constituent parts and relay them faithfully to higher CANS structures.

8. The three characteristics of continuous speech as listed by

Delgutte (1997) are: (1) strong vowels alternating with relatively weak consonants and resulting in an amplitude modulation at a frequency of approximately 3–4 Hz, corresponding to syllabic structure; (2) pronounced maxima that correspond to fundamental and formant frequencies; and (3) presence of both periodic (e.g., vowels, voiced consonants) and aperiodic (e.g., unvoiced consonants, fricatives) components.

9. *Cochlear nucleus (CN):* A primary function of the CN is contrast enhancement, particularly of modulations and transients (e.g., onsets) in the signal. The CN is also important for preliminary feature extraction via convergence, divergence, and differential cell responses.
    Superior olivary complex (SOC): The primary function of the SOC is coding of binaural cues via convergence and divergence from upsilateral and contralateral CN for purposes of localization, lateralization, and binaural integration.
    Lateral lemniscus (LL): The LL is the primary ascending auditory pathway. It receives both ipsilateral and contralateral projections and continues the bilateral representation from lower auditory structures.
    Inferior colliculus (IC): In the IC, further enhancement of amplitude modulations and binaural cues occurs. It is at this point in the CANS that the ascending pathway divides into primary and secondary (or diffuse) auditory systems.

10. The primary characteristics of acoustic signal encoding in the auditory thalamus include (1) serving as the primary way station for information between the brainstem and the cortex; (2) coding of stimuli with slowly changing acoustic parameters, such as vowels and syllable contrasts differing in duration; (3) additional binaural encoding; (4) further contrast and modulation enhancement; (5) complex signal encoding; (6) feature extraction; and (7) multimodality integration.

11. The *primary (cochleotopic) pathway* originates in the central nucleus of the inferior colliculus and is characterized by sharp tuning and tonotopic organization. The *diffuse (noncochleotopic) pathway* originates in the pericentral nucleus and exhibits broader frequency turning and little or no tonotopicity.

12. *supratemporal plane:* This is the upper surface of the temporal lobe. It is on the posterior portion of this area that Heschl's gyrus is located.

Heschl's gyrus: This is the primary auditory cortex, which is responsible for auditory sensation and perception.

planum temporal: This is the portion of the temporal lobe extending from Heschl's gyrus to the end of the lateral fissure. Some axonal connections between Heschl's gyrus and Wernicke's area travel along the planum temporal.

supramarginal gyrus: This gyrus curves around the posterior limit of the lateral fissure and makes up part of the auditory association cortex (Wernicke's area).

angular gyrus: Along with the supramarginal gyrus, which borders it posteriorly, the angular gyrus makes up part of the auditory association cortex (Wernicke's area).

insula: The insula, located medially to Heschl's gyrus, contains fibers responsive to acoustic stimuli. Some auditory nerve impulses arriving via the internal capsule are passed on to Heschl's gyrus by the insula.

arcuate fasciculus: This nerve fiber bundle provides communication between the auditory association cortex and Broca's area in the frontal lobe.

13.   **a.** anterior commissure
      b. rostrum
      c. genu
      d. body
      e. splenium

14.   The *corpus callosum* connects the two hemispheres of the brain and serves as the primary means of interhemispheric transfer and communication. Auditory tasks reliant on the corpus callosum include binaural hearing and localization, verbal labeling of dichotic stimuli presented to the left ear, verbal labeling of tonal patterns, auditory figure-ground abilities, phonological processing, and perception of auditory midline fusion. Multimodality tasks to which the corpus callosum contributes include language functions (linking of prosodic and linguistic information, lateralization of function, other language functions); other sensory functions (bilateral comparisons of tactile stimuli, verbal labeling of objects held in the nondominant hand, object formation, visual-spatial skills); motor functions such as bimanual and bipedal coordination; and higher-order cognitive functions, including selective and sustained attention, bilateral arousal levels, multimodality integration, and all other tasks requiring interhemispheric integration.

15.   The efferent auditory system is responsible for both excitato-

ry and inhibitory activity in the CANS. It is possible that the efferent system assists in detection of signals in noise. In addition, the olivocochlear bundle, which is the most caudal structure in the efferent auditory system, plays a role in auditory attention.

Chapter Two

1. Central auditory processes are the auditory system mechanisms and processes responsible for phenomena such as localization/lateralization, auditory discrimination, auditory pattern recognition, temporal aspects of audition, and auditory performance decrements with competing or degraded acoustic signals.

2. *Dichotic* refers to a condition in which different stimuli are presented to each ear simultaneously. *Diotic* refers to a situation in which identical stimuli are presented to both ears at the same time.

3. Kimura theorized that the contralateral pathways from the ear to the auditory cortex are stronger and more numerous than the ipsilateral pathways. For monotic stimuli, either type of pathway suffices for transmission of the signal. However, for dichotic stimuli, the contralateral pathways dominate and suppress the ipsilateral pathways. As a result, lesions in the right hemisphere or corpus callosum will result in a left-ear deficit on dichotic speech tasks, whereas lesions in the left (dominant) hemisphere will result in either a bilateral or right-ear deficit due to the contralateral processing condition that exists during dichotic listening.

4. The REA is the phenomenon in which performance for the right ear is better than that for the left ear among normal right-handed listeners during dichotic listening tasks. The REA is presumed to indicate a preexisting ear asymmetry, and provides evidence of left-hemisphere dominance for speech perception.

5. *right temporal lobe:* Lesions result in left-ear suppression or extinction.
    left temporal lobe: Lesions result in contralateral and/or bilateral suppression or extinction.
    corpus callosum: If only the anterior portion of the corpus callosum is lesioned, there will be no effect seen on dichotic listening performance. If the posterior portion is lesioned, how-

ever, left-ear extinction likely will occur during dichotic stimulation. Further, scores for the right ear may be enhanced due to a release from competition normally routed through the right hemisphere.

cochlea: Sensorineural hearing loss may affect the size and direction of the ear advantage depending on the stimuli used.

middle ear: Conductive hearing loss does not appear to affect performance on dichotic listening tasks as long as the stimuli are presented at a sufficient intensity level.

6. Temporal processing refers to the way in which the CANS deals with the time-related aspects of the acoustic signal.

7. At some level, virtually all auditory tasks are reliant on temporal processing. For example, the perception of melody in music requires perception of temporal order and frequency discrimination to determine whether the notes or chords are ascending or descending with respect to adjacent chords or notes. In speech perception, temporal processing is critical for discrimination of subtle time-based cues such as voice-onset time, minimally contrasting consonant pairs, and other spectro-temporal aspects of speech.

8. *temporal lobe:* Lesions of the right (nondominant) temporal lobe result in a bilateral deficit on temporal patterning tasks involving verbal or humming report, poor performance on two-tone ordering tasks when signals are delivered to different ears, and little or no effect on gap detection or two-tone ordering when signals are delivered to the right ear. Lesions of the left (dominant) temporal lobe result in significant contralateral and/or bilateral effects depending on the type of task, including a bilateral deficit on temporal patterning tasks involving verbal report, elevated gap detection thresholds, and poor performance on all two-tone ordering tasks.

corpus callosum: Lesions result in a bilateral deficit on temporal patterning tasks involving two or more successive stimuli when listeners are required to label verbally the stimuli.

brainstem: The effect of brainstem pathology on temporal processing is variable and depends upon the site of lesion and the type of task.

cochlea: Lesions of the cochlea do not appear to affect temporal patterning tasks when the stimulus is of sufficient intensity. Cochlear site-of-lesion may, however, result in a temporal integration function that is less steep than normal.

middle ear: Middle ear pathology resulting in conductive hearing loss has little or no impact on temporal processing.

9. Binaural interaction refers to the way in which the ears work together. This process depends primarily on the integrity of the brainstem auditory structures.

10. Auditory functions that rely on binaural interaction include localization and lateralization of auditory stimuli, binaural release from masking, detection of signals in noise, and binaural fusion.

11. The MLD is the difference in binaural masked thresholds for a signal between homophasic and antiphasic conditions. In the homophasic condition, both signal and noise are binaural and in phase, or binaural and out of phase. Consequently, both are perceived either at midline (in phase) or at the ear (out of phase). However, if one of the types of stimuli is in phase and the other is out of phase (antiphasic condition), they are perceived at different places, and the masked threshold improves. This improvement in masked threshold is the masking-level difference that occurs as a result of binaural release from masking.

> SπNπ: both signal and noise are binaural and out of phase.
> SøNø: both signal and noise are binaural and in phase.
> SπNø: signal is binaural and out of phase; noise is binaural and in phase.
> SøNπ: signal is binaural and in phase; noise is binaural and out of phase.

12. The antiphasic condition in which the signal delivered to the two ears is out of phase and the masking noise is in phase (SπNø) results in the largest MLDs. This occurs because the signal is perceived to be located at the ears while the noise is perceived to be located at midline.

13. *temporal lobe:* Lesions here may disrupt binaural perception, yet not directly affect binaural interaction. Binaural perceptual skills such as localization in the contralateral auditory field and interaural intensity differences required for lateralization may be affected.
corpus callosum: Lesions of the corpus callosum result in difficulty tracking auditory sources across the midline and generalized localization and auditory figure-ground difficulties.
brainstem: Lesions of the high brainstem have little or no effect on binaural interaction tests such as the MLD. However, gross lesions of the low brainstem will significantly disrupt all binaural interaction tasks.
cochlea: MLDs are abnormally reduced in cases involving

cochlear pathology. Localization and lateralization, on the other hand, are affected much less by cochlear pathology than by lesions occurring in other parts of the CANS. Indeed, even unilateral deafness does not necessarily destroy localization ability. There is, however, a great deal of variability in binaural interaction functions among listeners with cochlear lesions.

middle ear: Conductive hearing loss has been shown to degrade localization abilities, impair the ability to recognize speech in noise, and result in reduced MLDs. In cases of children with chronic otitis media, binaural interaction deficits may persist even after the conductive hearing loss is treated and hearing sensitivity returns to normal.

14. Multiple sclerosis causes focal lesions throughout the CANS. It slows neural transmission time, and may disrupt brainstem integration of binaural input. Individuals with multiple sclerosis may have difficulty processing interaural timing and intensity differences critical for localization of auditory stimuli, and with binaural fusion even in diotic listening conditions. Finally, individuals with multiple sclerosis are likely to exhibit reduced MLDs.

15. The speech sounds that are most vulnerable to disruption by auditory cortex dysfunction are consonants, especially stop consonants. This is because these sounds contain rapid spectro-temporal aacoustic changes that require precise cortical representation. Speech sounds with more slowly changing features, such as vowels, nasals, and glides, are not as reliant on precise temporal encoding at the level of the auditory cortex.

16. Top-down language, attention, and executive function will have a significant effect on auditory processing even at the basic sensory encoding level. Comprehension of spoken language is reliant on linguistic competence, short-term memory, familiarity with the subject matter and vocabulary, ability to attend, motivation, and a variety of other top-down factors. Even the perception of simple consonant-vowel syllables can be altered by visual input. Therefore, any definition or theory of CAPD must take into account the influence of top-down factors on sensory perception as well as the possibility that deficits in other sensory modalities may coexist with CAPD.

Chapter Three

1. The brain and spinal cord begin to develop during the third week after conception, with the appearance of the neural plate.
2. The primary cerebral lobes are clearly formed by 28 weeks gestational age.
3. *ectoderm:* gives rise to the outer skin, the nervous system (including the CANS), and the inner and outer ear.
    mesoderm: gives rise to the skeleton, including the bony structures of the middle ear, the circulatory system, and the reproductive organs.
    endoderm: gives rise to the digestive and respiratory systems.
4. The inner ear is functional and adult-like in size and structure by the end of 20 weeks gestational age. The brainstem auditory pathways are structurally complete by thirty weeks after conception.
5. Myelination is the progressive development of myelin, a sheath that insulates and protects nerve fibers and enhances the speed and efficiency of neural transmission. Myelination proceeds in a caudal-to-rostral fashion, with brainstem structures complete before the first year of age, while myelination of cortical communication areas continues until adolescence and early adulthood.
6. Dendritic branching refers to the process in which dendrites—extensions of nerve cells that transmit neural impulses—grow and branch out in different directions. This process increases the surface area available for connections with other nerve cells, with the result that more information can readily be transferred through the nervous system.
7. *ABR:* The ABR is an electrical, far-field recording of synchronous activity in the auditory nerve and brainstem in response to auditory stimuli. The ABR waveform is characterized by five to seven distinct waves that occur in the 10 msec following presentation of click or tone pip stimuli. Wave latencies, interwave intervals, and wave amplitudes reach adult values by age 2 to 3.
    MLR: The MLR is recorded in the same manner as the ABR; however, the MLR represents neural activity in the 10 to 90 msec following stimulus presentation. The MLR waveform

consists of three primary waves: Na, Pa, and Pb. Waves Na and Pa are present in nearly 100% of children by age 10 to 12. *LEP:* These are long latency, endogenous potentials which occur in response to internally generated processes related to attention to auditory stimuli. The auditory cortex is presumed to be the generator of this response. The three LEP waves, N1, P1, and P3, occur at 100, 200, and 300 msec, respectively, in adults. N1 and P2 reach adult values in adolescence. P3 latencies reach adult values in the early- to mid-teenage years.

8. Dichotic listening requires communication between the cerebral hemispheres via the corpus callosum, as well as proper functioning of both temporal lobes. In young children, a right-ear advantage (REA) is often observed on dichotic listening tasks due to incomplete myelination of the corpus callosum, which inhibits efficient interhemispheric transfer of information. The REA decreases as a function of increasing age.

9. When dichotic stimuli are less linguistically complex, the REA is less pronounced, even in the young child, and remains relatively constant with increasing age. When linguistically loaded stimuli such as sentences are utilized, however, young children exhibit a more pronounced REA which decreases with increasing age until approximately age 12.

10. Temporal processing abilities such as temporal patterning improve as a function of increasing age until approximately age 12. Gap detection thresholds appear to be adult-like by age 6 or 7, whereas temporal resolution abilities improve until age 8 to 10. While the peripheral mechanism responsible for encoding temporal aspects of the acoustic signal appear to be well developed in young children, the ability of the CANS to extract and process temporal cues improves as a function of increasing age.

11. As with dichotic listening and temporal processing, binaural interaction abilities appear to improve with increasing age. Localizing behaviors become progressively more accurate from a few months of age until approximately age 5. Integration and processing of binaural cues which occur in higher-level brainstem pathways do not reach maximum efficiency until approximately age 6. Finally, MLDs generally show an improvement in performance from infancy until age 6.

12. The ability to discriminate among all phonemes in any lan-

guage of the world is present at birth, but is mediated by experience. By 9 months of age, preferential responses are seen to those speech-sound components that occur in the native language. By one year of age, speech discrimination abilities are restricted to phonemic contrasts occurring in the native language only. Finally, the accuracy of speech-sound discrimination continues to improve until approximately age 8. Maturation of top-down factors such as attention, problem-solving, memory, and related executive abilities continues through puberty and beyond, and ongoing linguistic, cognitive, and experiential changes occur throughout the life span.

13. Performance on the majority of central auditory tests should reach adult values by age 11 or 12.

14. Abilities related to auditory processing change in a way that reflects the neuromaturation of the CANS from birth to age 12. Functioning that is normal for one stage of development or age group likely will be abnormal for a later stage or age. Therefore, age-appropriate normative data must be obtained in order to interpret performance on tests of central auditory processing accurately.

15. *Neuroplasticity* refers to the nervous system's ability to make organizational changes in response to internal and external changes. In essence, this term means that the CNS is able to form new connections as well as alter the functions that certain portions typically perform, in response to demands placed upon it.

16. Auditory deprivation may result in morphological changes within the CANS that impact auditory processing abilities. It has been shown that children with a history of chronic otitis media with effusion may exhibit reduced MLDs and difficulty hearing in noise even after PE tubes are in place and hearing sensitivity has returned to normal. These children also display abnormal ABR interwave intervals, suggesting dysfunction of structures in the brainstem. Similar results also have been seen in adults following otosclerosis-related auditory deprivation.

17. *Long-term potentiation* is the increase in synaptic activity and efficiency resulting from strong and repeated stimulation of a sensory system. It has been reported that long-term potentiation may involve an increase in nerve cell size and postsynaptic density.

18. If the nervous system has the ability to reorganize and

acquire new skills and behaviors, and if long-term potentiation represents an ability to improve neural transmission in sensory systems, then it may be hypothesized that increased auditory stimulation of inefficient CANS pathways may result in structural changes as well as concomitant functional changes such as improved auditory processing abilities.

Chapter Four

1. The purpose of screening for CAPD is to identify those children in need of further, comprehensive central auditory assessment while, at the same time, reducing the number of inappropriate referrals.

2. The four questions that should be answered by the multidisciplinary team through the screening process are: (1) Are the current evaluations sufficient in scope to address adequately the child's cognitive, academic, and speech/language abilities or strengths and weaknesses prior to addressing the issue of an auditory processing disorder? (2) Based on information obtained from the multidisciplinary team, is it likely that a CAPD exists that warrants further comprehensive auditory processing assessment? (3) Is the child able to participate in a comprehensive auditory processing assessment without the interference of confounding factors such as age, cognitive status, speech or language abilities, attention span, or others? (4) Would results of an auditory processing assessment add anything to the current management or intervention in the areas in which the child is having difficulty?

3. **a.** Prevalence of the disorder: 3–7% of school-aged children exhibit some form of learning disability. It is likely that the number of children with CAPD in this population is high, perhaps as many as half. Children in this subgroup must be properly identified if effective management is to be initiated for them.

   b. CAPD screening may help identify children in need of medical follow-up that might otherwise go undetected.

   c. CAPD screening would decrease the number of overreferrals for comprehensive central auditory evaluations.

   d. Identification of CAPD will help reduce the shopping around and anxiety on the parts of parents and children that result from efforts to identify the underlying causes of learning and listening difficulties.

    e. Identification of CAPD will allow for insightful educational planning based on individual children's auditory strengths and weaknesses.

    f. It is the audiologist's responsibility to evaluate all aspects of hearing.

4. A multidisciplinary team approach to CAPD screening provides more comprehensive information regarding the child's educational, social, communicative, cognitive, and medical characteristics than could be gathered by any one individual alone. This approach also reduces the time demand placed on any single individual and provides a more insightful answer to the question of whether additional testing is warranted.

5. *Audiologists:* manage and coordinate the screening effort and perform standard audiological evaluations in order to rule out hearing loss as a contributing factor to a given child's listening and learning difficulties.

    Speech-Language Pathologists: define children's receptive and expressive language abilities as well as oral and written language skills. Speech-language pathologists also provide results of auditory perceptual subtests of speech-language test tools.

    Educators: provide descriptive information regarding children's daily listening and learning behavior in the classroom environment. Educators also can illuminate areas of academic strengths and weaknesses for a given child.

    Psychologists: contribute information concerning children's cognitive skills and capacity for learning, help to identify attention-related disorders or emotional disturbances that may interfere with the learning process, and provide results of tests that tap auditory perceptual behaviors.

    Social Workers: responsible for reporting family dynamics, socioeconomic factors, and children's ability to socialize. This member is also the key link between school and family.

    Parents: provide information regarding family history of hearing or learning disorders, developmental milestones, auditory behaviors in the home environment, and medical history.

    Physicians: rule out pathological conditions for which medical intervention may be indicated and which may be a contributing factor to learning difficulties.

6. Although these tests may have subtests that tap auditory perceptual abilities, they seldom provide information related to the specific nature of an auditory deficit. Most of these

tests are confounded by language and other higher-level neurocognitive variables, do not provide for sufficient acoustic control, and have no documented validity in the identification of disorders of the CANS.

7. Speech-language, psychoeducational, cognitive tests that may provide valuable information to the CAP screening team may include but are not limited to:
   - Weschler Intelligence Scale for Children—Third Edition (WISC-III)
   - Woodcock-Johnson III Tests of Achievement (W-J III ACH) and Tests of Cognitive Ability (W-J III COG)
   - Auditory Discrimination Test—Second Edition (ADT)
   - Carrow Audiotory-Visual Abilities Test (CAVAT)
   - Clinical Evaluation of Language Fundamentals—Third Edition (CELF-3)
   - Comprehensive Test of Phonological Processing (CTOPP)
   - Goldman-Fristoe-Woodcock Test of Auditory Discrimination (G-F-W TAD)
   - Lindamood Auditory Conceptualization Test, Revised Edition (LAC-R)
   - The Listening Test
   - Phonological Awareness Profile
   - Phonological Awareness Test (PAT)
   - Test for Auditory Comprehension of Language—Third Edition (TACL-3)
   - Test of Auditory Perceptual Skills—Revised (TAPS-R)

8. Children with CAPD may behave as if they have a peripheral hearing loss even though hearing sensitivity is normal. In the classroom, these children are likely to perform more poorly in subjects requiring use of verbal language skills and may have difficulty with multistep directions. They may be distractible. Children with CAPD may refuse to participate in class dicussion or, conversely, may participate in a manner that indicates a lack of understanding of discussion content. They may or may not exhibit a language disorder. It is not uncommon to see decreased performance in areas such as vocabulary, sequencing, and auditory discrimination/phonemic decoding among children with CAPD. Although IQ may be normal or above normal, verbal scores often are markedly lower than performance scores, leading to a classification of "learning disability" for many children with CAPD. Music skills may be poor, but art and drawing skills often are good in these children. Overall, children with CAPD tend to show a

pattern in which skills and behaviors that rely on listening and verbal language are relatively depressed when compared to those which do not. Finally, many children with CAPD present with significant histories of chronic otitis media or family history of learning disorders. Some children with CAPD will exhibit patterns opposite of those discussed here, however. For example, children with CAPD arising from the right hemisphere may exhibit greater difficulty in nonverbal than in verbal tasks. Therefore, clinicians are cautioned not to place too much emphasis on symptom checklists as a guide to determining the likelihood of CAPD. Finally, children who exhibit *all* of the key indicators of CAPD probably do not have an underlying auditory deficit; instead, their difficulties are more likely due to a higher-order, more global processing deficit.

9   If a child is suspected of exhibiting a CAPD, but comprehensive central auditory assessment cannot be performed, first it should be acknowledged that CAPD can neither be ruled in or out. Second, although a deficit-specific management plan cannot be developed, intervention strategies that address the child's most salient complaints should be initiated.

10. The success of a CAPD screening program depends on the availability of resources for follow-through in the form of diagnostic assessment for those children for whom the need for further evaluation is indicated. The screening should be considered neither the starting place nor the end point of the assessment process. In addition, it is important to monitor the outcome of the screening program in terms of the number of children referred for screening, the number referred for comprehensive evaluation, and the number finally identified as exhibiting CAPD, in order to evaluate program efficacy. Finally, the success of any CAPD screening program depends upon the cooperative interaction among all individuals involved.

Chapter Five

1. A test battery approach to central auditory assessment is necessary because no single test is sufficient in scope to address the complexity of the CANS. Therefore, a number of tests that assess different processes should be utilized. Second, the outcome of central auditory assessment should

provide a description of children's auditory strengths and weaknesses, rather than simply indicating the presence or absence of a disorder, in order to allow for more effective, deficit-specific management. The differentiation of the site of dysfunction may influence recommendations made for management, particularly if medical referral is indicated. To identify the site of dysfunction accurately, it is critical that different tools that assess different levels of the central auditory system are used. Finally, it is the audiologist's responsibility to assess the central auditory system as part of overall hearing assessment, and a test battery approach to central auditory assessment represents the state-of-the-art in CAP evaluation and results in increased confidence in and validity of test results.

2. *false positive:* Also called a false alarm, this is a positive finding on a test when the disorder is not, in fact, present.

   false negative: Also known as a miss, this is a negative finding in a subject who does, in fact, have the disorder.

   true positive: Also referred to as a hit, this is a positive result for a subject in whom the disorder does exist, or the correct identification of the presence of a disorder.

   true negative: Also called a correct rejection, this is a negative result for a subject who does not have the disorder in question, or the correct identification of the absence of a disorder.

   sensitivity: refers to the test's ability to identify correctly the presence of a disorder. It is calculated by dividing the number of true positives (hits) by the total of true positives plus false negatives (misses).

   specificity: refers to the test's ability to identify correctly the absence of a disorder. It is calculated by dividing the number of true negatives (correct rejections) by the total of false positives (false alarms) and true negatives.

   efficiency: refers to the test's overall ability to identify both the presence and absence of a particular disorder correctly, or the overall degree of both sensitivity and specificity.

3. Reliability refers to the repeatability of test results, or the degree to which a test will yield the same results within the same test session or upon repeat testing. Procedural variables, or errors of measurement, that can affect reliability include calibration of equipment, practice effects, ceiling and floor effects, the use of too few items, and other factors directly related to the measurement being studied. Patient

variables that can affect reliability include patient age; degree and stability of peripheral hearing loss; stability of the disorder itself; overall health, attention, linguistic, and cognitive abilities; and the presence of additional, related disorders.

4. *Dichotic Digits Test:* Two digits from 1 to 10 (excluding 7) are presented to each ear simultaneously. Listeners are instructed to repeat all four digits heard. This test is sensitive to lesions of the brainstem, cortex, and corpus callosum and is relatively unaffected by peripheral hearing loss.

   Dichotic Consonant-Vowel Test: Stimuli consist of six CV segments. Different segments are presented to each ear simultaneously and subjects must choose both segments heard from a printed list. This test is sensitive to cortical lesions but does not identify laterality of dysfunction.

   Staggered Spondaic Word Test (SSW): This test involves the dichotic presentation of spondees in a manner such that the second syllable of the spondee presented to one ear overlaps the first syllable of the spondee presented to the other ear. The SSW is simple enough for use with a variety of ages and is relatively resistant to peripheral hearing loss. The SSW is sensitive to brainstem and cortical dysfunction.

   Competing Sentence Test (CST): The CST involves the dichotic presentation of sentences. Listeners are instructed to repeat the sentence heard in the target ear, while ignoring the sentence presented in the nontarget ear. This test is valuable in the investigation of neuromaturation and interhemispheric function.

   Synthetic Sentence Identification Test with Contralateral Competing Message (SSI-CCM): Stimuli consist of ten third-order approximations of English sentences. These sentences are presented to the target ear while ongoing competition in the form of continuous discourse is presented to the nontarget ear. Listeners choose which of the target sentences they hear from a printed list. This test assesses the process of binaural separation and is helpful in distinguishing brainstem from cortical pathology.

   Dichotic Sentence Identification Test (DSI): The DSI is similar to the SSI-CCM but is designed for use with hearing-impaired listeners. This test uses the SSI stimuli presented dichotically and requires listeners to choose from a printed list both sentences heard, thus tapping the process of binaural integration.

Dichotic Rhyme Test (DRT): Stimuli for this test consist of rhyming CVC words beginning with one of the stop consonants. Pairs of words differing only in the initial consonant are presented dichotically. Due to the close acoustical alignment of the stimuli, listeners hear and report only one word. This test taps the process of binaural integration and has been shown to be sensitive to dysfunction of the corpus callosum.

5. *Binaural separation:* Competing Sentences, SSI-CCM.
   Binaural integration: Dichotic Digits, Dichotic CVs, SSW, DSI, DRT.

6. *Frequency Patterns Test:* This test consists of 120 pattern sequences, each made up of three tone bursts in varying patterns of high- and low-frequency. Thirty items are presented to each ear, and listeners are required to report the pattern heard verbally (e.g., high-high-low; low-high-low). If performance in the verbal report condition is poor, listeners are then asked to hum the pattern heard, thus removing the linguistic labeling component of the task. This test is sensitive to disorders of the cerebral hemispheres and/or the corpus callosum.
   Duration Patterns Test: This test is similar to Frequency Patterns; however, the stimuli differ in terms of duration, rather than frequency. Again, subjects hum or verbally describe the pattern heard (e.g., long-short-long; short-long-short). This test is sensitive to disorders of the cerebral hemispheres and/or corpus callosum and is relatively resistant to peripheral hearing loss.
   Psychoacoustic Pattern Discrimination Test (PPDT): This test utilizes dichotically presented sequences of noise bursts or click trains. Listeners must indicate discrimination of a monaural change in the pattern by pressing a button. The PPDT is sensitive to disorders of the cerebral hemispheres.

7. Both Frequency Patterns and Duration Patterns tap the processes of discrimination (frequency or duration, respectively), temporal ordering, and linguistic labeling of auditory stimuli. The PPDT assesses temporal patterning abilities and discrimination of temporal changes in acoustic stimuli.

8. Methods of reducing the redundancy of a speech signal include low-pass filtering, in which high-frequency components of the word are filtered out; time compression, in which the temporal characteristics of a signal are altered without affecting the frequency characteristics; reverbera-

tion, which can be added to speech signals in order to reduce redundancy further; and the addition of background noise.

9. The lack of standardized test tools and material-specific normative data has resulted in conflicting findings for speech-in-noise tests. In addition, great variability is seen in speech-in-noise scores for both normal and lesioned subjects. Consequently, although speech-in-noise tests may be useful in describing auditory abilities, interpretation of results should be undertaken with caution.

10. Monaural low redundancy speech tasks assess the process of auditory closure.

11. *Rapidly Alternating Speech Perception (RASP):* In this test, speech is alternated quickly between the ears at periodic intervals. The sequential bursts fuse in the brainstem, and the target message is intelligible to normal listeners. Listeners with lesions of the low brainstem may have difficulty with this task; however, studies suggest that the RASP may not be sensitive to anything other than gross brainstem lesions.

    Binaural Fusion tests (BF): In these procedures, different portions of a signal are presented to each ear. The stimuli can be portioned via band-pass filtering with high-frequency information being delivered to one ear and low-frequency information being delivered to the other. Alternatively, CVC words can be used as stimuli, with the consonants presented to one ear and the vowels presented to the other. The test assesses listeners' ability to fuse the segmented stimuli into an intelligible whole. Research indicates that BF tasks have some limited utility in the identification of gross brainstem lesions.

    Interaural Difference Limen tasks: These procedures involve pairs of tonal stimuli that are presented to both ears simultaneously. Either the onset time or the intensity of the stimulus to one ear is manipulated relative to the other ear. Listeners are required to indicate when they perceive the signal as lateralizing to one side or the other. This type of task appears to provide some measure of brainstem integrity; however, it requires precise control of the acoustic stimuli and, therefore, its clinical availability is limited at this time.

    Masking Level Difference (MLD): This test involves the presentation of speech or tonal stimuli and noise while systematically varying the phase relationships between the ears.

The MLD examines the difference in masked thresholds of speech or tones across different phase relationships. The MLD has been shown to be sensitive to brainstem lesions.

12. In general, and with the exception of the MLD, binaural interaction tests in use today demonstrate questionable sensitivity. In addition, some tests of binaural interaction, such as interaural difference limen tasks, are difficult to administer and require more precise acoustic control of stimuli than is provided by standard audiological equipment. Finally, with the exception of the MLD, binaural interaction tests provide no more information regarding brainstem integrity than is currently available through procedures such as ABR.

13. Additional behavioral measures that may prove, with time, to be useful additions to central auditory assessment include but are not limited to parameter estimation sequential tracking (PEST) techniques for evaluating speech-sound *jnd*s, backward masking paradigms, and between-channel gap detection tests to assess temporal processing, auditory or visual continuous performance tests, and evaluation of analogous skills in other sensory modalities.

14. Electrophysiological testing can provide an objective supplement to behavioral procedures. In some cases, objective evidence of a processing disorder may be needed for legal or educational classification purposes, and electrophysiology may provide these objective data. In addition, behavioral data reflecting speech perception and other auditory processes may be provided by electrophysiological measures, particularly in hard-to-test populations. Finally, the ABR remains the most sensitive test of brainstem function in use today.

Chapter Six

1. Equipment needed for comprehensive behavioral central auditory assessment includes a two-channel audiometer, a good quality tape player or compact disc player, and a sound booth.

2. The first step in the evaluation process should be an interview with the children and accompanying caregivers to explain the evaluation procedure and to gather a thorough case history. The next step involves the actual adminstration of the selected test battery, during which children should be

monitored carefully for signs of fading attention or fatigue. Finally, assessment results should be explained to children and their caregiver(s) and preliminary recommendations for management made.

3. Because different tests of central auditory function assess different auditory processes, it is wise to include tests that tap each of these processes. The ages and cognitive ability of the children also will influence the choice of tests that will be included in the test battery, as will the desired outcome of the assessment procedure. Finally, through ongoing interpretation of test results during the assessment itself, it may be determined that additional tests need to be added to the battery in order to provide further clarification of dysfunctional areas.

4. Dichotic Digits:
   Presentation Level: 50 dB SL (re: spondee threshold) or at MCL
   Instructions: Listeners are informed that they will hear different numbers in each ear and should repeat all numbers heard.
   Scoring: Percent correct per ear
   Dichotic CVs:
   Presentation Level: 55 dBHL
   Instructions: Listeners are instructed to indicate, using a printed list, which two CV segments were heard.
   Scoring: Percent correct per ear
   SSW:
   Presentation Level: 50 dB SL (re: PTA or spondee threshold) is recommended; however, intensities as low as 25 dB SL may be used.
   Instructions: Listeners are instructed to repeat the words heard.
   Scoring: Raw SSW score indicates percentage of errors in each of four conditions (left and right competing and noncompeting), percentage of errors by ear, and total percentage of errors.
   Competing Sentences:
   Presentation Level: Target: 35 dB SL (re: PTA), Competing: 50 dB SL
   Instructions: Listeners are instructed to repeat the sentence heard in the target ear, while ignoring the message in the competing ear.
   Scoring: Percent correct per ear

SSI-CCM

Presentation Level: Primary message: 30 dB HL, Competing signal: varied from 30 to 50 dB HL

Instructions: Listeners are instructed to ignore the competing signal and to identify the sentence heard in the target ear from a printed list of items.

Scoring: Percent correct per ear

DSI:

Presentation Level: 50 dB SL (re: PTA of 500, 1000, and 2000 Hz)

Instructions: Listeners are to identify both sentences heard from a list of printed items.

Scoring: Percent correct per ear

Dichotic Rhyme Test:

Presentation Level: 50 dB SL (re: spondee threshold)

Instructions: Listeners are instructed to repeat the word that is heard.

Scoring: Percent correct per ear

Random Gap Detection Test (RGDT):

Presentation Level: 55 dB HL

Instructions: Listeners are instructed to either respond verbally or hold up the number of fingers corresponding to the number of tone stimuli heard.

Scoring: Average of gap detection thresholds for all stimuli

Frequency Patterns test:

Presentation Level: 50 dB SL (re: 1000 Hz threshold)

Instructions: Listeners should be instructed that they will hear sets of three tones that will vary in pitch, and are to describe the pattern of the tones heard in terms of high and low. When initially instructing the listeners, both visual and voiced pitch cues should be provided. Visual cues are then removed in order to ensure that listeners understand the task. In cases in which listeners perform poorly on the test, they can be instructed to hum or sing the patterns rather than label them verbally.

Scoring: Percent correct per ear

Duration Patterns test:

Presentation Level: 50 dB SL (re: 1000 Hz threshold)

Instructions: The instructions for this test are the same as for that of the Frequency Patterns test; however, listeners are instructed to label the patterns in terms of duration (e.g., long and short).

Scoring: Percent correct per ear

Low-Pass Filtered Speech:

Presentation Level: 50 to 70 dB HL

Instructions: Listeners are instructed to repeat the words heard, and to guess if unsure.

Scoring: Percent correct per ear

Time-Compressed Speech:

Presentation Level: 50 to 70 dB HL

Instructions: Listeners are instructed to repeat the words heard, and to guess if unsure.

Scoring: Percent correct per ear

SSI-ICM:

Presentation Level: Target: 30 dB HL, Competing signal: varied from 20 to 50 dB HL

Instructions: Listeners are instructed to select the target sentence heard from a printed list.

Scoring: The score is calculated by taking the average of percentages correct at 0 dB S/N and 20 dB S/N.

Band-pass Binaural Fusion:

Presentation Level: 20 dB SL (re: thresholds at 500 and 2000 Hz) for adults, and 30 dB SL for children

Instructions: Listeners are directed to repeat the words heard.

Scoring: Percent correct

Consonant-Vowel-Consonant (CVC) Fusion:

Presentation Level: 30 dB SL

Instructions: Listeners are directed to repeat the words heard.

Scoring: Percent correct

Masking Level Difference (MLD):

Presentation Level: Stimuli are presented at 16 different signal-to-noise ratios in 2 dB increments from 0 dB S/N to –30 dB S/N

Instructions: Listeners are asked to repeat the words heard.

Scoring: Thresholds are determined for both the SøNø and SπNø conditions. The MLD is calculated by determining the difference between the two thresholds.

5. The following tests may be suitable for use in cases of peripheral hearing loss: Dichotic Digits, SSW, DSI, Frequency Patterns, Duration Patterns, CVC Fusion

6. *Dichotic Digits, Dichotic CVs, SSW, DSI, DRT:* Binaural Integration

    Competing Sentences, SSI-CCM: Binaural Separation

    Frequency Patterns: Frequency Discrimination, Temporal Patterning Ordering, Linguistic Labeling

Duration Patterns: Duration Discrimination, Temporal Patterning Ordering, Linguistic Labeling
LPFS, Time Compressed Speech, SSI-ICM: Auditory Closure
Binaural Fusion, CVC Fusion, MLD: Binaural Interaction

Chapter Seven

1. The results of central auditory testing can help to answer questions related to the presence or absence of a disorder, the underlying processes affected, the site-of-dysfunction within the CANS, and the relationship of the CAPD to educational, cognitive, and communicative difficulties.
2. A lax criterion for identification of a disorder requires an abnormal finding on any single test in the battery. A strict approach demands abnormal findings on all tests utilized in order to identify the presence of a disorder positively.
3. The two components that should be present for finding the presence of a CAPD are an abnormal result on a test of central auditory processing and an indication of significant impact of the disorder upon learning or listening behavior.
4. Process-based interpretation refers to the assessment of a variety of specific auditory processes (i.e., auditory closure, binaural separation and integration, auditory temporal patterning, binaural interaction, auditory discrimination, temporal processing) with the goal of identifying areas of auditory strengths and weaknesses. This type of interpretation allows for a detailed description of children's underlying dysfunctional processes with an eye toward the development of deficit-specific management programs.
5. *Auditory Closure:* Individuals with deficits in this process may have difficulty understanding speech whenever the extrinsic redundancy of the message is reduced. They may have little or no problems understanding speech in a quiet environment; however, if the deficit is severe, even word recognition in quiet may be affected.
   Binaural Separation and Integration: As in auditory closure, a deficit in the areas of binaural separation or integration will manifest itself primarily in difficulty understanding speech-in-noise or when more than one person is talking at the same time. However, although the behavioral symptoms of auditory closure deficits and binaural separation/integration deficits are similar, the underlying processes that are dys-

functional are very different, as will be the recommendations for management.

Temporal Patterning: Individuals with deficits in temporal patterning may have difficulty in the recognition and use of prosodic aspects of speech, including the identification of key words, and subtle differences of meaning indicated by changes in stress and intonational patterns. Expressively, they may exhibit monotonic speech themselves. Finally, these individuals may have problems with sequencing critical elements, including sequencing individual sounds in words.

Binaural Interaction: The primary behavioral characteristic of a deficit in this process is difficulty in the detection of speech in a noisy background. Individuals with binaural interaction problems may also have impaired ability to localize auditory stimuli.

Temporal Processing: Temporal processing deficits have been hypothesized to cause a variety of speech, language, and learning difficulties. Because temporal processing is critical to a wide variety of auditory tasks, behavioral symptoms of temporal processing deficits may include difficulty with rapidly presented speech and auditory discrimination difficulties, among others.

Auditory Discrimination: This skill serves a vast number of auditory behaviors. Speech-sound discrimination difficulties can affect word recognition, auditory closure and speech-in-noise abilities, and many other behaviors. Children with deficits in speech-sound discrimination may behave as though they have a hearing loss, even if hearing is normal. Nonspeech auditory discrimination deficits may affect perception and use of prosodic elements of speech, music skills, and similar nonverbal abilities.

6. *Auditory Closure:* Poor performance on monaural low-redundancy speech tests and speech-in-noise tests. If the deficit is severe enough, even word recognition in quiet may be affected.

Binaural Separation and Integration: Poor performance on dichotic listening tasks. Individuals with binaural separation deficits also will perform poorly on tests of speech-in-noise.

Temporal Patterning: Poor performance on tests of temporal patterning (e.g., Frequency and Duration Patterns), in both the linguistic labeling and humming response conditions.

Binaural Interaction: Abnormally reduced MLDs, poor performance on speech-in-noise and binaural fusion tests, and abnormal ABR results.

Temporal Processing: Individuals with deficits in temporal processing typically exhibit poor performance on tests of temporal resolution, such as gap detection testing and backward masking paradigms. In addition, they may demonstrate bilateral deficits on some monaural low-redundancy speech tasks, especially those that involve time-compressed speech, and auditory discrimination tasks involving rapidly changing spectro-temporal acoustic features and/or frequency, intensity, or duration difference limens.

Auditory Discrimination: Individuals with auditory discrimination deficits may perform poorly on speech and language measures that involve phonological awareness or similar abilities. In addition, they may demonstrate bilateral deficits on tests of monaural low-redundancy speech and elevated *jnd*s for phonemes or nonverbal auditory stimuli.

7. *Auditory-Closure (Decoding):* Environmental modifications to improve access to auditory information, activities designed to improve auditory closure from phonemic to sentence levels, preteaching of new concepts and vocabulary, and frequent repetition of key messages. In addition, consonant and vowel discrimination training may be indicated.

    Binaural Separation and Integration: Environmental modifications to enhance auditory information while decreasing background noise; compensatory strategies focusing on direction of attention and selective listening.

    Temporal Patterning: Prosody training and key word extraction. Reading aloud daily with particular emphasis on intonation, stress, and rhythm characteristics of speech may help develop awareness of prosodic aspects of speech.

    Binaural Interaction: Environmental modifications to enhance access to auditory signals. Training in localization of auditory stimuli may be warranted. Additionally, the need for medical intervention should be ruled out.

    Temporal Processing: Environmental modifications focused on slowing down the speaking rate. Direct remediation activities to improve temporal resolution and related abilities.

    Auditory Discrimination: Direct therapy involving minimal contrast speech or nonspeech pairs. Environmental modifications to improve acoustic access to the speech signal. Recruitment of top-down auditory closure compensatory mechanisms.

8. When site of dysfunction has been determined through a comprehensive central auditory assessment, clinicians are better able to make informed decisions regarding the need for medical referral, and the management approach selection is likely to be more efficient. Finally, knowing the site of dysfunction facilitates monitoring the efficacy of rehabilitation in terms of tracking changes in the effects of lesions. It should be noted, however, that site of dysfunction may not be identifiable with any degree of certainty in many cases.

9. *Brainstem:* Abnormal findings on the Synthetic Sentence Identification Test with Ipsilateral Competing Message, binaural fusion, and masking-level difference are indicative of lesions in this area. Also, Dichotic Digits, SSW, Competing Sentences, and Low-Pass Filtered Speech appear to be sensitive to brainstem dysfunction. Finally, brainstem dysfunction also can be identified through abnormalities in acoustic reflex testing, speech audiometry, and auditory brainstem response testing.

    Cerebral: Left-hemisphere cerebral lesions tend to affect performance on monaural low-redundancy speech tests either bilaterally or contralaterally (i.e., right worse than left). Similarly, bilateral and/or right-ear deficits are often seen on dichotic speech tasks. Scores on Frequency and Duration Patterns testing usually are depressed when linguistic labeling is required; however, performance typically is in the normal range with a humming response. Finally, speech-sound auditory discrimination and temporal processing abilities likely will be areas of deficit for individuals with left-hemisphere lesions. In contrast, right-hemisphere lesions tend to affect Frequency and Duration Patterns testing in both the linguistic labeling and humming conditions. Left-ear deficits on dichotic speech tasks are common, and nonspeech auditory discrimination may be an area of deficit. Performance on monaural low-redundancy speech tasks, temporal processing, and speech-sound auditory discrimination is often normal for individuals with right-hemisphere lesions.

    Interhemispheric: Findings in cases of corpus callosum lesions include left-ear deficits on dichotic speech tasks and bilateral deficits on temporal patterning tasks when listeners are required to label verbally what was heard. However, performance on temporal patterning tasks tends to improve when listeners are asked to hum or sing the response.

Performance on tests of monaural low-redundancy speech is generally normal with this type of lesion.

10. *Auditory Decoding Deficit:* Children characterized in this subprofile will experience difficulty understanding speech in noise. Sound blending, discrimination, and retention of phonemes often are poor. Reading, speech-to-print skills, vocabulary, syntax, and semantic skills may be weak. These children tend to perform poorly on dichotic listening tasks and tests of monaural low- redundancy speech, with right-ear performance often worse than left-ear performance. Electrophysiology may show decreased responses over left hemisphere; MMNs may be absent to consonant-vowel contrasts but may be present to tonal stimuli. Speech-sound (especially consonant) discrimination and temporal processing abilities are likely to be poor.

Integration Deficit: Children in this subprofile may have difficulty with multimodality tasks that require interhemispheric cooperation. Binaural hearing skills may be poor, linking linguistic elements of speech with prosodic tone-of-voice cues may be an area of difficulty, and a variety of learning sequelae may be present. Children with Integration Deficit may also demonstrate difficulty with activities requiring bimanual or bipedal coordination, and may perform more poorly when the spoken message is augmented with multimodality cues. On tests of central auditory function, integration deficit is characterized by left-ear suppression on dichotic listening tasks, combined with bilateral deficits on tests of temporal patterning in the linguistic labeling condition only.

Prosodic Deficit: Children with Prosodic Deficit may have frequent misunderstandings due to difficulty perceiving humor, sarcasm, and other forms of communication that rely on subtle prosodic cues, difficulty comprehending the *intent* of communication, difficulty identifying key words in a message, and difficulty comprehending abstract communicative exchanges or topics. They may exhibit poor pragmatic and social communication abilities, poor sight word reading and spelling abilities, difficulty with nonverbal tasks, poor visual-spatial and gestalt patterning abilities, and difficulty staying on topic during conversation. Children with Prosodic Deficit may be at risk for depressive disorder secondary to right-hemisphere dysfunction, and may perform better with concrete, rather than abstract information. On tests of central auditory function, Prosodic Deficit is characterized by left-ear deficit on dichotic speech tasks combined with deficits on temporal patterning tasks in both the linguistic labeling and humming conditions. Electrophysiology may show decreased responses over right hemisphere; MMN are typically present to consonant-vowel contrasts but may be absent to tonal stimuli. Nonspeech discrimination skills may be poor. Binaural interaction, temporal processing, monaural low-redundancy speech, and speech-sound discrimination abilities are typically normal; however, some difficulty with vowel discrimination may be present.

Associative Deficit: Children in this category often exhibit receptive language deficits. Although early academic achievement may be age-appropriate, increasing linguistic demands in the classroom by approximately the third grade often precipitate general academic difficulties. Associative Deficit is characterized by the inability to apply the rules of language to incoming auditory stimuli. At its most severe, this dysfunction can result in the inability to attach linguistic meaning to phonemic units. On central auditory tests, children in this subprofile tend to exhibit bilateral deficits on dichotic listening tasks. Temporal patterning performance and speech sound discrimination usually are good; however, word recognition may be poor.

Output-Organization Deficit: This subprofile involves an impaired ability to sequence, plan, and organize responses. Children with Output-Organization Deficit may present with poor organizational skills, difficulty following directions, reversals, and poor word recall and retrieval abilities. Sequencing errors and sound blending difficulties also may be demonstrated. Children in this category may show good reading comprehension abilities, whereas writing and spelling skills may be poor due to the multi-element nature of these tasks. On central auditory testing, these children often have difficulty with any task that requires report of more than two critical elements. Therefore, performance on monaural low-redundancy speech tests may be good; however, tests such as Frequency and Duration Patterns, Dichotic Digits, Competing Sentences, and Staggered Spondaic Words likely will indicate poor performance.

11. *Auditory Decoding Deficit:* An effective management approach for this deficit may resemble traditional aural rehabilitation, including consonant and vowel training, instruction in speech to print skills, vocabulary building and other auditory

closure activities, and environmental modifications designed to enhance access to auditory information. Finally, preteaching of new information and vocabulary will increase the extrinsic redundancy of the learning environment, and repetition of key information may be helpful, but only if the repetition is clearer acoustically than the original presentation of the message.

Integration Deficit: Management approaches aimed at improving interhemispheric transfer of information are likely to be beneficial for children in this subprofile. The use of multimodality cues, unless appropriately implemented, may be contraindicated for individuals with Integration Deficit.

Prosodic Deficit: Management for children with Prosodic Deficit should include placement with animated teachers who make generous use of prosodic cues and multimodality augmentation, avoidance of "hinting" and abstract communications, and reading aloud with exaggerated prosodic features. Direct remediation to address prosody and temporal patterning training may be indicated. Compensatory strategies should include social communication and judgment intervention, role-playing activities, and other tasks directed at comprehension of underlying intent and topic maintenance. Children with Prosodic Deficit may also require intervention from other professionals, including possible psychological counseling.

Associative Deficit: Management approaches for children with Associative Deficit should include elements of speech-language intervention. Metacognitive techniques aimed at strengthening the memory trace associated with item recall are helpful. Further, preteaching of new information and the imposition of external organization within the classroom are appropriate classroom-based strategies. Finally, frequent checks for understanding should be made by asking children to paraphrase or demonstrate what is expected, rather than requesting simple repetition of instructions. Repetition is rarely effective for a child with Associative Deficit. Instead, information should be rephrased using simpler language and smaller linguistic units.

Output-Organization Deficit: As with Associative Deficit, children with Output-Organization Deficit likely will benefit from intervention designed to aid in the development of organizational skills. Speech-language intervention often is indicated for remediation of the expressive language component found in this subprofile. Finally, both repetition and rephrasing of key information may be useful for the child with Output-Organization Deficit, but only if the message and required response are broken down into linguistic units of no more than two critical elements.

12. The most important factor to look for when attempting to differentially diagnose CAPD and other disorders is the presence of *patterns* indicative of dysfunction in auditory areas of the brain. Thus, for example, the ability to differentially diagnose AD/HD and CAPD is dependent on one's familiarity with the diagnostic indicators of the two disorders. Children with AD/HD typically do not show patterns of performance on behavioral tests of central auditory function that are consistent with dysfunction in an underlying CANS region (or adjacent CANS regions) or that suggest a particular subprofile of CAPD. Children with AD/HD most often do poorly on all tests administered, or may perform normally on behavioral central auditory test batteries, particularly if the AD/HD is being controlled for. Cognitive disorders are conceptualized as higher-order, supramodal disorders that affect function across sensory modalities. Therefore, the presence of relatively equally developed skills across language, auditory visual, motor, and related areas would argue against CAPD as the primary diagnosis. CAPD does not underlie more pervasive, higher-order disorders. Instead, the auditory difficulties should be considered a symptom rather than a cause of the cognitive deficit. CAPD can and does coexist with hearing loss in some children, and certainly in aging adults. It is important to realize that there are several issues to consider when testing a child with a hearing loss for CAPD, particularly when we know that peripheral hearing dysfunction changes the input provided to the CANS for processing and thereby affects the structural and functional reorganization of the central auditory pathways. When evaluating a child with a hearing loss for CAPD, clinicians should be aware that the hearing loss may affect the central test results. Therefore, clinicians must be careful in analyzing the results and look for specific deficiencies in those applicable tests in order to give appropriate treatment plans for management. Finally, there are very few tests of central auditory function that are appropriate for use with children younger than approximately age 7, not only due to their abilities to participate in the testing but also due to the variability in brain function and maturation. Therefore, it is

essential that we attempt to estimate, as accurately as possible, the type or types of auditory deficit that may be present. It is important to use the information from the multidisciplinary team accumulated during the screening process to look for patterns of strengths and weaknesses that may be indicative of a specific subtype of CAPD or a combination of subtypes.

13. At present, there is no evidence at present to support modality-specific memory or attention. Although different types of memory have been shown to have distinct neurophysiologic substrates, these memory categories are delineated on the basis of type of information, not whether the information is presented visually, auditorily, or through another modality. Similarly, attention is a more global top-down deficit that is not sensory-modality-specific and thus cannot be described as affecting only one sensory system, such as audition. Therefore, because both memory and attention are not sensory-modality-specific, these terms cannot effectively be used to describe or discuss CAPD. Instead, it is more likely that the presence of bottom-up auditory processing difficulties leaves little energy for attending to or remembering auditory information, thus creating the appearance of "auditory memory" or "auditory attention" deficits in children with CAPD.

Chapter Eight

1. The three main categories of CAPD management in the educational setting are (a) environmental modifications and classroom-based strategies designed to improve the child's access to auditory information; (b) remediation techniques designed to provide direct intervention for deficit areas; and (c) compensatory strategies designed to teach the child how to overcome residual dysfunction and maximize the use of auditory information.

2. The clinician should be cautious when asked to make "general recommendations" for all children with CAPD, as some suggestions will not be appropriate for children with certain types of auditory deficits. However, the following suggestions are helpful for all listeners in general: reduction in or elimination of adverse noise sources, education of significant individuals regarding listening and the nature of auditory disor-

ders, and optimization of the learning environment based on the individual child's needs.

3. *Auditory Decoding Deficit:* Environmental modifications and classroom-based management strategies for children with Auditory Decoding Deficit may include use of an assistive listening device, preferential seating, employment of multimodality cues, repetition, provision of a notetaker or recoding information in pictorial form, general suggestions for improving S/N ratio, preteaching new information/vocabulary, checking frequently for comprehension, gaining attention, use of positive reinforcement, and avoidance of auditory fatigue.

Prosodic Deficit: Environmental modifications and classroom-based management strategies for children with Prosodic Deficit may include placement with an "animated" teacher, preferential seating, employment of multimodality cues, repetition or rephrasing (but only if prosodic cues are made more perceptually salient), provision of a notetaker, general suggestions for improving S/N ratio, preteaching new information/vocabulary, checking frequently for comprehension, gaining attention, use of positive reinforcement, and avoidance of auditory fatigue.

Integration Deficit: Environmental modifications and classroom-based management strategies for children with Integration Deficit may include use of an assistive listening device, repetition, provision of a notetaker, general suggestions for improving S/N ratio, preteaching new information/vocabulary, checking frequently for comprehension, gaining attention, use of positive reinforcement, and avoidance of auditory fatigue.

Associative Deficit: Environmental modifications and classroom-based management strategies for children with Associative Deficit may include preferential seating, employment of multimodality cues, rephrasing using smaller linguistic units, provision of a notetaker or recoding information into pictorial form, general suggestions for improving S/N ratio, preteaching new information/vocabulary, checking frequently for comprehension, gaining attention, use of positive reinforcement, and avoidance of auditory fatigue.

Output-Organization Deficit: Environmental modifications and classroom-based management strategies for children with Output-Organization Deficit may include preferential seating, employment of multimodality cues, rephrasing using smaller linguistic units, provision of a notetaker, and general suggestions for improving S/N ratio, preteaching new information/vocabulary, checking frequently for comprehension, gaining attention, use of positive reinforcement, and avoidance of auditory fatigue. In particular, methods of enhancing organizational skills will be of great benefit.

4. Compensatory strategies useful for children with CAPD include metalinguistic, metacognitive, and linguistic strategies designed to aid children in actively monitoring and self-regulating their own comprehension abilities and developing general problem-solving skills. Included are metacognitive skills (active listening techniques, self-instruction and reauditorization, self-regulation and problem solving, self-reflection and journaling), metamemory strategies (chunking, elaboration, recoding information, setting auditory information to music, verbal rehearsal), and linguistic/metalinguistic strategies (training in the rules of language, discourse cohesion and other formal schema induction, content schema induction).

5. Children with CAPD tend to be passive rather than active listeners. Steps need to be taken to increase children's internal motivation to implement compensatory strategies and other management suggestions, thus returning the locus of control back to the student. In this way, children take responsibility for their own listening behavior and are able to self-monitor and problem-solve in cases in which comprehension is troublesome. Only through the inclusion of children as active participants in their own management program will the success of that program be ensured.

Chapter Nine

1. Three primary assumptions underlie the rationale for deficit-specific CAPD intervention. They are (1) fundamental auditory mechanisms and processes underlie and are important to more complex listening, learning, and communication behaviors; (2) we are able, at present, to isolate and identify those processes that are dysfunctional in a given child; and (3) improvement in fundamental auditory processes will lead to concomitant improvement in functional listening, learning, and communication behaviors.

2. *Auditory Closure Activities:* These activities focus on the use of context to fill in missing elements of a message. They may

include a variety of missing word/syllable/phoneme exercises, speech-in-noise training, and context-based vocabulary building. Auditory closure activities are particularly appropriate for children with Auditory Decoding Deficit.

Binaural Separation/Integration Activities: These activities are designed to improve message comprehension in the presence of competing messages, and may include both dichotic listening training and localization training. They are most appropriate for children with Integration Deficit.

Temporal Patterning Activities: Temporal patterning activities focus on auditory pattern recognition and sequencing. They may include either basic temporal patterning skills (such as identification, discrimination, or imitation of auditory patterns that differ in rhythm or stress) as well as higher-level prosody training activities. These activities are most appropriate for children with Prosodic Deficit.

Auditory Discrimination and Temporal Processing Activities: Auditory discrimination activities can use either speech or nonspeech stimuli. Speech-sound (phoneme) discrimination training is most appropriate for children with Auditory Decoding Deficit. Speech-to-print skills should also be included to improve word-attack reading and spelling abilities. Nonspeech discrimination training, including difference limens for frequency, intensity, and duration, and discrimination of direction of tonal glides, may be indicated for children with Prosodic Deficit. Finally, temporal processing activities to bolster temporal resolution abilities, including gap detection and flutter fusion tasks, may be most appropriate for children with Auditory Decoding Deficit who demonstrate elevated temporal gap detection thresholds or other signs of dysfunctional processing of very fine temporal aspects of audition.

Interhemispheric Exercises: These activities require the two hemispheres of the brain to work cooperatively, and can consist of linguistic or nonlinguistic activities. Examples include grab-bag games in which verbal report of objects held in the left hand is required, piano or other music lessons, video games requiring auditory/visual integration and bimanual coordination, sports activities requiring bimanual and bipedal coordination, singing or listening to music with an eye toward comprehension of the lyrics, and any other activity that requires interhemispheric transfer.

3. Management approaches appropriate for very young chil-

dren could include virtually any activity used with older children. Phoneme training, reading aloud with selective listening goals, interhemispheric exercises, "guess the emotion" games to identify prosodic cues, and games designed to improve direction-following skills can all be fun and useful for very young children suspected of exhibiting CAPD.

4. **a.** Yes. Johnny appears to exhibit deficits in the areas of binaural separation, binaural integration, and linguistic labeling of tonal patterns. When taken in combination, this pattern suggests a deficit in the interhemispheric transfer of auditory information.

   b. Integration Deficit.

   c. Environmental modifications: Possible use of assistive listening device, repetition of key information, provision of a notetaker, preteach new information/vocabulary, check frequently for comprehension. Avoid use of multimodality cues if their addition confuses Johnny. Similarly, allow for preferential seating away from visual cues if he seems to do better that way. Compensatory strategies: Attribution training, choose from metalinguistic, metacognitive, and metamemory strategies appropriate for Johnny's functional difficulty areas. Recoding information in pictorial form will probably not be a beneficial memory strategy for Johnny. Direct remediation activities: Interhemispheric exercises, dichotic listening training, localization training.

5. Yes. Mary appears to be exhibiting a primary deficit in auditory closure, especially for rapid speech. It would be interesting to see Mary's performance on more fine-grained auditory discrimination and temporal processing tests. Dichotic listening findings may be reflective of a left-hemisphere site of dysfunction rather than specific binaural separation/integration difficulties per se.

   b. Auditory Decoding Deficit.

   c. Environmental modifications: Use of assistive listening device, preferential seating, employment of multimodality cues, repetition (not rephrasing) of key information, provision of a notetaker or recoding information in pictorial form, preteaching new information/vocabulary, and other general strategies to enhance motivation and avoid auditory fatigue. Compensatory strategies: Active listening techniques and attribution training will be very beneficial. Choose from metalinguistic, metacognitive, and metamemory strategies appropriate for Mary's functional difficulty areas. Direct remediation activities: Auditory closure activities, phoneme discrimination and speech-to-print skills, temporal processing training if needed.

6. **a.** Yes. Fred's test results suggest a deficit in binaural separation and integration. However, his other findings indicate that his dichotic listening performance may be the result of a more generalized left-hemisphere involvement not affecting primary auditory cortex. Therefore, determination of a precise auditory process/mechanism that is dysfunctional is difficult.

    b. Associative Deficit.

    c. Environmental modifications: These should be programmed to fit Fred's particular academic complaints. It will be very important for Fred's teacher to rephrase information using smaller linguistic units. Compensatory strategies: Strategies designed to train metalinguistic skills, including rules of language, discourse cohesion devices, and formal/content schema induction, will likely be of great benefit for Fred. Other strategies may be chosen as needed as well. Direct remediation activities: Speech-language intervention for receptive language difficulties is indicated.

7. **a.** Yes. Alex exhibits deficits in the area of auditory temporal patterning. Secondary deficits appear to be apparent in binaural separation/integration; however, dichotic listening findings may be indicative of right-hemisphere involvement when taken in combination with temporal patterning findings.

    b. Prosodic Deficit.

    c. Environmental modifications: Placement with an "animated" teacher, preferential seating, employment of multimodality cues, repetition or rephrasing of key information (only if prosodic cues are rendered more perceptually salient), provision of a notetaker, and general recommendations related to maximizing S/N ratios, making frequent checks for comprehension, and providing positive reinforcement. Recoding information in pictorial format would probably not be a good strategy for Alex. Compensatory strategies: In particular, content schema induction may be indicated to improve Alex's interpretation of social situations. Active listening techniques and attribution training will probably be of value, as will methods of enhancing Alex's memory trace and improving sequencing. Direct remediation activities: Prosody training, temporal patterning training, nonspeech discrimination activities. In addition, speech-language intervention may be needed for pragmatic and social language concerns. Finally, Alex should be evaluated for the need for possible intervention by other professionals, including psychologic counseling.

8. **a.** Yes. Lexy exhibits a deficit confined to binaural separation of auditory information.

   b. It is difficult to place Lexy within a specific subprofile of CAPD, as she exhibits only one isolated (albeit significant) finding on central auditory testing. If pressed, it is likely that Lexy falls loosely within the category of Integration Deficit based on her functional complaints. However, that cannot be determined at the present time.

   c. Intervention should be designed that specifically addresses message comprehension in the presence of competing signals. Thus, dichotic listening training is indicated, as are many of the environmental modifications and compensatory strategies that enhance the ability to attend to and/or hear the signal in noisy or competing environments.

9. **a.** No. Caleb appears to exhibit deficits in all processing areas, which is highly suggestive of a higher-order, more global cognitive or attention confound.

   b. Caleb does not exhibit characteristics of a CAPD subprofile. Instead, his test findings and behavioral sequelae are highly suggestive of a possible attention confound.

   c. Caleb should undergo follow-up and evaluation for possible attention or other higher-level deficit. In the meantime, compensatory strategies to improve active listening behaviors and attribution training may be useful behavioral management tools for Caleb.

Chapter Ten

1. Education of key individuals involved in CAP service delivery will serve to inform them of the current issues surrounding the topic of CAPD in the educational setting, and to help ensure their cooperation in the service delivery effort. In addition, education of these individuals will delineate each person's role and expected contribution to the effort, and

facilitate provision of quality identification and follow-through services.

2. *Audiologists:* Key topics important in the education of the audiologist include specific training in the scientific under-pinnings of central auditory processing; practical application of scientific theory; identification, assessment, and management issues; and time management.

   Speech-Language Pathologists: Speech-language pathologists will benefit from education in the areas of appropriate methods of diagnosing CAPD, as well as implementation of CAPD management approaches.

   Educators: Classroom and special education teachers likely will be particularly interested in information regarding the educational impact of CAPD and methods of CAPD management, particularly classroom-based management techniques.

   Psychologists: Psychologists will require information regarding appropriate methods of diagnosing CAPD, as well as the need for their contribution of information regarding cognitive capacities and psychoeducational abilities of the child in question. In addition, a discussion of the neurophysiological bases of CAPD should be included in any educational program aimed at psychologists.

   Parents: Parents of children with CAPD should be informed as to the general nature of CAPD, types of management approaches useful for children with CAPD, and prognosis for success.

   Private Practitioners: Private practitioners and other physicians will need specific education regarding appropriate methods of diagnosing CAPD and the need for diagnosticians to work closely with educational personnel in the assessment and management process.

3. Components of any diagnostic CAP report should include background information, results of audiological evaluation, results of central auditory assessment, impressions, and recommendations for management or follow-up.

4. If results of a central auditory assessment yield no significant findings, clinicians should state clearly in the diagnostic report that the presence of a CAPD is not likely in those areas specifically assessed. In this manner, readers can be led to the understanding that auditory difficulties may exist in areas not specifically addressed by the evaluation process.

5. The use of handouts in imparting CAP-related information

will allow clinicians to provide detailed information regarding management activities and other CAP-related topics, while saving valuable time that might otherwise be used in the repetitive relay of the same information to multiple sources.

6. A child study is a meeting in which all of the key service providers involved in the education of a given child are brought together to discuss educational options and methods of addressing the child's needs. This meeting can be a particularly useful forum for clinicians engaged in CAP service delivery to impart diagnostic information and suggestions for management in such a way as to ensure understanding and cooperation among persons involved, and to answer questions in a timely fashion.

7. The primary components of any CAP service delivery program include education and training, screening, comprehensive CAP assessment, management, and follow-through, and a procedure for monitoring program efficacy through data collection and research.

8. Knowledge of data collection and scientific methodology will serve to provide clinicians with a means of monitoring program efficacy, as well as answering pertinent questions regarding treatment efficacy and other timely topics.

9. The primary purpose of outcome measures is to document the impact of treatment. More specifically, outcome measures will provide further knowledge in the field, determine efficacy of various therapeutic approaches, and influence third-party reimbursement companies, legislators, and others as to the value and cost-effectiveness of services. Speech-language pathologists and audiologists should be involved in the collection of outcomes data to help them develop and implement service-delivery programs, plan diagnostic and intervention services, prioritize clients in their caseloads, and obtain third-party reimbursement. In addition, under the ASHA Code of Ethics, clinicians must engage in data collection as part of their professional duties. Clinicians have an ethical obligation to demonstrate the effectiveness of their services and to share the information obtained with others in the field.

10. This question should be addressed by individual readers in their own way, paying particular attention to those areas cited in this chapter.

Chapter Eleven

1. By functioning in the dual role of scientist and practitioner, clinicians will be able to approach clinical decision making from a scientific perspective, thus improving the effectiveness of their clinical skills. In addition, job satisfaction and stimulation will likely increase, and clinicians will be in a position to add important information to the body of CAPD-related literature concerning diagnostic and remediation techniques.

2. The process of engaging in diagnostic activities, as well as in choosing therapy techniques and monitoring their effectiveness, relies upon the scientific method. There-fore, the activities that every clinician engages in on a daily basis involve the incorporation of scientific methodology into the clinical setting.

3. *data:* attributes or events observed during research activities.

   variable: an outcome that can take on more than one value. Variables can be independent or dependent.

   independent variable: a condition controlled by the researcher in order to test its effect upon the outcome.

   dependent variable: a variable that measures the outcome of a research study.

   sample: the group chosen from the general population for study in a given research project.

   inferential method: the process of inferring the results from a sample to a population.

   variability: the degree of spread or dispersion that characterizes a group of scores within a sample or a population.

   significance: a finding that two experimental groups are different. Significance is expressed in terms of probability that the findings were due to chance.

   correlation: a relationship between two or more variables. The finding that two or more variables are correlated does not imply cause and effect.

4. Factors that help to determine the degree to which the results of a study can be generalized to the population as a whole include the representativeness of the sample chosen, the sample size, and the significance of the findings.

5. Statistical significance refers to a finding that two experimental groups are different. The degree to which such findings

will be clinically significant, however, depends on whether the findings can be utilized in the real-life, clinical setting.

6. A negative correlation is one in which the inverse relationship exists, or one in which the value of one variable increases as the value of another decreases. Conversely, a positive correlation indicates that changes in two or more related variables occur in the same direction (e.g., as one increases, so does the other).

7. *Experimental Research:* This type of research is designed to determine the effect of a given variable on the outcome variable and involves manipulation of an independent, or "treatment," variable.

   Descriptive Research: The goal of descriptive research is to describe the characteristics of a selected phenomenon and involves the collection of data without manipulation of variables.

   Correlational Research: The purpose of this type of research is to determine if and how two or more variables are related to one another, without implying cause and effect.

   Historical Research: Historical research is concerned primarily with describing the nature of events that have occurred in the past for the purpose of examining trends in data.

8. In experimental research design, clinicians have complete control over the assignment of subjects to sample groups and manipulation of the primary independent variable under study. In contrast, causative-comparative research is useful when the independent variable is already established and cannot be manipulated by the researcher. In this type of research, the assignment of subjects to sample groups is essentially out of the hands of the researcher.

9. Mean = 86.8

10. Median = 93.5; Mode = 99

11. Tests of significance determine whether two or more groups are different and, if so, the probability that the differences found are due to chance.

12. t tests are designed to determine whether scores for two groups are significantly different. ANOVA (F tests) serve the same function; however, these tests of significance are designed for use with more than two groups.

13. The primary purpose of measures of association or correlation is to determine whether a significant relationship exists between two or more variables.

References

Abel, S., Bert, B., & McLean, J. (1978). Sound localization: Value in localizing lesions of the auditory pathway. *Journal of Otolaryngology, 7*, 132–140.

Ackerman, S. (1992). *Discovering the Brain.* Washington, DC: National Academy Press.

Aiello, I., Sotgiu, S., Sau, G. F., Manca, S., Conti, M., & Rosati, G. (1995). Long latency evoked potentials in a case of corpus callosum agenesia. Italian *Journal of Neurological Sciences, 15*, 497–505.

American Speech-Language-Hearing Association (1990). Audiological assessment of central auditory processing: an annotated bibliography. *Asha, 32* (Suppl. 1), 13–30.

American Speech-Language-Hearing Association (1995). *Central auditory processing: current status of research and implications for clinical practice. A report from the ASHA task force on central auditory processing.* Rockville, MD: Author.

American Speech Language Hearing Association. (1996). Central auditory processing: Current status of research and implications for clinical practice. *American Journal of Audiology, 5*, 41–54.

Anderson, K., & Matkin, N. H. (1996). *Screening Instrument for Targeting Educational Risk (S.I.F.T.E.R.).* Tampa, FL: Educational Audiology Association.

Anderson, K., & Smaldino, J. (1998). *Listening Inventory for Education (L.I.F.E.).* Tampa, FL: Educational Audiology Association.

Anderson, K. L., & Smaldino, J. J. (2000). *Children's Home Inventory of Listening Difficulties (CHILD).* Tampa, FL: Educational Audiology Association.

Aoki, C., & Siekevitz, P. (1988). Plasticity in brain development. *Scientific American, 259*, 56–64.

Arnst, D. J. (1982). SSW test results with peripheral hearing loss. In D. Arnst & J. Katz (Eds.), *The SSW test: Development and clinical use* (pp. 287–293). San Diego, CA: College-Hill Press.

Ashmead, D., Davis, D., Whalen, T., & Odom, R. (1991). Sound localization and

489

sensitivity to interaural time differences in human infants. *Child Development, 61,* 1211–1226.

Auerbach, S., Allard, T., Naeser, M., Alexander, M., & Albert, M. (1982). Pure word deafness. Analysis of a case with bilateral lesions and a defect at the prephonemic level. *Brain, 105,* 271–300.

Ballesteros, M. C., Hansen, P. E., & Soila, K. (1993). MR imaging of the developing human brain. Part 2. Postnatal development. *RadioGraphics, 13,* 611–622.

Baran, J. A., & Musiek, F. E. (1991). Behavioral assessment of the central auditory nervous system. In W. Rintelmann (Ed.), *Hearing assessment* (2nd ed., pp. 549–602). Austin, TX: PRO-ED.

Baran, J. A., Musiek, F. E., & Reeves, A. G. (1986). Central auditory function following anterior sectioning of the corpus callosum. *Ear and Hearing, 7,* 359–362.

Baran, J. A., Verkest, S., Gollegly, K., Kibbe-Michal, K., Rintelmann, W. F., & Musiek, F. E. (1985). Use of compressed speech in the assessment of central nervous system disorder. *Journal of the Acoustical Society of America, 78* (Suppl. 1), S41.

Barkley, R. A. (1999). Attention-deficit hyperactivity disorder. In *The Scientific American book of the brain* (pp. 219–228). New York: Lyons Press.

Barkovich, A. J., & Kios, B. O. (1988). Normal postnatal development of the corpus callosum as demonstrated by MR imaging. *American Journal of Neuroradiology, 9,* 487–491.

Barrett, M., Huisingh, R., Bowers, L., LoGiudice, C., & Orman, J. (1992). *The Listening Test.* East Moline, IL: LinguiSystems, Inc.

Bashford, J. A., Reinger, K. R., & Warren, R. M. (1992). Increasing the intelligibility of speech through multiple phonemic restorations. *Perception and Psychophysics, 51,* 211–217.

Beasley, D. S., Forman, B., & Rintelmann, W. F. (1972). Intelligibility of time-compressed CNC monosyllables by normal listeners. *Journal of Auditory Research, 12,* 71–75.

Beasley, D. S., Schwimmer, S., & Rintelmann, W. F. (1972). Intelligibility of time-compressed monosyllables. *Journal of Speech and Hearing Research, 15,* 340–350.

Bellis, T. J. (1985). Middle latency and 40 Hz. responses during complete nights of natural sleep. Unpublished Masters thesis. Santa Barbara, CA: University of California.

Bellis, T. J. (1996). *Assessment and management of central auditory processing disorders in the educational setting: From science to practice.* San Diego, CA: Singular Publishing Group.

Bellis, T. J. (1999). Subprofiles of central auditory processing disorders. *Educational Audiology Review, 2,* 9–14.

Bellis, T. J. (1999). *The effects of age and gender on behavioral and temporal indices of corpus callosum function across the life-span of the normal adult.* Unpublished Doctoral Dissertation. Northwestern University, Evanston, IL.

Bellis, T. J. (2002). *When the brain can't hear: Unraveling the mystery of auditory processing disorder.* New York: Pocket Books.

Bellis, T. J. (in press). Developing deficit-specific intervention plans for individuals with auditory processing disorders. *Seminars in Hearing.*

Bellis, T. J., & Ferre, J. M. (1996). Assessment and management of CAPD in children. *Educational Audiology Association Monograph.*

Bellis, T. J., & Ferre, J. M. (1999). Multidimensional approach to the differential diagnosis of central auditory processing disorders in children. *Journal of the American Academy of Audiology, 10,* 319–328.

Bellis, T. J., Nicol, T., & Kraus, N. (2000). Aging affects hemispheric asymmetry in the neural representation of speech sounds. *Journal of Neuroscience, 20,* 791–797.

Bellis, T. J., & Wilber, L. A. (2001). Effects of aging and gender on interhemispheric function. *Journal of Speech, Language, and Hearing Research, 44,* 246–263.

Belmont, I., & Handler, A. (1971). Delayed information processing and judgement of temporal order following cerebral damage. *Journal of Nervous and Mental Disease, 152,* 353–361.

Bergman, M. (1957). Binaural hearing. *Archives of Otolaryngology, 66,* 572–588.

Berlin, C. I. (1999). *The efferent auditory system: Basic science and clinical applications.* San Diego, CA: Singular Publishing Group.

Berlin, C. I., Cullen, J. K., Hughes, L. F., Berlin, J. L., Lowe-Bell, S. S., & Thompson, C. L. (1975). Dichotic processing of speech: Acoustic and phonetic variables. In M.D. Sullivan (Ed.), *Central auditory processing disorders* (pp. 36–46). Proceedings of a conference at the University of Nebraska Medical Center, Omaha.

Berlin, C., Hughes, L., Lowe-Bell, S., & Berlin, H. (1973). Dichotic right ear advantage in children 5 to 13. *Cortex, 9,* 393–401.

Berlin, C. I., Lowe-Bell, S. S., Jannetta, P. J., & Kline, D. G. (1972). Central auditory deficits after temporal lobectomy. *Archives of Otolaryngology, 96,* 4–10.

Bhatnagar, S. C., & Andy, O. J. (1995). *Neuroscience for the study of communicative disorders.* Baltimore: Williams & Wilkins.

Blaettner, U., Scherg, M., & Von Cramon, D. (1989). Diagnosis of unilateral telencephalic hearing disorders: Evaluation of a simple psychoacoustic pattern discrimination test. *Brain, 112,* 177–195.

Bliss, T., & Lomo, T. (1973). Long-lasting potentiation of synaptic transmission in the dentate area of the anaesthetized rabbit following stimulation of the perforant path. *Journal of Physiology, 232,* 331–356.

Blumstein, S., & Cooper, W. (1974). Hemisphere processing of intonation contours. *Cortex, 10,* 146–158.

Bocca, E., Calearo, C., & Cassinari, V. (1954). A new method for testing hearing in temporal lobe tumors. *Acta Otolaryngologica (Stockholm), 44,* 219–221.

Bornstein, S. P. (1994). Time compression and release from masking in adults and children. *Journal of the American Academy of Audiology, 5,* 89–98.

Bornstein, S. P., Wilson, R. H., & Cambron, N. K. (1994). Low- and high-pass filtered Northwestern University Auditory Test No. 6 for monaural and binaural evaluation. *Journal of the American Academy of Audiology, 5*, 259–264.

Bradlow, A. R., & Pisoni, D. B. (1999). Recognition of spoken words by native and non-native listeners: Talker-, listener-, and item-related factors. *Journal of the Acoustical Society of America, 106*, 2074–2085.

Bradlow, A. R., Pisoni, D. B., Akahane-Yamada, R., & Tokhura, Y. (1999). Training Japanese listeners to identify English /r/ and /l/: IV. Some effects of perceptual learning on speech production. *Journal of the Acoustical Society of America, 101*, 2299–2310.

BrainTrain. (2001). *SoundSmart™*. Richmond, VA: BrainTrain.

Brazelton, T. B. (1973). *Neonatal behavioral assessment scale*. London: Spastics International Medical Publications.

Broadbent, D. E. (1954). The role of auditory localization in attention and memory span. *Journal of Experimental Psychology, 47*, 191–196.

Bryden, M. (1963). Ear preference in auditory perception. *Journal of Experimental Psychology, 16*, 359–360.

Buchwald, J. S., Hinman, C., Norman, R. S., Huang, C. M., & Brown, K. A. (1981). Middle and long-latency auditory evoked potentials recorded from the vertex of normal and chronically lesioned cats. *Brain Research, 205*, 91–109.

Butterworth, G., & Castillo, M. (1976). Coordination of auditory visual space in newborn human infants. *Perception, 5*, 155–160.

Cacace, A. T., & McFarland, D. J. (1998). Central auditory processing disorder in school-aged children: A critical review. *Journal of Speech, Language, and Hearing Research, 41*, 355–373.

Caird, D. M., & Klinke, R. (1987). The effect of inferior colliculus lesions on auditory evoked potentials. *Electroencephalography and Clinical Neurophysiology, 68*, 237–240.

Calvert, G. A., Bullmore, E. T., Brammer, M. J., Campbell, R., Williams, S. C. R., McGuire, P. K., Woodruff, P. W. R., Iverson, S. D., & David, A. S. (1997). Activation of auditory cortex during silent lipreading. *Science, 276*, 593–596.

Carmon, A., & Nachshon, I. (1971). Effect of unilateral brain damage on perception of temporal order. *Cortex, 7*, 410–418.

Carrow-Woolfolk, E. (1981). *Carrow auditory-visual abilities test*. Austin, TX: PRO-ED.

Carrow-Woolfolk, E. (1998). *Test for Auditory Comprehension of Language—3rd Edition*. Austin, TX: PRO-ED.

Cedrus Corporation. (1997). *SuperLab experimental laboratory software*. Phoenix, AZ: Cedrus.

Cervette, M. J. (1984). Auditory brainstem response testing in the intensive care unit. *Seminars in Hearing, 5*, 57–68.

Cheour-Luhtanen, M., Alho, K., Sainio, K., Rinne, T., Reinikainen, K., Pohjavuori, M., Renlund, M., Aaltonen, O., Eerola, O., & Naatanen, R. (1996). The ontogenetically earliest discriminative response of the human brain. *Psychophysiology, 33*, 478–481.

Chermak, G. D. (1992, February). Central auditory processing disorders (CAPD): Key concepts and clinical considerations. Paper presented at the American Speech-Language-Hearing Association Workshop on Central Auditory Processing, Orlando, FL.

Chermak, G. D. (1998). Managing central auditory processing disorders: Metalinguistic and metacognitive approaches. *Seminars in Hearing, 19,* 379–392.

Chermak, G. D., & Musiek, F. E. (1997). *Central auditory processing disorders: New perspectives.* San Diego, CA: Singular Publishing Group.

Chermak, G. D., & Musiek, F. E. (1995). Managing central auditory processing disorders in children and youth. *American Journal of Audiology,* 61–65.

Chermak, G. D., Vonhof, M. R., & Bendel, R. B. (1989) Word identification performance in the presence of competing speech and noise in learning disabled adults. *Ear and Hearing, 10,* 90–93.

Cherry, R. S. (1980). *Selective auditory attention test.* St. Louis, MO: Auditec.

Chiappa, K. H. (1980). Brainstem auditory evoked potentials in 200 patients with multiple sclerosis. *Annals of Neurology, 7,* 135–143.

Chiappa, K. H., (1983.) *Evoked potentials in clinical medicine.* New York: Raven Press.

Clarkson, M., Clifton, R., & Morongiello, B. (1985). The effects of sound duration on newborns' head orientation. *Journal of Experimental Child Psychology, 39,* 20–36.

Clarkson, M., Clifton, R., Swain, I., & Perris, E. (1989). Stimulus duration and repetition rate influence newborns' head orientation toward sound. *Developmental Psychobiology, 22,* 683–705.

Clopton, B., & Silverman, M. (1978). Changes in latency and duration of neural responding following developmental auditory deprivation. *Experimental Brain Research, 32,* 39–47.

Cognitive Concepts. (1998). *Earobics™.* Evanston, IL: Cognitive Concepts, Inc.

Colavita, F. B., Szeligo, F. V., & Zimmer, S. D. (1974). Temporal pattern discrimination in cats with insular-temporal lesions. *Brain Research, 79,* 153–156.

Cole, R. A., & Rudnicky, A. I. (1983). What's new in speech perception? The research ideas of William Chandler Bagley, 1874–1946. *Psychological Review, 90,* 94–104.

Conners, C. K. (1996). *Conners' Rating Scales—Revised.* San Antonio, TX: The Psychological Corporation.

Courchesne, E., (1978). Neurophysiological correlates of cognitive development: Changes in long-latency event-related potentials from childhood to adulthood. *Electroencephalography and Clinical Neurophysiology, 45,* 468–482.

Cowell, P. E., Allen, L. S., Zaltimo, N. S., & Dennenberg, V. H. (1992). A developmental study of sex and age interactions in the human corpus callosum. *Developmental Brain Research, 66,* 187–192.

Cox, L. C. (1985). Infant assessment: Developmental and age related considerations. In Jacobsen, J. (Ed.) *The auditory brainstem response* (pp. 298–316). San Diego, CA: College-Hill Press.

Crandell, C., & Smaldino, J. (2001). An update on classroom acoustics. *The ASHA Leader, 6,* 5, 20.

Cranford, J. L. (1984). Brief tone detection and discrimination tests in clinical audiology with emphasis on their use in central nervous system lesions. *Seminars in Hearing, 5,* 263–275.

Cranford, J. L., Stream, R. W., Rye, C. V., & Slade, T. L. (1982). Detection versus discrimination of brief-duration tones: Findings in patients with temporal lobe damage. *Archives of Otolaryngology, 108,* 350–356.

Dalebout, S. D., & Fox, L. G. (2000). Identification of the mismatch negativity in the responses of individual listeners. *Journal of the American Academy of Audiology, 11,* 12–22.

Dalebout, S. D., & Fox, L. G. (2001). Reliability of the mismatch negativity in the responses of individual listeners. *Journal of the American Academy of Audiology, 12,* 245–253.

Damasio, H., & Damasio, A. (1979). "Paradoxic" ear extinction in dichotic listening: Possible anatomic significance. *Neurology, 29,* 644–653.

Davis, H., & Onishi, S. (1969). Maturation of auditory evoked potentials. *International Audiology, 8,* 24–33.

Davis, P. A. (1939). Effects of acoustic stimuli on the waking human brain. *Journal of Neurophysiology, 2,* 494–499.

Dayal, V. S., Tarantino, L., & Swisher, L. P. (1966). Neuro-otologic studies in multiple sclerosis. *Laryngoscope, 76,* 1798–1809.

DeCharms, R. C., & Merzenich, M. M. (1996). Primary cortical representation of sounds by the coordination of action-potential timing. *Nature, 381,* 610–613.

Delgutte, B. (1997). Auditory neural processing of speech. In W. J. Hardcastle & J. Laver (Eds.), *Handbook of phonetic sciences.* Cambridge, MA: Blackwell Publishers.

Delgutte, B., & Kiang, N. Y. S. (1984). Speech encoding in the auditory nerve: I. Vowel-like sounds. *Journal of the Acoustical Society of America, 75,* 866–878.

Dennis, M. (1976). Impaired sensory and motor differentiation with corpus callosum agenesis: A lack of callosal inhibition during ontogeny? *Neuropsychologia, 14,* 455–469.

Despland, P. A. & Galambos, R. (1980). The auditory brainstem response (ABR) is a useful tool in the intensive care nursery. *Pediatric Research, 14,* 154–158.

Diagnostic and statistical manual of mental disorders, fourth edition, text revision (DSM-IV-TR). (1999). Washington, DC: American Psychiatric Association.

Dirks, D. (1964). Perception of dichotic and monaural verbal material and cerebral dominance for speech. *Acta Oto-laryngology, 58,* 78–80.

Dirks, D., & Wilson, R. (1969). binaural hearing of speech for aided and unaided conditions. *Journal of Speech and Hearing Research, 12,* 650–664.

DiSimoni, F. (1978). *The Token Test for Children.* Hingham, MA: Teaching Resources Corp.

Disterhoft, J. F., & Stuart, D. K. (1976). Trial sequence of changed unit activity in auditory system of alert rat during conditioned response acquisition and extinction. *Journal of Neurophysiology, 39,* 266–281.

Domitz, D. M., & Schow, R. L. (2000). A new CAPD battery—Multiple auditory processing assessment (MAPA): Factor analysis and comparisons with SCAN. *American Journal of Audiology, 9,* 101–111.

Drulovic, B., Ribaric-Jankes, K., Kostic, V., & Sternic, N. (1994). Multiple sclerosis as the cause of sudden "pontine" deafness. *Audiology, 33,* 195–201.

Durlach, N. I., Thompson, C. L., & Colburn, H. S. (1981). Binaural interaction in impaired listeners: A review of past research. *Audiology, 20,* 181–211.

Durston, S., Hulshoff Pol, H. E., Casey, B. J., Giedd, J. N., Buitelaar, J. K., & van Engeland, H. (2001). Anatomical MRI of the developing human brain: What have we learned? *Journal of the American Academy of Child and Adolescent Psychiatry, 40,* 1012–1020.

Eberling, C., Bak, C., Kofoed, B., Lebech, J., & Saermark, K. (1982). Auditory magnetic fields. Source location and tonotopical organization of the right hemisphere of the human brain. *Scandinavian Audiology, 9,* 203–207.

Efron, R. (1963). Temporal perception, aphasia and deja vu. *Brain, 86,* 403–424.

Efron, R. (1985). The central auditory system and issues related to hemispheric specialization. In M.L. Pinheiro & F.E. Musiek (Eds.), *Assessment of central auditory dysfunction: Foundations and clinical correlates* (pp. 143–154). Baltimore: Williams & Wilkins.

Efron, R. (1990). *The decline and fall of hemispheric specialization.* Hillsdale, NJ: Lawrence Erlbaum.

Efron, R., & Crandall, P. H. (1983). Central auditory processing: Effects of anterior temporal lobectomy. *Brain and Language, 19,* 237–253.

Efron, R., Crandall, P. H., Koss, D., Divenyi, P. L., & Yund, E. W. (1983). Central auditory processing. III. The "Cocktail Party" effect and anterior temporal lobectomy. *Brain and Language, 19,* 254–263.

Efron, R., Dennis, M., & Yund, E. W. (1977). The perception of dichotic chords by hemispherectomized subjects. *Brain and Language, 4,* 537–549.

Efron, R., Yund, E. W., Nichols, D., & Crandall, P. H. (1977). An ear asymmetry for gap detection following anterior temporal lobectomy. *Neuropsychologia, 23,* 43–50.

Elliott, L. L. (1979). Performance of children aged 9 to 17 years on a test of speech intelligibility in noise using sentence material with controlled word predictability. *Journal of the Acoustical Society of America, 66,* 651–653.

Elliott, L. L. (1995). Verbal auditory closure and the Speech Perception in Noise (SPIN) test. *Journal of Speech, Language, and Hearing Research, 38,* 1363–1376.

Erikkson, P. S., Perfilieva, E., Bjork-Eriksson, T., Alborn, A. M., Nordborg, C., Peterson, D. A., & Gage, F. H. (1998). Neurogenesis in the adult human hippocampus. *Nature Medicine, 4,* 1313–1317.

Fairbanks, G., Everitt, W., & Jaeger, R. (1954). Methods for time or frequency compression-expansion of speech. *Trans IRE-PGA, AU-2,* 7–12.

Farmer, M. E., & Klein, R. (1995). The evidence for a temporal processing deficit linked to dyslexia: A review. *Psychonomic Bulletin & Review, 2,* 460–493.

Ferre, J. (1987). Pediatric central auditory processing disorder: Considerations for diagnosis, interpretation, and remediation. *Journal of the Academy of Rehabilitative Audiology, 20,* 73–81.

Ferre, J. (1992, November). CATfiles: Improving the clinical utility of central auditory function tests. Paper presented at the American Speech-Language-Hearing Association Annual Convention, San Antonio, TX.

Ferre, J. (1994, March). The clinical utility of the concept of central auditory processing—a commentary. Paper presented at the American Speech-Language-Hearing Association Task Force on Central Auditory Processing Consensus Development Conference, Albuquerque, NM.

Ferre, J. M. (1997). *Processing power: A guide to CAPD assessment and management.* San Antonio, TX: Communication Skill Builders.

Field, J., Muir, D., Pilon, R., Sinclair, M., & Dodwell, P. (1980). Infants' orientation to lateral sounds from birth to 3 months. *Child Development, 51,* 295–298.

Fifer, R., Jerger, J., Berlin, C., Tobey, E., & Campbell, J. (1983). Development of a dichotic sentence identification test for hearing impaired adults. *Ear and Hearing, 4,* 300–305.

Fischer, C., Bognar, L., Turjman, F., & Lapras, C. (1995). Auditory evoked potentials in a patient with a unilateral lesion of the inferior colliculus and medial geniculate body. *Electroencephalography and Clinical Neurophysiology, 96,* 261–267.

Fisher, L. I. (1985). Learning disabilities and auditory processing. In R. J. Van Hattum (Ed.), *Administration of speech-language services in the schools* (pp. 231–292). San Diego, CA: College Hill Press.

Flowers, A., Costello, M., & Small, V. (1973). *Flowers-Costello Tests of Central Auditory Abilities.* Dearborn, MI: Perceptual Learning Systems.

Franzen, M. D. (1989). *Reliability and validity in neuropsychological assessment.* New York: Plenum Press.

Futai, K., Okada, M., Matsuyama, K., & Takahashi, T. (2001). High-fidelity transmission acquired via a developmental decrease in NMDA receptor expression at an auditory synapse. *Journal of Neuroscience, 21,* 3342–3349.

Gabriele, M. L., Brunso-Bechtold, J. K., & Henkel, C. K. (2000). Plasticity in the development of afferent patterns in the inferior colliculus of the rat after unilateral cochlear ablation. *Journal of Neuroscience, 20,* 6939–6949.

Galambos, R., Wilson, M. J., & Silva, P. D. (1994). Identifying hearing loss in the intensive care nursery: A 20-year summary. *Journal of the American Academy of Audiology, 5,* 151–162.

Gardner, M. R. (1996). *Test of auditory perceptual skills—Revised.* Hydesville, CA: Psychological and Educational Publications, Inc.

Gardner, M. R. (1994). *Test of auditory perceptual skills: Upper level.* Hydesville, CA: Psychological and Educational Publications, Inc.

Gatehouse, R. (1976). *Further research in localization of sound by completely monaural subjects.* Journal of Auditory Research, 16, 265–273.

Gazzaniga, M. S. (1995). Principles of human brain organization derived from split-brain studies. *Neuron, 14,* 217–228.

Gazzaniga, M. S., & Hillyard, S. A. (1973). Attention mechanisms following brain bisection. In A. F. Sanders (Ed.), *Attention and performance IV* (pp. 221–238). Amsterdam: North Holland.

Gazzaniga, M. S., Ivry, R. B., & Mangun, G. R. (1998). *Cognitive neuroscience: The biology of the mind.* New York. W. W. Norton & Company, Inc.

Gazzaniga, M., & Sperry, R. (1967). Language after section of the cerebral commissures. *Brain, 90,* 131–148.

Geisler, C., Frishkopf, L., & Rosenblith, W. (1958). Extracranial responses to acoustic clicks in man. *Science, 128,* 1210–1211.

Geschwind, N., & Levitsky, W. (1968). Human brain: left-right asymmetries in temporal speech region. *Science, 161,* 186–187.

Gillam, R. B., Crofford, J. A., Gale, M. A., & Hoffman, L. M. (2001a). Language change following computer-assisted language instruction with Fast ForWord or Laureate Learning Systems software. *American Journal of Speech-Language Pathology, 10,* 231–247.

Gillam, R. B., Loeb, D. F., & Friel-Patti, S. (2001b). Looking back: A summary of five exploratory studies of Fast ForWord. *American Journal of Speech-Language Pathology, 10,* 269–273.

Girard, N., Raybaud, C., & DuLac, P. (1991). MRI study of brain myelination. *Canadian Journal of Neuroradiology, 18,* 291–307.

Gold, J. I., & Knudsen, E. I. (2000). A site of auditory experience-dependent plasticity in the neural representation of auditory space in the barn owl's inferior colliculus. *Journal of Neuroscience, 20,* 3469–3486.

Goldman, R., Fristoe, M., & Woodcock, R. W. (1970). *Goldman-Fristoe-Woodcock Test of Auditory Discrimination.* Circle Pines, MN: American Guidance Service, Inc.

Goldenberg, G., Oder, W., Spatt, J., & Podreka, I. (1992). Cerebral correlates of disturbed executive function and memory in survivors of severe closed head injury: A SPECT study. *Journal of Neurology, Neurosurgery and Psychiatry, 55,* 362–368.

Goldstein, R. (1972). Presidential address: 1971 national convention. *Asha, 14,* 58–62.

Goldstone, R. L. (1994). Influences of categorization on perceptual discrimination. *Journal of Experimental Psychology, 123,* 178–200.

Goodin, D., Squires, K., Henderson, B, & Starr, A. (1978). Age related variations in evoked potentials to auditory stimuli in normal human subjects. *Electroencephalography and Clinical Neurophysiology, 44,* 447–458.

Green, D. M. (1966). Interaural phase effects in the masking of signals of different durations. *Journal of the Acoustical Society of America, 39,* 720–724.

Greene, T. (1929). The ability to localize sound. *Archives of Surgery: Chicagy, 6,* 1825–1841.

Groenen, P. (1997). *Central auditory processing disorders: A psycholinguistic approach.* Nijmegen: University Hospital of Nijmegen.

Grose, J. H., Hall, J. W., & Gibbs, C. (1993). Temporal analysis in children. *Journal of Speech and Hearing Research, 36*, 351–356.

Grote, C. L., Pierre-Louis, S. J., Smith, M. C., Roberts, R. H., & Varney, N. R. (1995). Significance of unilateral ear extinction on the dichotic listening test. *Journal of Clinical and Experimental Neuropsychology, 17*, 108.

Gustafsson, B., & Wigstrom, H. (1988). Physiological mechanisms underlying long-term potentiation. *Trends in Neuroscience, 11*, 156–162.

Haggard, M. P., & Hughes, E. A. (1991). Screening children's hearing: A review of the literature and implications of otitis media. *London: HMSO.*

Hall, J. W., & Derlacki, E. D. (1986). Binaural hearing after middle ear surgery. *Journal of Otology Rhinology and Laryngology, 95*, 118–124.

Hall, J. W., & Derlacki, E. D. (1988). Binaural hearing after middle ear surgery: MLD for interaural time and level cues. *Audiology, 27*, 89–98.

Hall, J. W., & Grose, J. H. (1990). The masking-level difference in children. *Journal of the American Academy of Audiology, 1*, 81–88.

Hall, J. W., & Grose, J. H. (1993). The effect of otitis media with effusion on the masking-level difference and the auditory brainstem response. *Journal of Speech and Hearing Research, 36*, 210–217.

Hall, J. W., & Grose, J. H. (1994). Development of temporal resolution in children as measured by the temporal modulation transfer function. *Journal of the Acoustical Society of America, 96*, 150–154.

Hall, J. W., Grose, J. H., & Pillsbury, H. C. (1990.) Predicting binaural hearing after stapedectomy from pre-surgery results. *Archives of Otolaryngology, Head and Neck Surgery, 116*, 946–950.

Hall, J. W., Grose, J. H., & Pillsbury, H. C. (1995). Long-term effects of chronic otitis media on binaural hearing in children. *Archives of Otolaryngology, 121*, 857–862.

Hall, J. W., Tyler, R. S., & Fernandez, M. A. (1984). Factors influencing the masking level difference in cochlear hearing-impaired and normal-hearing listeners. *Journal of Speech and Hearing Research, 27*, 145–154.

Hamre, C. E. (1972). Research and clinical practice: A unifying model. *Asha, 14*, 542–545.

Harris, J. D. (1960). Combinations of distortions in speech: The twenty-five per cent safety factor by multiple-cueing. *Archives of Otolaryngology, 72, 227–232.*

Hashimoto, I., Ishiyama, Y., Yoshimoto, T., & Nemoto, S. (1981). Brainstem auditory-evoked potentials recorded directly from the human brainstem and thalamus. *Brain, 104*, 841–859.

Hausler, R., Colburn, H. S., & Marr, E. (1983). Sound localization in subjects with impaired hearing. *Acta Oto-laryngology* (Suppl. 400), Monograph.

Hausler, R., & Levine, R. A. (1980). Brainstem auditory evoked potentials are related to interaural time discrimination in patients with multiple sclerosis. *Brain Research, 191*, 589–594.

Hayakawa, K., Konishi, Y., Matsuda, T., Kuriyama, M., Konishi, K., Yamashita, K., Okumura, R., & Hamanaka, D. (1989). Development and aging of brain midline structures: Assessment with MR imaging. *Radiology, 172*, 171–177.

Hebb, D. O. (1949). *The organization of behavior.* New York: John Wiley & Sons.

Heffner, H. E., & Heffner, R. S. (1986). Effect of unilateral and bilateral auditory cortex lesions on the discrimination of vocalizations by Japanese macaques. *Journal of Neurophysiology, 35,* 683–701.

Heilman, K. M., Hammer, L. C., & Wilder, B. J. (1973). An audiometric defect in temporal lobe dysfunction. *Neurology (NY), 3,* 384–386.

Heise, D. R. (1969). Separating reliability and stability in test-retest correlation. *American Sociological Review, 34,* 93–104.

Helfer, K. S., & Wilber, L. A. (1990). Hearing loss, aging, and speech perception in reverberation and noise. *Journal of Speech and Hearing Research, 33,* 149–155.

Hendler, T., Squires, N. K., & Emmerich, D. S. (1990). Psychophysical measures of central auditory dysfunction in multiple sclerosis: Neurophysiological and neuroanatomical correlates. *Ear and Hearing, 11,* 403–415.

Hexamer, M., & Bellis, T. J. (2000, April). A comparison of dichotic sentence procedures: The Willeford and Auditec versions of the Competing Sentence Test. Poster presented at the South Dakota Speech-Language-Hearing Association Annual Meeting, Sioux Falls, SD.

Hirsh, I. J. (1948). The influence of interaural phase on interaural summation and inhibition. Journal of the Acoustical Society of America, 20, 536–544.

Hirsh, I. J. (1959). Auditory perception of temporal order. *Journal of the Acoustical Society of America, 31,* 759–767.

Hirsh, I. J., Reynolds, E. G., & Joseph, M. (1954). Intelligibility of different speech materials. *Journal of the Acoustical Society of America, 31,* 759–767.

Hirsh, I. J., & Sherrick, Jr., C. E. (1961). Perceived order in different sense modalities. *Journal of Experimental Psychology, 62,* 423–432.

Hood, L. J. (1998). *Clinical applications of the auditory brainstem response.* San Diego, CA: Singular Publishing Group.

Hoptman, M. J., & Davidson, R. J. (1994). How and why do the two cerebral hemispheres interact? *Psychological Bulletin, 116,* 195–219.

Hugdahl, K., Bronnick, K., Kyllingsbaek, S., Law, I., Gade, A., & Paulson, O. B. (1999). Brain activation during dichotic presentations of consonant-vowel and musical instrument stimuli: A 150-PET study. *Neuropsychologia, 37,* 431–440.

Hughes, J. W. (1946). The threshold of audition for short periods of stimulation. *Procedures of the Research Society of London, 133B,* 486–490.

Hurley, R., & Singer, J. (April, 1989). The effectiveness of selected auditory processing tests as screening tests with children. Paper presented at the American Academy of Audiology Annual Conference, Kiawah, S.C.

Huttenlocher, P. R., & Dabholkar, A. S. (1977). Regional differences in synaptogenesis in human cerebral cortex. *Journal of Comparative Neurology, 387,* 167–178.

Hynd, G. W., Semrud-Clikeman, M., Lorys, A. R., Novey, E. S., & Eliopulos, D. (1990). Brain morphology in developmental dyslexia and attention deficit disorder/hyperactivity. *Archives of Neurology, 47,* 916–919.

Irvine, D. R. F., Rajan, R., Wize, L. Z., & Heil, P. (1991). Reorganization in auditory cortex of adult cats with unilateral restricted cochlear lesions. *Society for Neuroscience, 17* (Abstract), 1485.

Irwin, R. J., Ball, A. K., Kay, N., Stillman, J. A., & Bosser, J. (1985). The development of auditory temporal acuity in children. *Child Development, 56,* 614–620.

Ivey, R. G. (1969). *Tests of CNS auditory function.* Unpublished Master's Thesis. Ft. Collins, CO: Colorado State University.

Jacobson, J. (Ed.) (1985). *The auditory brainstem response.* San Diego, CA: College-Hill Press.

Jacobson, J. T., Deppe, U., & Murray, T. J. (1983). Dichotic paradigms in multiple sclerosis. *Ear and Hearing, 3,* 311–317.

Jensen, J. K., Neff, D. L., & Callaghan, B. P. (1987). Frequency, intensity, and duration discrimination in young children. *Asha, 29,* 88.

Jerger, J. (1963). Viewpoint. *Journal of Speech and Hearing Research, 6,* 203–206.

Jerger, J., Greenwald, R., Wambacq, I., Seipel, A., & Moncrieff, D. (2000). Toward a more ecologically valid measure of speech understanding in background noise. *Journal of the American Academy of Audiology, 11,* 273–282.

Jerger, J. (1997). Functional asymmetries in the auditory system. *Annals of Otology, Rhinology, and Laryngology, 106,* 23–30.

Jerger, S., Jerger, J., & Abrams, S. (1983). Speech audiometry in the young child. *Ear and Hearing, 4,* 56–66.

Jerger, J., Brown, D., & Smith, S. (1984). Effect of peripheral hearing loss on the MLD. *Archives of Otolaryngology, 110,* 290–296.

Jerger, J., & Jerger, S. W. (1974). Auditory findings in brainstem disorders. *Archives of Otolaryngology, 99,* 342–349.

Jerger, J., & Jerger, S. (1975). Clinical validity of central auditory tests. *Scandinavian Audiology, 4,* 147–163.

Jerger, S., Jerger, J., Alford, B. R., & Abrams, S. (1983). Development of speech intelligibility in children with recurrent otitis media. *Ear and Hearing, 4,* 138–145.

Jerger, J., Lovering, L., & Wertz, M. (1972). Auditory disorder following bilateral temporal lobe insult: Report of a case. *Journal of Speech and Hearing Disorders, 37,* 524–535.

Jerger, J., Moncrieff, D., Greenwald, R., Wambacq, I., & Seipel, A. (2000). Effect of age on interaural asymmetry of event-related potentials in a dichotic listening task. *Journal of the American Academy of Audiology, 11,* 383–389.

Jerger, J., & Musiek, F. (2000). Report of the consensus conference on the diagnosis of auditory processing disorders in school-aged children. *Journal of the American Academy of Audiology, 11,* 467–474.

Jewitt, D., & Williston, J. (1971). Auditory-evoked far fields averaged from the scalp of humans. *Brain, 94,* 618–696.

Jirsa, R. E. (1992). The clinical utility of the P3 AERP in children with auditory processing disorders. *Journal of Speech and Hearing Research, 35,* 903–912.

Johnson, S. C., Farnsworth, T., Pinkston, J. B., Bigler, E. D., & Blatter, D. D. (1994). Corpus callosum surface area across the human adult life span: Effect of age and gender. *Brain Research Bulletin, 35,* 373–377.

Jongkees, L., & Van der Veer, R. (1957). Directional hearing capacity in hearing disorders. *Acta Oto-laryngology, 48,* 465–474.

Jusczyk, P. W., Cutler, A., & Redanz, N. J. (1993). Infants' preference for the predominant stress patterns of English words. *Child Development, 64,* 675–687.

Kalikow, D. N., Stevens, K. N., & Elliott, L. L. (1977). Development of a test of speech intelligibility in noise using sentence materials with controlled word predictability. *Journal of the Acoustical Society of America, 61,* 1337–1351.

Kalil, R. E. (1989, December). Synapse formation in the developing brain. *Scientific American,* 76–85.

Kalil, R. E., Dubin, M. W., Scott, G., & Stark, L. A. (1986). Elimination of action potentials blocks the structural development of retinogeniculate synapses. *Nature, 323,* 156–158.

Kandel, E. R., & Hawkins, R. D. (1999). The biological basis of learning and individuality. In *The Scientific American book of the brain* (pp. 139–154). New York: Lyons Press.

Kaplan, E. (1995). *Weschsler Intelligence Scale for Children—Third Edition.* San Antonio, TX: The Psychological Corporation.

Karaseva, T. A. (1972). The role of the temporal lobe in human auditory perception. *Neuropsychologia, 10,* 227–231.

Katz, J. (1962). The use of staggered spondaic words for assessing the integrity of the central auditory nervous system. *Journal of Auditory Research, 2,* 327–337.

Katz, J. (1968). The SSW test: An interim report. *Journal of Speech and Hearing Disorders, 33,* 132–146.

Katz, J. (1977). The staggered spondaic word test. In R.W. Keith (Ed.), *Central auditory dysfunction* (pp. 103–121). New York: Grune & Stratton.

Katz, J. (1986). *SSW Test User's Manual.* Vancouver, WA: Precision Acoustics.

Katz, J. (1992). Classification of auditory processing disorders. In J. Katz, N. Stecker, & D. Henderson (Eds.), *Central auditory processing: A transdisciplinary view* (pp. 81–91). St. Louis, MO: Mosby Year Book.

Katz, J. (1994). *Handbook of clinical audiology* (4th ed.). Baltimore: Williams & Wilkins.

Katz, J. (Ed.) (2002). *Handbook of clinical audiology, fifth edition.* New York: Lippincott Williams & Wilkins.

Katz, J., Smith, P., & Kurpita, B. (1992). Categorizing test findings in children referred for auditory processing deficits. *SSW Reports, 14,* 1–6.

Katz., J., Stecker, N., & Masters, M. G. (1994, March). Central auditory processing: A coherent approach. Paper presented at the American Speech-Language-Hearing Association Task Force on Central Auditory Processing Consensus Development Conference, Albuquerque, NM.

Keith, R. (1977). Synthetic sentence identification test. In R.W. Keith (Ed.), *Central auditory dysfunction* (pp. 73–102). New York: Grune & Stratton.

Keith, R. (1984). Dichotic listening in children. In D. Beasley (Ed.), *Audition in childhood: Methods of study* (pp. 1–23). San Diego, CA: College Hill Press.

Keith, R. (1986). *SCAN: A screening test for auditory processing disorders.* San Antonio,TX: The Psychological Corporation.

Keith, R. (1994a). *ACPT: Auditory continuous performance test.* San Antonio,TX: The Psychological Corporation.

Keith, R. (1994b). *SCAN-A: A test for auditory processing disorders in adolescents and adults.* TX: The Psychological Corporation, Harcourt Brace Jovanovich, Inc.

Keith, R. W. (2000a). *SCAN-C Test for Auditory Processing Disorders in Children—Revised.* San Antonio, TX: Psychological Corporation.

Keith, R. W. (2000b). Development and standardization of SCAN-C Test for Auditory Processing. *Journal of the American Academy of Audiology, 11,* 438–445.

Keith, R. W. (2000c). *Random gap detection test.* St. Louis, MO: Auditec.

Keith, R. W., Rudy, J., Donahue, P. A., & Katbamna, B. (1989). Comparison of SCAN results with other auditory and language measures in a clinical population. *Ear and Hearing, 10,* 382–386.

Kelly, J. (1986). The development of sound localization of auditory processing in mammals. In R.N. Aslin (Ed.), *Advances in neural and behavioral development: Vol. 2* (pp. 202–234). Norwood, NJ: Ablex.

Kiang, N. Y. S. (1975). Stimulus representation in the discharge patterns of auditory neurons. In D.B. Tower (Ed.), *The nervous system. Volume 3: Human communication and its disorders* (pp. 81–96). New York: Raven Press.

Kileny, P., Paccioretti, D., & Wilson, A. F. (1987). Effects of cortical lesions on middle-latency auditory evoked responses (MLR). *Electroencephalography and Clinical Neurophysiology, 66,* 108–120.

Kimura, D. (1961a). Some effects of temporal-lobe damage on auditory perception. *Canadian Journal of Psychology, 15,* 156–165.

Kimura, D. (1961b). Cerebral dominance and the perception of verbal stimuli. *Canadian Journal of Psychology, 15,* 166–171.

King, C., McGee, T., Rubel, E. W., Nicol, T., & Kraus, N. (1995). Acoustic features and acoustic change are represented by different central pathways. *Hearing Research, 85,* 45–52.

King, C., Nicol, T., McGee, T., & Kraus, N. (1999). Thalamic asymmetry is related to acoustic signal complexity in guinea pigs. *Neuroscience Letters, 267,* 89–92.

King, F., & Kimura, D. (1972). Left-ear superiority in dichotic perception of vocal, non-verbal sounds. *Canadian Journal of Psychology, 26,* 111–116.

Kitzes, L. M., Farley, G. R., & Starr, A. (1978). Modulation of auditory cortex unit activity during the performance of a conditioned response. *Experimental Neurology, 62,* 678–697.

Knudsen, E. J. (1983). Early auditory experience aligns the auditory map of space in the optic tectum of the barn owl. *Science, 222,* 939–942.

Knudsen, E. J. (1987). Early auditory experience shapes auditory localization behavior and the spatial tuning of auditory units in the barn owl. In

J. Rauschecker & P. Marler (Eds.), *Imprinting and cortical plasticity* (pp. 7–23). New York: John Wiley & Sons.

Knudsen, E. J., Esterly, S. D., & Knudsen, P. F. (1984). Monaural occlusion alters sound localization during a sensitive period in the barn owl. *Journal of Neuroscience, 4,* 1001–1011.

Knudsen, E., & Knudsen, P, (1985). Vision guides the adjustment of auditory localization in young barn owls. *Science, 230,* 545–548.

Koch, D. B., McGee, T. J., Bradlow, A. R., & Kraus, N. (1999). Acoustic-phonetic approach toward understanding neural processes and speech perception. *Journal of the American Academy of Audiology, 10,* 304–318.

Kolata, G. (1984). Studying learning in the womb: Behavioral scientists are using established experimental methods to show that fetuses can and do learn. *Science, 20,* 302–303.

Kolb, B., & Whishaw, I. Q. (1996). *Fundamentals of human neuropsychology.* New York: W. H. Freeman and Company.

Kraus, N., Koch, D. B., McGee, T. J., Nicol, T. G., & Cunningham, J. (1999). Normal development of speech-sound discrimination in school-age children: Psychophysical and neurophysiologic measures. *Journal of Speech, Language, and Hearing Research, 42,* 1042–1060.

Kraus, N., McGee, T., Micco, A., Sharma, A., Carrell, T., & Nicol, T. (1993). Mismatch negativity in school-age children to speech stimuli that are just perceptibly different. *Electroencephalography and Clinical Neurophysiology, 88,* 123–130.

Kraus, N., McGee, T., Carrell, T., King, C., Littman, T., & Nicol, T. (1994). Discrimination of speech-like contrasts in the auditory thalamus and cortex. *Journal of the Acoustical Society of America, 96,* 2758–2767.

Kraus, N., McGee, T., Littman, T., Nicol, T., & King, C. (1994). Nonprimary auditory thalamic representation of acoustic change. *Journal of Neurophysiology, 72,* 1270–1277.

Kraus, N., McGee, T., Littman, T., Nicol, T., & King, C. (1994). Nonprimary auditory thalamic representation of acoustic change. *Journal of Neurophysiology, 72,* 1270–1277.

Kraus, N., McGee, T., Carrell, T., King, C., Tremblay, K., & Nicol, T. (1995). Central auditory system plasticity associated with speech discrimination training. *Journal of Cognitive Neuroscience, 7,* 25–32.

Kraus, N., McGee, T., Carrell, T. D., & Sharma, A (1995). Neurophysiologic bases of speech discrimination. *Ear and Hearing, 16,* 19–37.

Kraus, N., McGee, T. J., Carrell, T. D., Zecker, S. D., Nicol, T. G., & Koch, D. B. (1996). Auditory neurophysiologic responses and discrimination deficits in children with learning problems. *Science, 273,* 971–973.

Kraus, N., McGee, T., & Comperatore, C. (1989). MLRs in children are consistently present during wakefulness, stage 1 and REM sleep. *Ear and Hearing, 10,* 339–345.

Kraus, N., Ozdamar, O., Hier, D., & Stein, L. (1982). Auditory middle latency responses in patients with cortical lesions. *Electroencephalography and Clinical Neurophysiology, 54,* 247–287.

Kraus, N., Ozdamar, O., Krier, D., & Stein, L. (1982). Auditory middle latency response in patients with cortical lesions. *Electroencephalography and Clinical Neurophysiology, 88,* 247–287.

Kraus, N. Smith, D., Reed, N., Stein, L., & Cartee, C. (1985). Auditory middle latency responses in children: Effects of age and diagnostic category. *Electroencephalography and Clinical Neurophysiology, 62,* 343–351.

Kraus, N., Smith, D. I., McGee, T., Stein, L., & Cartee, C. (1987). Development of the middle latency response in an animal model and its relation to the human response. *Hearing Research, 27,* 165–176.

Kraus, N., Smith, D. I., & McGee, T. (1988). Midline and temporal lobe MLRs in the guinea pig originate from different generator systems: A conceptual framework for new and existing data. *Electroencephalography and Clinical Neurophysiology, 70,* 541–558.

Kuhl, P. K. (1979). Models and mechanisms in speech perception. Species comparisons provide further contributions. *Brain, Behavior and Evolution, 16,* 374–408.

Kuhl, P. K. (2000). A new view of language acquisition. *Proceedings of the National Academy of Sciences, 97,* 11850–11857.

Kuhl, P. K., & Miller, J. D. (1978). Speech perception by the chinchilla: Identification function for synthetic VOT stimuli. *Journal of the Acoustical Society of America, 63,* 905–917.

Kurdziel, S. A., Noffsinger, P. D., & Olsen, W. (1976). Performance by cortical lesion patients on 40 and 60 percent time-compressed materials. *Journal of the Americal Audiological Society, 2,* 3–7.

Kurtzberg, D., Vaughan, H. G., Kreuzer, J. A., & Fliegler, K. Z. (1995). Developmental studies and clinical application of mismatch negativity: Problems and prospects. *Ear and Hearing, 16,* 104–117.

Lackner, J. R., & Teuber, H. L. (1973). Alterations in auditory fusion thresholds after cerebral injury in man. *Neuropsychologia, 11,* 409–415.

Lecours, A. R. (1975). Myelogenetic correlates of development of speech and language. In E. H. Lenneberg and E. Lenneberg (Eds), *Foundation of language development, Vol. 1* (pp. 121–135). New York: Academic Press.

Lenneberg, E. H. (1967). *Biological foundations of language.* New York: John Wiley & Sons.

Lepore, F., Lassonde, M., Poirier, P., Schiavetto, A., & Veillette, N. (1994). Midline sensory integration in callosal agenesis. In M. Lassonde & M. A. Jeeves (Eds.), *Callosal agenesis: A natural split brain?* (pp. 155–169). New York: Plenum Press.

Lepore, F., Ptito, M., & Guillemot, J-P. (1986). The role of the corpus callosum in midline fusion. In F. Lepore, M. Ptito, & H. H. Jasper (Eds.), *Two hemispheres—one brain. Functions of the corpus callosum* (pp. 211–229). New York: Alan R. Liss, Inc.

Lessler, K. (1972, February). Health and educational screening of school-age children: Definition and objectives. *American Journal of Public Health, 62,* 191–198.

Levine, R. A., Gardner, J. C., Stufflebeam, S. M., Fullterton, B. C., Carlisle, E. W.,

Furst, M., Rosen, B. R., & Kiang, N. Y. S. (1993a). Binaural auditory processing in multiple sclerosis subjects. *Hearing Research, 68*, 59–72.

Levine, R. A., Gardner, J. C., Stufflebeam, S. M., Fullterton, B. C., Carlisle, E. W., Furst, M., Rosen, B. R., & Kiang, N. Y. S. (1993b). Effects of multiple sclerosis brainstem lesions on sound lateralization and brainstem auditory evoked potentials. *Hearing Research, 68*, 73–88.

Lewellen, M. J., Goldinger, S. D., Pisoni, D. B., & Greene, B. G. (1993). Lexical familiarity and processing efficiency: Individual differences in naming, lexical decision, and semantic categorization. *Journal of Experimental Psychology, 122*, 316–330.

Lewis, M. (1986). *Learning disabilities and prenatal risks.* Urbana, IL: University of Illinois Press.

Liberman, A. M. (1996). *Speech: A special code.* Cambridge, MA: MIT Press.

Licklider, J. C. R. (1948). The influence of interaural phase relations upon the masking of speech by white noise. *Journal of the Acoustical Society of America, 20*, 150–159.

Liegeois-Chauvel, C., Musolino, A., Badier, J. M., Marquis, P., & Chauvel, P. (1994). Evoked potentials recorded from the auditory cortex in man: Evaluation and topography of the middle latency components. *Electroencephalography and Clinical Neurophysiology, 92*, 204–214.

Lindamood, C., & Lindamood, P. (1971). *The Lindamood Auditory Test of Cenceptualization (LAC).* Boston: Teaching Resources Corp.

Lindamood, C. H., & Lindamood, P. C. (1979). *Lindamood Auditory Conceptualization Test, Revised Edition.* Itasca, IL: Riverside Publishing Company.

Litovsky, R. (1991). *Developmental changes in sound localization precision under conditions of the precedence effect.* Unpublished doctoral dissertation, University of Massachusetts, Amherst. As reported in Clifton, R. K. (1992). The development of spatial hearing in infants. In L. A. Werner & E. W. Rubel (Eds.), *Developmental psychoacoustics* (pp. 135–157). Washington, DC: American Psychological Association.

Luce, P. A., & Pisoni, D. B. (1998). Recognizing spoken words: The neighborhood activation model. *Ear and Hearing, 19*, 1–36.

Luria, A. (1973). *The working brain: An introduction to neuropsychology.* New York: Basic Books.

Lynn, G. E., & Gilroy, J. (1972). Neuro-audiological abnormalities in patients with temporal lobe tumors. *Journal of Neurological Sciences, 17,* 167–184.

Lynn, G. E., & Gilroy, J. (1975). Effects of brain lesions on the perception of monotic and dichotic speech stimuli. In M. D. Sullivan (Ed.), *Central auditory processing disorders* (pp. 47–83). Proceedings of a conference at the University of Nebraska Medical Center, Omaha.

Lynn, G. E., Gilroy, J., Taylor, P. C., & Leiser, R. P. (1981). Binaural masking-level differences in neurological disorders. *Archives of Otolaryngology, 107*, 357–362.

Magavi, S. S., Leavitt, B. R., & Macklis, J. D. (2000). Induction of neurogenesis in the neocortex of adult mice. *Nature, 405*, 951–955.

Makela, J. P., & McEvoy, L. (1996). Auditory evoked fields to illusory sound source movements. *Experimental Brain Research, 110*, 446–454.

Marshall, L., Brandt, J. F., Marston, L. E., & Ruder, K. (1979). Changes in the number and types of errors on repetition of acoustically distorted sentences as a function of age in normal children. *Journal of the Americal Audiology Society, 4*, 218–225.

Marvel, J. B., Jerger, J. F., & Lew, H. L. (1992). Asymmetries in topographic brain maps of auditory evoked potentials in the elderly. *Journal of the American Academy of Audiology, 3*, 361–368.

Massaro, D. W. (1972). Preperceptual images, processing time, and perceptual units in auditory perception. *Psychological Review, 79*, 124–145.

Massaro, D. W. (1975). *Understanding language: An information-processing analysis of speech perception, reading, and psycholinguistics.* New York: Academic Press.

Masters, M., Stecker, N., & Katz, J. (1993, November). CAP disorders, language difficulty, and academic success: A team approach. Paper presented at the American Speech-Language-Hearing Association annual convention, Los Angeles, CA.

Matzker, J. (1959). Two new methods for the assessment of central auditory functions in cases of brain disease. *Annals of Otology, Rhinology and Laryngology, 68*, 1155–1197.

Maue-Dickson, W. (1981). The auditory nerve and central auditory pathways: Prenatal development. In Martin, F. N. (Ed.), *Medical Audiology. Disorders of Hearing* (pp. 371–392). Englewood Cliffs, NJ: Prentice-Hall.

McCroskey, R. L., & Keith, R. W. (1996). *Auditory Fusion Test-Revised.* St. Louis, MO: Auditec.

McFarland, D. J., & Cacace, A. T. (1995). Modality specificity as a criterion for diagnosing central auditory processing disorders. *American Journal of Audiology, 4*, 36–48.

McFarland, D. J., Cacace, A. T., & Setzen, G. (1998). Temporal-order discrimination for selected auditory and visual stimulus dimensions. *Journal of Speech-Language-Hearing Research, 41*, 300–314.

McGee, T., Kraus, N., Comperatore, C., & Nicol, T. (1991). Subcortical and cortical components of the MLR generating system. *Brain Research, 544*, 211–220.

McGee, T., Kraus, N. King, C., & Nicol, T. (1996). Acoustic elements of speechlike stimuli are reflected in surface recorded responses over the guinea pig temporal lobe. *Journal of the Acoustical Society of America, 90*, 3606–3614.

McGee, T., Kraus, N., & Nicol., T. (1997). Is it really a mismatch negativity? An assessment of methods for determining response validity in individual subjects. *Electroencephalography and Clinical Neurophysiology, 104*, 359–368.

McGurk, H., Turnure, C., & Creighton, S. (1977). Auditory-visual coordination in neonates. *Child Development, 48*, 138–143.

Medin, D. L., & Ross, B. H. (1997). *Cognitive Psychology (2nd edition).* Orlando, FL: Harcourt Brace & Company.

Merzenich, M. M., Jenkins, W. M., Johnston, P., Schreiner, C., Miller, S. L., & Tallal, P. (1996). Temporal processing deficits of language-learning impaired children ameliorated by training. *Science, 271*, 77–81.

Merzenich, M. M., & Haas, J. H. (1982, December). Reorganization of mammalian somatosensory cortex following peripheral nerve injury. *Trends in Neuroscience*, 434–436.

Merzenich, M. M., Rencanzone, G., Jenkins, W. M., Allard, T. T., & Nudo, R. J. (1988). Cortical representational plasticity. In P. Rakic & W. Singer (Eds.), *Neurobiology of neocortex* (pp. 41–67.) New York: John Wiley & Sons.

Miller, E. (1971). Handedness and the pattern of human ability. *British Journal of Psychology, 62*, 111–112.

Miller, G. A., & Gildea, P. M. (1987). How children learn words. *Scientific American, 257*, 94–99.

Miller, G. A., & Licklider, J. C. R. (1950). The intelligibility of interrupted speech. *Journal of the Acoustical Society of America, 22*, 167–173.

Milner, B., Taylor, S., & Sperry, R. (1968). Lateralized suppression of dichotically presented digits after commissural section in man. *Science, 161*, 184–185.

Moller, A. R., Jannetta, P. J., & Moller, M. B. (1981). Neural generators of brainstem evoked potentials. Results from human intracranial recordings. *Annals of Otology, 90,* 591–596.

Moore, D. R., Hutchings, M. E., King, A. J., & Kowalchuk, N. E. (1989). Auditory brainstem of the ferret: Some effects of rearing with unilateral ear plug on the cochlea, cochlear nucleus, and projections to the inferior colliculus. *Journal of Neuroscience, 9*, 1213–1222.

Moore, D. R., & Irvine, D. R. F. (1981). Plasticity of binaural interaction in the cat inferior colliculus. *Brain Research, 208,* 198–202.

Morales-Garcia, C., & Poole, J. O. (1972). Masked speech audiometry in central deafness. *Acta Otolaryngologica (Stockholm), 74*, 307–316.

Morongiello, B., & Clifton, R. (1984). Effects of sound frequency on behavioral and cardiac orienting in newborn and five-month-infants. *Journal of Experimental Child Psychology, 38*, 429–446.

Morrongiello, B. A., & Trehub, S. E. (1987). Age-related changes in auditory temporal perception. *Journal of Experimental Child Psychology, 44,* 413–426.

Moscovitch, M. (1992). Language and the cerebral hemispheres: Reaction-time studies and their implications for models of cerebral dominance. In F. Craik & T. A. Salthouse (Eds.), *Handbook of aging and cognition* (pp. 283–299). Mahway, NJ: Lawrence Erlbaum and Associates.

Mueller, H. G., Beck, W. G., & Sedge, R. K. (1987). Comparison of the efficiency of cortical level speech tests. *Seminars in Hearing, 8,* 279–298.

Mueller, H. G., & Bright, K. E. (1994). Monosyllabic procedures in central testing. In J. Katz (Ed.), *Handbook of clinical audiology*, (4th ed., pp. 222–238). Baltimore: Williams & Wilkins.

Muir, D., Abraham, W., Forbes, B., & Harris, L. (1979) The ontogenesis of an auditory localization response from birth to 4 months of age. *Canadian Journal of Psychology, 43,* 199–216.

Muir, D., & Clifton, R. (1985). Infants' orientation to the localization of sound sources. In G. Gottlieb & N. Krasnegor (Eds.), *The measurement of audition and vision during the first year of postnatal life: A methodological overview* (pp. 171–194). Norwood, NJ: Ablex.

Musiek, F. E. (1983a). Assessment of central auditory dysfunction: The Dichotic Digits Test revisited. *Ear and Hearing, 4,* 79–83.

Musiek, F. E. (1983b). Assessment of three dichotic speech tests on subjects with intracranial lesions. *Ear and Hearing, 4,* 318–323.

Musiek, F. E. (1983c). The evaluation of brainstem disorders using ABR and central auditory tests. *Monographs in Contemporary Audiology, 4,* 1–24.

Musiek, F. E. (1986). Neuroanatomy, neurophysiology, and central auditory assessment. Part III: Corpus callosum and efferent pathways. *Ear and Hearing, 7,* 349–358.

Musiek, F. E. (1999). Habilitation and management of auditory processing disorders: Overview of selected prodecures. *Journal of the American Academy of Audiology, 10,* 329–342.

Musiek, F. E. (1994). Frequency (pitch) and duration pattern tests. *Journal of the American Academy of Audiology, 5,* 265–268.

Musiek, F. E., Baran, J. A., & Pinheiro, M. L. (1990). Duration pattern recognition in normal subjects and patients with cerebral and cochlear lesions. *Audiology, 29,* 304–313.

Musiek, F. E., Gollegly, K. M., Lamb L. E., & Lamb, P. (1990). Selected issues in screening for central auditory processing dysfunction. *Seminars in Hearing, 11,* 372–384.

Musiek, F. E., Baran, J. A., & Pinheiro, M. L. (1994). *Neuroaudiology case studies.* San Diego, CA: Singular Publishing Group.

Musiek, F. E., & Chermak, G. D. (1994). Three commonly asked questions about central auditory processing disorders: Assessment. *American Journal of Audiology, 3,* 23–27.

Musiek, F. E., & Chermak, G. D. (1995). Three commonly asked questions about central auditory processing disorders: Managment. *American Journal of Audiology, 4,* 15–18.

Musiek, F. E., Gollegly, K. M., & Baran, J. A. (1984.) Myelination of the corpus callosum and auditory processing problems in children: Theoretical and clinical correlates. *Seminars in Hearing, 5,* 231–241.

Musiek, F., Gollegly, K., Kibbe, K., & Reeves, A. (1985). Electrophysiologic and behavioral auditory findings in multiple sclerosis. *American Journal of Otology, 10,* 343–350.

Musiek, F. E., Gollegly, K. M., Kibbe, K. S., & Verkest-Lenz, S. B. (1991). Proposed screening test for central auditory disorders: Follow-up on the Dichotic Digits Test. *American Journal of Otology, 12,* 109–113.

Musiek, F. E., & Lamb, L. (1994). Central auditory assessment: An overview. In J. Katz (Ed.), *Handbook of clinical audiology,* (4th ed., pp. 197–211). Baltimore: Williams & Wilkins.

Musiek, F. E., Gollegly, K. M., Lamb, L. E., & Lamb, P. (1990). Selected issues in screening for central auditory processing dysfunction. *Seminars in Hearing, 11,* 372–384.

Musiek, F., Gollegly, K., & Ross, M. (1985). Profiles of types of auditory processing disorders in children with learning disabilities. *Journal of Children with Communication Disorders, 9*, 43.

Musiek, F., & Guerkink, N. (1982). Auditory brainstem response and central auditory test findings for patients with brainstem lesions. *Laryngoscope, 92*, 891–900.

Musiek, F. E., & Hoffman, D. W. (1990). An introduction to the functional neurochemistry of the auditory system. *Ear and Hearing, 11*, 395–402.

Musiek, F. E., Kibbe, K., & Baran, J. A. (1984). Neuroaudiological results from split-brain patients. *Seminars in Hearing, 5*, 219–229.

Musiek, F. E., Kurdziel-Schwan, S., Kibbe, K. S., Gollegly, K. M., Baran, J. A., & Rintelmann, W. F. (1989). The dichotic rhyme task: Results in split-brain patients. *Ear and Hearing, 10*, 33–39.

Musiek, F. E., & Lee, W. (1995). Auditory brainstem response in patients with cochlear pathology. *Ear and Hearing, 16*, 631–636.

Musiek, F. E., & Pinheiro, M. L. (1987). Frequency patterns in cochlear, brainstem, and cerebral lesions. *Audiology, 26*, 79–88.

Musiek, F. E., Pinheiro, M. L., & Wilson, D. H. (1980). Auditory pattern perception in "split-brain" patients. *Archives of Otolaryngology, 106*, 610–612.

Musiek, F. E., & Reeves, A. (1986). Effects of partial and complete corpus callosotomy of central auditory function. In F. Lepore, M. Ptito, & H. H. Jasper (Eds.), *Two hemispheres—one brain. Functions of the corpus callosum* (pp. 423–433). New York: Alan R. Liss, Inc.

Musiek, F. E., & Reeves, A. G. (1990). Asymmetries of the auditory areas of the cerebrum. *Journal of the American Academy of Audiology, 1*, 240–245.

Musiek, F. E., Reeves, A. G., & Baran, J. A. (1985). Release from central auditory competition in the split-brain patient. *Neurology, 35*, 983–987.

Musiek, F. E., Verkest, S. B., & Gollegly, K. M. (1988). Effects of neuro-maturation on auditory-evoked potentials. *Seminars in Hearing, 9*, 1–13.

Musiek, F. E., Weider, D. J., & Mueller, R. (1982). Audiological findings in Charcot-Marie-Tooth syndrome. *Archives of Otolaryngology, 109*, 595–599.

Musiek, F., Wilson, D., & Pinheiro, M. (1979). Audiological manifestations in split-brain patients. *Journal of the American Audiology Society, 5*, 25–29.

Myers, R. E. (1959). Localization of function in the corpus callosum: Visual gnostic transfer. *Archives of Neurology, 1*, 74–77.

Myers, R. E., & Ebner, F. F. (1976). Localization of function in the corpus callosum: Tactile information transmission in macaca mulatta. *Brain Research, 103*, 455–462.

Myklebust, H. (1954). *Auditory disorders in children.* New York: Grune & Stratton.

Naatanen, R., & Alho, K. (1997). Mismatch negativity—the measure for central sound representation accuracy. *Audiology and Neuro-Otology, 2*, 341–353.

Naatanen, R., & Gaillard, A. W. K. (1983). The N2 deflection of ERP and the orienting reflex. In A. W. K. Gaillard & W. Ritter (Eds.), *EEG correlates of information processing: Theoretical issues* (pp. 119–141). Amsterdam: North Holland.

Naatanen, R., Gaillard, A. W. K., & Montysalo, S. (1978). Early selective-attention effect on evoked potential reinterpreted. *Acta Psychologica, 42,* 313–329.

Naatanen, R., & Kraus, N. (Eds.) (1995). Special issue: Mismatch negativity as an index of central auditory function. *Ear and Hearing, 16,* 1–146.

Naatanen, R., Lehtokoski, A., Lennes, M., Cheour, M., Huotilainen, M., Iivonen, A., Vainio, M., Allik, J., Sinkkonen, J., & Alho, K. (1997). Language-specific phoneme representations revealed by electric and magnetic brain responses. *Nature, 385,* 432–434.

Naatanen, R., & Picton, T. W. (1987). The N1 wave of the human electric and magnetic response to sound: A review and analysis of the component structure. *Psychophysiology, 24,* 375–425.

Naatanen, R., Schroger, E., Karakas, S., Tervanieme, M., & Paavilainen, P. (1993). Development of neural representations for complex sound patterns in the human brain. *NeuroReport, 4,* 503–506.

Nebes, R. D. (1971). Handedness and the perception of port-while relationships. *Cortex, 7,* 350–356.

Niccum, N., Rubens, A., & Speaks, C. (1981). Effects of stimulus material on the dichotic listening performance of aphasic patients. *Journal of Speech and Hearing Research, 24,* 526–534.

Niccum, N., Speaks, C., Katsuki-Nakamura, J., & Van Tassell, D. (1987). Effects of simulated conductive hearing loss on dichotic listening performance for digits. *Journal of Speech and Hearing Disorders, 52,* 313–318.

Noback, C. R., (1985). Neuroanatomical correlates of central auditory function. In M. L. Pinheiro and F. E. Musiek (Eds.), *Assessment of central auditory dysfunction: Foundations and clinical correlates* (pp. 7–21). Baltimore: Williams & Wilkins.

Noffsinger, D., Martinez, C., & Schaefer, A. (1982). Auditory brainstem responses and masking level differences from persons with brainstem lesions. *Scandinavian Audiology, 15,* 81–93.

Noffsinger, D., Martinez, C. D., & Wilson, R. H. (1994). Dichotic listening to speech. Background and preliminary data for digits, sentences, and nonsense syllables. *Journal of the American Academy of Audiology, 5,* 248–254.

Noffsinger, D., Olsen, W. O., Carhart, R., Hart, C. W., & Sahgal, V. (1972). Auditory and vestibular aberrations in multiple sclerosis. *Acta Oto-Laryngology* (Suppl. 303), 1–63.

Noffsinger, D., Schaefer, A. B., & Martinez, C. D. (1984). Behavioral and objective estimates of auditory brainstem integrity. *Seminars in Hearing, 5,* 337–349.

Noffsinger, D., Wilson, W. H., & Musiek, F. E. (1994). Department of Veterans Affairs compact disc recording for auditory perceptual assessment: Background and introduction. *Journal of the American Academy of Audiology, 5,* 231–235.

Nordlund, B. (1964). Directional audiometry. Acta Oto-Laryngology, 57, 1–18.

Nordlund, B., & Fritzel, B. (1963). The influence of azimuth on speech signals. *Acta Oto-Laryngology, 56,* 632–642.

Nozza, R. J. (1987). The binaural masking level difference in infants and adults: Developmental change in binaural hearing. *Infant Behavior Development, 10*, 105–110.

Nozza, R. J., Wagner, E. F., & Crandall, M. A. (1988). Binaural release from masking for a speech sound in infants, preschoolers, and adults. *Journal of Speech and Hearing Research, 31*, 212–218.

Olds, J., Disterhoft, J. F., Segal, M., Kornblith, C. L., & Hirsh, R. (1972). Learning centers of rat brain mapped by measuring latencies of conditioned unit responses. *Journal of Neurophysiology, 35*, 202–219.

Olsen, W. O. (1983). Dichotic test results for normal subjects and for temporal lobectomy patients. *Ear and Hearing, 4*, 324–330.

Olsen, W., & Noffsinger, D. (1976). Masking level differences for cochlear and brainstem lesions. *Annals of Otology, 85*, 820–825.

Olsen, W. O., Noffsinger, D., & Carhart, R. (1976). Masking level differences encountered in clinical populations. *Audiology, 15*, 287–301.

Olsen, W. O., Noffsinger, P. D., & Kurdziel, S. A. (1975). Speech discrimination in quiet and in white noise by patients with peripheral and central lesions. *Acta Otolaryngologica (Stockholm), 80*, 375–382.

Osterhammel, P. A., Shallop, J. K., & Terkildsen, K. (1985). The effect of sleep on the auditory brainstem response (ABR) and the middle latency response (MLR). *Scandinavian Audiology, 14*, 47–50.

Ozdamar, O., & Kraus, N. (1983). Auditory middle latency responses in humans. *Audiology, 22*, 34–49.

Palmer, T. D., Markakis, E. A., Willhoite, A. R., Safar, F., & Gage, F. H. (1999). Fibroblast growth factor-2 activates a latent neurogenic program in neural stem cells from diverse regions of the adult CNS. *Journal of Neuroscience, 19*, 8487–8497.

Palva, A., & Jokinen, K. (1975). Undistorted and filtered speech audiometry in children with normal hearing. *Acta Otolaryngologica, 80*, 383–388.

Pandya, D. N. (1995). Anatomy of the auditory cortex. *Revue Neurologique, 151*, 486–494.

Pandya, D. N., & Kuypers, H. G. J. M. (1969). Cortico-cortical connections in the rhesus monkey. *Brain Research, 13*, 13–36.

Pantev, C., Ross, B., Berg, P., Elbert, T., & Rockstroh, B. (1998). Study of the human auditory cortices using a whole-head magnetometer: Left vs. right hemisphere and ipsilateral vs. contralateral stimulation. *Audiology and Neuro-Otology, 3*, 183–190.

Papsin, B. C., & Abel, S. M. (1988). Temporal summation in hearing-impaired listeners. *Journal of Otolaryngology, 17*, 93–100.

Parthasarathy, T. K. (2000). Electrophysiologic assessment of CAPD: A review of the basics. *The Hearing Journal, 53*, 52–60.

Perrault, N., & Picton, T. W. (1984). Event-related potentials recorded from the scalp and nasopharyns. I. N1 and P2. *Electroencephalography and Clinical Neurophysiology, 47*, 637–647.

Phillips, D. P. (1990). Neural representation of sound amplitude in the auditory cortex: Effects of noise making. *Behavioural Brain Research, 37*, 197–214.

Phillips, D. P. (1995). Central auditory processing: A view from neuroscience. *American Journal of Otology, 16,* 338–352.

Phillips, D. P. (1999). Auditory gap detection, perceptual channels, and temporal resolution. *Journal of the American Academy of Audiology, 10,* 343–354.

Phillips, D. P., & Farmer, M. E. (1990). Acquired word deafness and the temporal grain of sound discrimination in the primary auditory cortex. *Behavioural Brain Research, 40,* 85–94.

Phillips, D. P., & Hall, S. E. (1987). Responses of single neurons in cat auditory cortex to time-varying stimuli: Linear amplitude modulations. *Experimental Brain Research, 67,* 479–492.

Phillips, D. P., & Hall, S. E. (1990). Response timing constraints on the cortical representation of sound time structure. *Journal of the Acoustical Society of America, 88,* 1403–1411.

Phillips, D. P., & Hall, S. E. (2000). Independence of frequency channels in auditory temporal gap detection. *Journal of the Acoustical Society of America, 108,* 2957–2963.

Phillips. J. L. (1996). *How to think about statistics.* New York: W. H. Freeman and Company.

Pickles, J. O. (1985). Physiology of the cerebral auditory system. In M. L. Pinheiro & F. E. Musiek (Eds.), *Assessment of central auditory dysfunction: Foundations and clinical correlates* (pp. 67–86). Baltimore: Williams & Wilkins.

Picton, T., Woods, D., Baribeau-Braun, J., & Healey, T. (1977). Evoked potential audiometry. *Journal of Otolaryngology, 6,* 90–119.

Picton, T. W., & Hillyard, S. H. (1988). Endogenous event-related potentials. In T. W. Picton (Ed.), *Human event-related potentials (Vol. 3,* pp. 98–123). Amsterdam: Elsevier Science Publishers.

Pillsbury, H. C., Grose, J. H., & Hall, J. W. (1991.) Otitis media with effusion in children. *Archives of Otolaryngology, Head and Neck Surgery, 117,* 718–723.

Pinheiro, M. L. (1976). Auditory pattern perception in patients with right and left hemisphere lesions. *Ohio Journal of Speech and Hearing, 2,* 9–20.

Pinheiro, M. L., & Musiek, F. E. (1985). Sequencing and temporal ordering in the auditory system. In M. L. Pinheiro & F. E. Musiek (Eds.), *Assessment of central auditory dysfunction: Foundations and clinical correlates* (pp. 219–238). Baltimore: Williams & Wilkins.

Pinheiro, M. L., & Ptacek, P. H. (1971). Reversals in the perception of noise and tone patterns. *Journal of the Acoustical Society of America, 49,* 1778–1782.

Pinheiro, M. L., & Tobin, H. (1969). Interaural intensity difference for intracranial localization. *Journal of the Acoustical Society of America, 46,* 1482–1487.

Pinheiro, M. L., & Tobin, H. (1971). The interaural intensity difference as a diagnostic indicator. *Acta Oto—Laryngology, 71,* 326–328.

Pisoni, D. B. (2000). Cognitive factors and cochlear implants: Some thoughts on perception, learning, and memory in speech perception. *Ear and Hearing, 21,* 70–78.

Polich, J., Howard, L., & Starr, A. (1985). Effects of age on the P-300 component of the event related potential from auditory stimuli: Peak definition, variation, and measurement. *Journal of Gerontology, 40,* 721–726.

Ponton, C. W., Don, M., Eggermont, J. J., & Kwong, B. (1997). Integrated mismatch negativity (MMN): A noise-free representation of evoked responses allowing single-point distribution-free statistical tests. *Electroencephalography and Clinical Neurophysiology, 104,* 143–150.

Ponton, C. W., Eggermont, J. J., Kwong, B., & Don, M. (2000). Maturation of human central auditory system activity: Evidence from multi-channel evoked potentials. *Clinical Neurophysiology, 111,* 220–236.

Porter, R., & Berlin, C. (1975). On interpreting developmental change in the dichotic right ear advantage. *Brain and Language, 2,* 186–200.

Preilowski, B. F. B. (1972). Possible contribution of the anterior forebrain commissures to bilateral motor coordination. *Neuropsychologia, 10,* 267–277.

Preilowski, B. F. B. (1975). Bilateral motor interaction: Perceptual-motor performance of partial and complete "split brain" patients. In K. T. Zulch, O. Creutzfeldt, & G. C. Galbraith (Eds.), *Cerebral localization* (pp. 115–132). Berlin: Springer.

Ptacek, P. H., & Pinheiro, M. L. (1971). Pattern reversal in auditory perception. *Journal of the Acoustical Society of America, 49,* 493–498.

Pujol, J., Vendrell, P., Junque, C., Marti-Vilalta, J. L., & Capdevila, A. (1993). When does human brain development end? Evidence of corpus callosum growth up to adulthood. *Annals of Neurology, 34,* 71–75.

Quaranta, A., & Cervellera, G. (1974). Masking level differences in normal and pathological ears. *Audiology, 13,* 428–431.

Quine, D. B., Regan, D., & Murray, T. J. (1983). Delayed auditory tone perception in multiple sclerosis. *Canadian Journal of Neurological Sciences, 10,* 183–186.

Rasmussen, T., & Milner, B. (1977). The role of early left brain injury in determining lateralization of cerebral speech functions. *Annals of the New York Academy of Sciences, 299,* 355–369.

Rauschecker, J. P., & Marler, P. (1987). Cortical plasticity and imprinting: Behavioral and physiological contrasts and parallels. In J. P. Rauschecker & P. Marler (Eds.), *Imprinting and cortical plasticity* (pp. 349–366). New York: John Wiley & Sons.

Recanzone, G., Merzenich, M., & Schreiner, C. (1992). Changes in the distributed temporal response properties of SI cortical neurons reflect improvements in performance on a temporally-based tactile discrimination task. *Journal of Neurophysiology, 67,* 1071–1091.

Recanzone, G., Schreiner, C., & Merzenich, M. (1993). Plasticity in the frequency representation of primary auditory cortex following discrimination training in adult owl monkeys. *Journal of Neuroscience, 13,* 37–104.

Rees, N. (1973). Auditory processing factors in language disorders: The view from Procrustes' bed. *Journal of Speech and Hearing Disorders, 38,* 308–315.

Rencanzone, G. H., Schreiner, C. E., & Merzenich, M. M. (1993.) Plasticity in the frequency representation of primary auditory cortex following discrimination training in adult owl monkeys. *Journal of Neuroscience, 13,* 87–103.

Restak, R. M. (1986). *The Infant Mind.* Garden City, NY: Doubleday & Company.

Restak, R. (2001). *The secret life of the brain.* Washington, DC: Joseph Henry Press.

Reynolds, C. R., & Kamphaus, R. W. (1998). *Behavioral Assessment System for Children.* Circle Pines, MN: American Guidance Service.

Reynolds, W. M. (1987). *Auditory Discrimination Test* (2nd ed.). Los Angeles: Western Psychological Services.

Ringo, J. L., Doty, R. W., Demeter, S., & Simard, P. Y. (1994). Time is of the essence: A conjecture that hemispheric specialization arises from inter-hemispheric conduction delay. *Cerebral Cortex, 4,* 791–798.

Rintelmann, W. F. (1985). Monaural speech tests in the detection of central auditory disorders. In M. L. Pinheiro & F. E. Musiek (Eds.), *Assessment of central auditory dysfunction: Foundations and clinical correlates* (pp. 173–200). Baltimore: Williams & Wilkins.

Ritter, W., Simson, R., Vaughan, H. G., & Macht, M. (1982). Manipulation of event-related potential manifestations of information processing stages. *Science, 218,* 909–911.

Robertson, C., & Salter, W. (1995). *The Phonological awareness profile.* East Moline, IL: LinguiSystems, Inc.

Robertson, C., & Salter, W. (1997). *The Phonological awareness test.* East Moline, IL: LinguiSystems, Inc.

Robertson, D., & Irvine, D. R. F. (1989). Plasticity of frequency organization in auditory cortex of guinea pigs with partial unilateral deafness. Journal of Comparative Neurology, 282, 456–471.

Roeser, R. J., Johns, D. F., & Price, L. L. (1976). Dichotic listening in adults with sensorineural hearing loss. *Journal of the American Audiology Society, 2,* 19–25.

Roeser, R. J., Millay, K. K., & Morrow, J. M. (1983). Dichotic Consonant-Vowel (CV) perception in normal and learning-impaired children. *Ear and Hearing, 4,* 293–299.

Romand, R. (Ed.), (1983). *Development of auditory and vestibular systems.* New York: Academic Press.

Roser, D. (1966). Directional hearing in persons with hearing disorders. *Journal of Laryngology and Rhinology, 45,* 423–440.

Roush, J., & Tait, C. A., (1984). Binaural fusion, masking level differences, and auditory brainstem responses in children with language-learning disabilities. *Ear and Hearing, 5,* 37–41.

Rubens, A. B., Froehling, B., Slater, G., & Anderson, D. (1985). Left ear suppression on verbal dichotic tests in patients with multiple sclerosis. *Annals of Neurology, 18,* 459–463.

Rugg, M. D. (1984a). Event-related potentials and the phonological processing of words and non-words. *Neuropsychologia, 22,* 435–443.

Rugg, M. D., (1984b). Event-related potentials in phonological matching tasks. *Brain and Language, 23,* 225–240.

Ryugo, D. K., & Weinberger, N. M. (1978). Differencial plasticity of morphologically distinct populations in the medial geniculate body of the cat during classical conditioning. *Behavioral Biology, 22*, 275–301.

Sahley, T. L., Nodar, R. H., & Musiek, F. E. (1997). *Efferent auditory system: Structure and function.* San Diego, CA: Singular Publishing Group.

Sahley, T. L., Kalish, R. B., Musiek, F. E., & Hoffman, D. W. (1991). Effects of opioid drugs on auditory evoked potentials suggest a role of lateral olivocochlear dynorphins in auditory function. *Hearing Research, 55*, 133–142.

Salamy, A. (1978). Commissural transmission: Maturational changes in humans. *Science, 200*, 1409–1410.

Salamy, A. (1984). Maturation of the auditory brainstem response from birth through early childhood. *Journal of Clinical Neurophysiology, 1*, 293–329.

Salamy, A., Mendelson, T., Tooley, W., & Chaplin, E. (1980). Differential development of brainstem potentials in healthy and high-risk infants. *Science, 210*, 553–555.

Salasoo, A., & Pisoni, D. B. (1985). Interaction of knowledge sources in spoken word identification. *Journal of Memory and Language, 24*, 210–231.

Salkind, N. J. (1991). *Exploring research.* New York: Macmillan.

Sams, M., Aulanko, R., Hamalainen, M., Hari, R., Lounasmaa, O. V., Lu, S. T., & Simola, J. (1991). Seeing speech: Visual information from lip movements modifies activity in the human auditory cortex. *Neuroscience Letters, 127*, 141–145.

Sams, M., Paavilainen, P., Alho, K., & Naatanen, R. (1985). Auditory frequency discrimination and event-related potentials. *Electroencephalography and Clinical Neurophysiology, 62*, 437–448.

Sanchez-Longo, L., & Forster, F. (1958). Clinical significance of impairments in sound localizations. *Neurology, 8*, 119–125.

Sanchez-Longo, F., Forster, F., & Auth, T. (1957). A clinical test for sound localization and its applications. *Neurology, 7*, 655–663.

Satz, K., Achenback, E., Pattishall, E., & Fennell, E. (1965). Order of report, ear asymmetry and handedness in dichotic listening. *Cortex, 1*, 377–395.

Sauerwein, H. C., & Lassonde, M. (1997). Neuropsychological alterations after split-brain surgery. *Journal of Neurosurgical Sciences, 41*, 59–66.

Scherg, M., Vasjar, J., & Picton, T. (1989). A source analysis of the late human auditory evoked potentials. *Journal of Cognitive Neuroscience, 1*, 336–355.

Schneider, B. A., Trehub, S. E., Morrongiello, B. A., & Thorpe, L. A. (1989). Developmental changes in masked thresholds. *Journal of the Acoustical Society of America, 86*, 1733–1741.

Schopler, E., Reichler, R., & Renner, B. R. (1988). *Child Autism Rating Scale.* Los Angeles, CA: Western Psychological Services.

Schow, R. L., & Chermak, G. D. (1999). Implications from factor analysis for central auditory processing disorders. *American Journal of Audiology, 8*, 137–142.

Schow, R. L., Seikel, J. A., Chermak, G. D., & Berent, M. (2000). Central auditory processes and test measures: ASHA 1996 revised. *American Journal of Audiology, 9*, 1–6.

Schreiner, C. E. (1995). Order and disorder in auditory cortical maps. *Current Opinion in Neurobiology, 5,* 489–496.

Schreiner, C. E., & Mendelson, J. R. (1990). Functional topography of cat primary auditory cortex: Distribution of integrated excitation. *Journal of Neurophysiology, 64,* 1442–1459.

Schoeny, Z. G., & Carhart, R. (1971). Effects of unilateral Meniere's disease on masking-level differences. *Journal of the Acoustical Society of America, 50,* 1143–1150.

Scientific Learning Corporation. (1997). *Fast ForWord*™. Berkeley, CA: Scientific Learning Corporation.

Semel, E., Wiig, E. H., & Secord, W. (1987). *Clinical Evaluation of Language Fundamentals—Revised: Examiner's manual.* San Antonio, TX: The Psychological Corporation.

Semiel, E., Wiig, E. H., & Secord, W. A. (1995). *Clinical Evaluation of Language Fundamentals—3rd Edition.* San Antonio, TX: Psychological Corporation.

Sharma, A., Kraus, N., McGee, T. J., & Nicol, T. G. (1997). Developmental changes in P1 and N1 central auditory responses elicited by consonant-vowel syllables. *Electroencephalography and Clinical Neurophysiology, 104,* 540–545.

Shehata-Dieler, W., Shimizu, H., Soliman, S., & Tusa, R. (1991). Middle latency auditory evoked potentials in temporal lobe disorders. *Ear & Hearing, 12,* 377–388.

Sidtis, J. (1982). Predicting brain organization from dichotic listening performance: Cortical and subcortical functional asymmetries contribute to perceptual asymmetries. *Brain and Language, 17,* 287–300.

Sidtis, J. J., Volpe, B. T., Holtzman, J. D., Wilson, D. H., & Gazzaniga, M. S. (1981). Cognitive interaction after staged callosal section: Evidence for transfer of semantic activation. *Science, 212,* 344–346.

Silverman, F. H. (1977). *Research design in speech pathology and audiology.* Englewood Cliffs, NJ: Prentice-Hall.

Sinha, S. O. (1959). *The role of the temporal lobe in hearing.* Unpublished master's thesis, Montreal, Quebec, Canada: McGill University.

Sloan, C. (1995). *Treating auditory processing difficulties in children.* San Diego, CA: Singular Publishing Group.

Smith, A. (1966). Speech and other functions after left (dominant) hemispherectomy. *Journal of Neurology, Neurosurgery and Psychiatry, 29,* 167–171.

Smith, B. B., & Resnick, D. M. (1972). An auditory test for assessing brain stem integrity: Preliminary report. *Laryngoscope, 82,* 414–424.

Smoski, W. J., Brunt, M. A., & Tanahill, J. C. (1998). *Children's Auditory Performance Scale.* Tampa, FL: Educational Audiology Association.

Sparks, R., & Geschwind, N. (1968). Dichotic listening in man after section of neocortical commissures. *Cortex, 4,* 3–16.

Sparks, R., Goodglass, H., & Nickel, B. (1970). Ipsilateral versus contralateral extinction in dichotic listening resulting from hemispheric lesions. *Cortex, 6,* 249–260.

Speaks, C., Gray, T., Miller, J., & Rubens, A. (1975). Central auditory deficits and temporal-lobe lesions. *Journal of Speech and Hearing Disorders, 40,* 192–205.

Speaks, C., Niccum, N., & Van Tasell, D. (1985). Effects of stimulus material on the dichotic listening performance of patients with sensorineural hearing loss. *Journal of Speech and Hearing Research, 28,* 16–25.

Squires, K., & Hecox, K. (1983). Electrophysiological evaluation of higher level auditory processing. *Seminars in Hearing, 4,* 415–432.

Staffel, J. G., Hall, J. W., Grose, J. H., & Pillsbury, H. C. (1990). NøSø and NøSπ detection as a function of masker bandwidth in normal-hearing and cochlear-impaired listeners. *Journal of the Acoustical Society of America, 87,* 1720–1727.

Starr, A., Amlie, R. N., Martin, W. H., & Sanders, S. (1977). Development of auditory function in newborn infants revealed by auditory brainstem potentials. *Pediatrics, 60,* 831–839.

Streeter, G. L. (1906). On the development of the membranous labyrinth and the acoustic and facial nerves in the human embryo. *American Journal of Anatomy, 6,* 139–165.

Stryker, M. P., & Harris, W. A. (1986). Binocular impulse blockade prevents the formation of ocular dominance columns in cat visual cortex. *Journal of Neuroscience, 6,* 2117–2133.

Studdert-Kennedy, M., & Mody, M. (1995). Auditory temporal perception in the reading impaired: A critical review of the evidence. *Psychonomic Bulletin & Review, 2,* 508–514.

Sugishita, M., Otomo, K., Yamazaki, K., Shimizu, H., Yoshioka, M., & Shinohars, A. (1995). Dichotic listening in patients with partial section of the corpus callosum. *Brain, 118,* 417–427.

Sutton, S., Braren, M., Zubin, J., & John, E. R. (1965). Evoked-potential correlates of stimulus uncertainty. *Science, 155,* 1436–1439.

Suzuki, T., Hirabayashi, M., & Kobayashi, K. (1983). Auditory middle responses in young children. *British Journal of Audiology, 17,* 5–9.

Swadlow, H. (1979). Interhemispheric communication between neurons in visual cortex of the rabbit. In I. S. Russell, M. W. VanHof, & G. Berlucchi (Eds.), *Structure and function of the cerebral commissures* (pp. 211–223). London: Macmillan.

Sweetow, R. W., & Reddell, R. C. (1978). The use of masking level differences in the identification of children with perceptual learning problems. *Journal of the American Auditory Society, 4,* 52–56.

Swisher, L., & Hirsh, I. J. (1972). Brain damage and the ordering of two temporally successive stimuli. *Neuropsychologia, 10,* 137–152.

Tallal, P., Miller, S. L., Bedl, G., Byma, G., Wang, X., Nagarajan, S. S., Schreiner, C., Jenkins, W. M., & Merzenich, M. M. (1996). Language comprehension in language-learning impaired children improved with acoustically modified speech. *Science, 271,* 81–84.

Tallal, P., Miller, S., & Fitch. R. H. (1993). Neurobiological basis of speech: A case for the preeminence of temporal processing. *Annals of the New York Academy of Sciences, 682,* 27–47.

Technical Committee on Architectural Acoustics of the Acoustical Society of America. (2000). Classroom acoustics: A resource for creating learning environments with desirable listening conditions. Melville, NY: Acoustical Society of America.

Thompson, M. E., & Abel, S. M. (1992a). Indices of hearing in patients with central auditory pathology. I: Detection and discrimination. *Scandinavian Audiology, 21* (Suppl. 35), 3–15.

Thompson, M. E., & Abel, S. M. (1992b). Indices of hearing in patients with central auditory pathology. II: Choice response time. *Scandinavian Audiology, 21* (Suppl. 35), 17–22.

Tobin, H. (1985). Binaural interaction tasks. In M. L. Pinheiro & F. E. Musiek (Eds.), *Assessment of central auditory dysfunction: Foundations and clinical correlates* (pp. 155–172). Baltimore: Williams & Wilkins.

Tonal and speech materials for auditory perceptual assessment (1992). Long Beach, CA: Research and Development Service, Veterans' Administration Central Office.

Tonning, F. (1971). Directional audiometry. II. The influence of azimuth on the perception of speech. *Acta Oto-Laryngology, 72,* 352–357. Tonning, F. (1973). Directional audiometry. VIII. The influence of hearing aids on the localization of white noise. *Acta Oto-Laryngology, 76,* 114–120.

Tonning, F. (1975). Auditory localization and its clinical applications. *Audiology, 14,* 368–380.

Townsend, T. H., & Goldstein, D. P. (1972). Supra-threshold binaural unmasking. *Journal of the Acoustical Society of America, 51,* 621–624.

Trehub, S. E., Schneider, B. A., & Henderson, J. L. (1995). Gap detection in infants, children, and adults. *Journal of the Acoustical Society of America, 98,* 2532–2541.

Tremblay, K., Kraus, N., Carrell, T. D., & McGee, T. (1997). Central auditory system plasticity: Generalization to novel stimuli following listening training. *Journal of the Acoustical Society of America, 102,* 3762–3773.

Tremblay, K., Kraus, N., & McGee, T. (1998). The time course of auditory perceptual learning: Neurophysiological changes during speech-sound training. *NeuroReport, 9,* 3557–3560.

Tremblay, K., Kraus, N., McGee, T., Ponton, C., & Otis, B. (2001). Central auditory plasticity: Changes in the N1-P2 complex after speech-sound training. *Ear and Hearing, 22,* 79–90.

Turner, R. G., & Nielsen, D. W. (1984). Application of clinical decision analysis to audiological tests. *Ear and Hearing, 5,* 125–133.

Vaughan Jr., H. G., & Ritter, W. (1970). The sources of auditory evoked responses recorded from the human scalp. *Electroencephalography and Clinical Neurophysiology, 28,* 360–367.

Viehweg, R., & Campbell, R. (1960). Localization difficulty in monaurally impaired listeners. *Annals of Otology, Rhinology and Laryngology, 69,* 622–634.

Voigt, T., LeVay, S., & Stamnes, M. A. (1988). Morphological and immunocytochemical observations on the visual callosal projections in the cat. *Journal of Comparative Neurology, 272,* 450–460.

Walsh, E. (1957). An investigation of sound localization in patients with neurological abnormalities. *Brain, 80,* 222–250.

Wagner, R. K., Torgesen, J. K., & Rashotte, C. A. (1999). *Comprehensive Test of Phonological Processing.* Austin, TX: PRO-ED.

Watson, B. U., & Miller, T. K. (1993). Auditory perception, phonological processing, and reading ability/disability. *Journal of Speech and Hearing Research, 36,* 850–863.

Wedenberg, E. (1965). Prenatal Test of Hearing. *Acta Otolaryngology, Suppl. 206,* 27–32.

Weinberger, N. M. (1993). Learning-induced changes of auditory receptive fields. *Current Opinion in Neurobiology, 3,* 570–577.

Weiss, M., Zelazo, P., & Swain, I. (1988). Newborn response to auditory stimulus discrepancy. *Child Development, 59,* 1530–1541.

Welsh, L. W., Welsh, J. J., & Healy, M. (1980). Central auditory testing and dyslexia. *Laryngoscope, 90,* 972–984.

Welsh, L. W., Welsh, J. J., Healy, M., & Cooper, B. (1982). Cortical, subcortical, and brainstem dysfunction: A correlation in dyslexic children. *Annals of Otology, Rhinology and Laryngology, 91,* 310–315.

Wepman, J. M., & Morency, A. (1973). *Auditory sequential memory test.* Los Angeles: Western Psychological Services.

Wepman, J. M., & Reynolds, W. M. (1986). *Auditory Discrimination Test.* Los Angeles, CA: Western Psychological Services.

Werker, J. F., & Tees, R. C. (1999). Influences on infant speech processing: Toward a new synthesis. *Annual Review of Psychology, 50,* 509–535.

Werner, L. A., Marean, G. C., Halpin, C. F., Spetner, N. B., & Gillenwater, J. M. (1992). Infant auditory temporal acuity: Gap detection. *Child Development, 63,* 260–272.

Wertheimer, M. (1961). Psychomotor coordination of auditory and visual space at birth. *Science, 134,* 1692.

Wexler, B., & Hawles, T. (1983). Increasing the power of dichotic methods: The fused rhymed words test. *Neuropsychologia, 21,* 59–66.

White, E. J. (1977). Children's performance on the SSW test and Willeford battery: Interim clinical data. In R. W. Keith (Ed.), *Central auditory dysfunction* (pp. 319–340). New York: Grune & Stratton.

Wightman, F., Allen, P., Dolan, T., Kistler, D., & Jamieson, D. (1989). Temporal resolution in children. *Child Development, 60,* 611–624.

Willeford, J. (1976). Differential diagnosis of central auditory dysfunction. In L. Bradford (Ed.), *Audiology: An audio journal for continuing education* (Vol. 2). New York: Grune & Stratton.

Willeford, J. (1977). Assessing central auditory behavior in children: A test battery approach. In R. W. Keith (Ed.), *Central auditory dysfunction* (pp. 43–72). New York: Grune & Stratton.

Willeford, J. A., & Bilger, J. M. (1978). Auditory perception in children with learning disabilities. In J. Katz (Ed.), *Handbook of clinical audiology (2nd ed.)* (pp. 410–425). Baltimore: Williams & Wilkins.

Willeford, J. A., & Burleigh, J. M. (1985). *Handbook of central auditory processing disorders in children.* New York: Grune & Stratton.

Willeford, J. A., & Burleigh, J. M. (1994). Sentence procedures in central testing. In J. Katz (Ed.), *Handbook of clinical audiology, fourth edition* (pp. 256–268). Baltimore: Williams & Wilkins.

Wilson, L., & Mueller, H. G. (1984). Performance of normal hearing individuals on Auditec filtered speech tests. *Asha, 27,* 189.

Wilson, R. H. (1994). Word recognition with segmented-alternated CVC words: Compact disc trials. *Journal of the American Academy of Audiology, 5,* 255–258.

Wilson, R. H., Arcos, J. T., & Jones, H. C. (1984). Word recognition with segmented-alternated CVC words: A preliminary report on listeners with normal hearing. *Journal of Speech and Hearing Disorders, 47,* 111–112.

Wilson, R. H., Preece, J. P., Salamon, D. L., Sperry, J. L., & Bornstein, S. P. (1994). Effects of time compression and time compression plus reverberation on the intelligibility of the Northwestern University Auditory Test No. 6. *Journal of the American Academy of Audiology, 5,* 269–277.

Wilson, R. H., Zizz, C. A., & Sperry, J. L. (1994). Masking-level difference for spondaic words in 2000-msec bursts of broadband noise. *Journal of the American Academy of Audiology, 5,* 236–242.

Wioland, N., Rudolf, G., Metz-Lutz, M. N., Mutschler, V., & Marescaux, C. (1999). Cerebral correlates of hemispheric lateralization during a pitch discrimination task: An ERP study in dichotic situation. *Clinical Neurophysiology, 110,* 516–523.

Woodcock, R. (1976). *Goldman-Fristoe-Woodcock Auditory Skills Test Battery—Technical manual.* Circle Pines, MN: American Guidance Service.

Woodcock, R. (1977). *Woodcock-Johnson Psycho-educational Test Battery: Technical report.* Allen, TX: DLM Teaching Resources.

Woodcock, R. W., & Johnson, M. B. (1989). *Woodcock-Johnson—Revised.* Itasca, IL: Riverside Publishing.

Woodcock, R., McGraw, K., & Mather, N. (2001). *Woodcock-Johnson III.* Itasca, IL: Riverside Publishing.

Wright, B. A., Lombardino, L. J., King, W. M., Puranik, C. S., Leonard, C. M., & Merzenich, M. M. (1997). Deficits in auditory temporal and spectral resolution in language-impaired children. *Nature, 387,* 176–178.

Yakovlev, P. I., & Lecours, A. R. (1967). The myelogenetic cycles of regional maturation of the brain. In A. Minkowski (Ed.), *Regional development of the brain in early life* (pp. 3–70). Oxford, England: Blackwell.

Yencer, K. A. (1998). Is auditory integration training an effective treatment for children with central auditory processing disorders? In M. G. Masters, N. A. Stecker, & J. Katz (Eds.), *Central auditory processing disorders: Mostly management* (pp. 151–173). Needham Heights, MA: Allyn & Bacon.

Yingling, C. D., & Skinner, J. E. (1997). Gating of thalamic input to cerebral cortex by nucleus reticularis laminaris. In J. E. Desmedt (Ed.), *Attention, voluntary contraction, and event-related cerebral potentials. Progress in clinical neurophysiology* (pp. 70–96). Basel: Karger.

Zurif, E. (1974). Auditory lateralization: Prosodic and syntactic factors. *Brain and Language, 1*, 391–401.

Index

('i' indicates an illustration; 't' indicates a table)